BIRTH DEFECTS

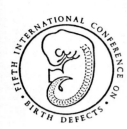

BIRTH DEFECTS

PROCEEDINGS OF
THE FIFTH INTERNATIONAL CONFERENCE
MONTREAL, CANADA, 21-27 AUGUST, 1977

SPONSORED BY
THE NATIONAL FOUNDATION-MARCH OF DIMES
AND ORGANIZED BY INTERNATIONAL
BIRTH DEFECTS CONGRESS, LTD.

Editors:

JOHN W. LITTLEFIELD
The Children's Medical and Surgical Center,
The Johns Hopkins Hospital,
Baltimore, Md., U.S.A.

JEAN DE GROUCHY
Laboratoire de Cytogénétique,
Hôpital des Enfants-Malades,
Paris, France

Co-editor:

F.J.G. EBLING
Department of Zoology,
University of Sheffield, U.K.

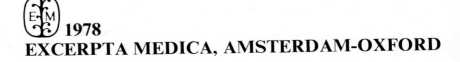

1978
EXCERPTA MEDICA, AMSTERDAM-OXFORD

International Congress Series No. 432

ISBN 0444 90024 1

Library of Congress Cataloging in Publication Data

International Conference on Birth Defects, 5th,
    Montreal, Quebec, 1977.
    Birth defects.

    (International congress series: no. 432)
    Includes indexes.
    1. Abnormalities, Human–Congresses.
I. Littlefield, John W., 1925–   II. Grouchy,
Jean de. III. Ebling, Francis John Govier, 1918–
IV. National Foundation. V. International Birth
Defects Congress. VI. Title. VII. Series.
[DNLM: 1. Abnormalities–Congresses.   W3 EX89 no. 432
1977 / QS675 I5922 1977b]
RG626.I47   1977   616'.043   78–1487
ISBN 0-444-90024-1

Publisher
Excerpta Medica
305 Keizersgracht
Amsterdam
P.O. Box 1126

Sole Distributors for the USA and Canada
Elsevier/North-Holland Inc.
52 Vanderbilt Avenue
New York, N.Y. 10017

Printed in The Netherlands by Drukkerij Casparie, IJsselstein

THE NATIONAL FOUNDATION is dedicated to the long-range goal of preventing birth defects. Our interim goal is to search for ways to ameliorate those birth defects which cannot be prevented.

As part of our efforts to achieve these goals, we sponsor, or participate in, a variety of scientific meetings and symposia where all questions relating to birth defects are freely discussed. Through our professional educational program we speed the dissemination of information by publishing the proceedings of these meetings and symposia. From time to time, we also reprint pertinent journal articles to help achieve our goal. Now and then, in the course of these articles or discussions, individual viewpoints may be expressed which go beyond the purely scientific and into controversial matters. It should be noted, therefore, that personal viewpoints about such matters will not be censored but this does not constitute an endorsement of them by The National Foundation.

Fifth International Conference on Birth Defects

Committee of Honor

Dr. Robert Bell
Principal, McGill University

Dr. Pierre Bois
Doyen de la Faculté de Médecine,
Université de Montréal

Dr. Malcolm Brown *
President, Medical Research Council, Canada

Dr. R. F. P. Cronin
Dean of Medicine, McGill University

M. Jean Drapeau
Maire de Montréal

Dr. Gustave Gingras
Chancellor of the University of Prince Edward
Island, Director of Rehabilitation Services,
Prince Edward Island

M. Paul Lacoste
Recteur, Université de Montréal

Honorable Denis Lazure
Ministre des Affaires Sociales, Province de Quebec

* deceased

Fifth International Conference on Birth Defects

Officers of the Conference

F. Clarke Fraser	Honorary President
Arno G. Motulsky	General Chairman
Mary Ellen Avery	Co-Chairman
John W. Littlefield	Scientific Program Committee Chairman
Jean de Grouchy	Vice-Chairman
Richard C. Gedney	Secretary General
Mrs. Alice Jacoby	Conference Coordinator
Mrs. Norma Pelatti	Secretarial Assistant
Ms. Debbie Siegert	Assistant

Executive Committee

Arno G. Motulsky, U.S.A.	Chairman
Mary Ellen Avery, U.S.A.	Co-Chairman

Members

Nikolay P. Bochkov, U.S.S.R.
Cedric O. Carter, Great Britain
Louis Dallaire, Canada
F. Clarke Fraser, Canada
J. Heinrich Holzner, Austria
Widukind Lenz, Federal Republic of Germany
Victor A. McKusick, U.S.A.
Hideo Nishimura, Japan
Paul E. Polani, Great Britain
Norman H. Topping, U.S.A.
Heinrich Ursprung, Switzerland

Fifth International Conference on Birth Defects

Scientific Program Committee

John W. Littlefield, U.S.A.   *Chairman*
Jean de Grouchy, France   *Vice-Chairman*

Members

Mary Ellen Avery, U.S.A.
Dorothea Bennett, U.S.A.
Daniel Bergsma, U.S.A.
David H. Comings, U.S.A.
James D. Ebert, U.S.A.
Charles J. Epstein, U.S.A.
Douglas M. Fambrough, U.S.A.
M. A. Ferguson-Smith, Scotland
Robert M. Herndon, U.S.A.
Norman Kretchmer, U.S.A.
Robert W. Miller, U.S.A.
Leon E. Rosenberg, U.S.A.
Stephen Roth, U.S.A.
Joseph Warshaw, U.S.A.

Ex-Officio

F. Clarke Fraser, Canada
Victor A. McKusick, U.S.A.
Arno G. Motulsky, U.S.A.

Fifth International Conference on Birth Defects

Conference Interpreters

Mrs. Thérèse Romer, Saint-Eustache, Canada *(chief interpreter)*
Mrs. Simone Trenner, Montreal, Canada
Mrs. Eliane Gerstein, Montreal, Canada

Advisory and executive assistance

Holland Organizing Centre
International Congress Consultants
16, Lange Voorhout, The Hague
The Netherlands

The National Foundation–March of Dimes 1938–1977

The history of The National Foundation–March of Dimes is closely interwoven with that of medical research in the last four decades, as is seen in the programs of international conferences that the Foundation has sponsored, first in polio, later in birth defects. The Foundation's goals and research programs have coincided with the most dynamic areas of research.

In the 1940s, it was the rise of virology. This set the stage for the conquest of polio and prevention of measles, rubella and, perhaps soon, hepatitis B. Researchers also learned to use the virus as a tool of molecular genetics and apply techniques developed in bacterial viruses to animal viruses. It was phage that confirmed DNA as genetic material.

The 1950s saw triumphs of molecular biology and the coming of cell culture. From Zinder and Lederberg's transduction, through Watson and Crick's double helix, to the operon of Jacob and Monod, molecular biology owes much to the methods and insights of virologists, particularly the phage coterie. Phage pioneer Alfred Hershey put it thus: ·Perhaps the first main point to emerge from the study of . . . phages is that phage heredity and bacterial heredity are interwoven quite as closely as phage and bacterial functions; then the second main point would be that the interweaving is not inextricable.' From this intellectual ground, cancer virologists were to launch into the realm of oncogenes and proviruses.

Cell culture arose from tissue culture in the early '50s when a way was found to free cells from tissues. It became possible to count cells, grow them, clone them, and before long, hybridize them. Cell culture enabled geneticists to see human chromosomes one by one, and to find that many well-established and hitherto nameless birth defects had specific karyotypic abnormalities; cytogenetics thus entered clinical practice. Soon biochemists noted that cells in culture are like a man in miniature which can be metabolically dissected to reveal the molecular characteristics of the donor. What *E. coli* did for molecular biology, the fibroblast was to do for human genetics.

In the 1960s we saw explosive growth in immunology. The take-off point was probably the clonal selection theory, an attempt to explain how we distinguish self from not-self and how this information is continuously applied. The thymus was 'discovered' and the two-component theory brought conceptual order to study of immune response. The end of the decade saw victories of cellular engineering to correct immune deficiencies with bone marrow, fetal thymus or liver, thymus extracts, transfer factor, or combinations of these. These attempts focused the immunologists' search for ways to bypass the xenophobic rigor of immune surveillance, to make immune mechanism an obedient servant of man, and to make transplantation practical.

By 1960, biochemical geneticists were on the eve of a great adventure, though few could have foreseen what their efforts would bring in 10 years. Molecular characterization of gene products soon showed that humans differ in biochemical make-up as in physical appearance and that whenever known inborn errors of metabolism are examined, genetic variants are likely to be found. Said Barton Childs, *circa* 1959:

> Gene effects . . . are infinitely modifiable and indeed, in each individual, in greater or lesser degree, must be unique; but they are all traceable to that relationship of specificity between the genetic material and those molecules which exert qualitative and quantitative control over the metabolism of the living cell . . . The genetic method can isolate and circumscribe the problems to be studied with a high degree of refinement, but it remains for the biochemist to elucidate them.

Elucidate he did, and the results profoundly affected notions of evolution and conduct of genetic research.

By 1969, McKusick could say at the 3rd International Conference that molecular biology had freed genetics of its former dependence on pedigrees of obvious hereditary variations. We can now study genes directly in man by studying their products, proteins. Applied at the clinical level, this led to prenatal diagnosis, carrier detection, screening of newborns and high risk groups, and predictive counseling for an increasingly large number of birth defects.

By the early 1970s developmental biology was emerging as the core science of birth defects. The term refers not to a specific discipline but to a way of looking at things. It adds to medical thinking the element of time: life is development, it says, and birth defects are developmental anomalies. We need to know when genes act and in what sequences, and what can change the timetable. Each of the stages of man is an act in a scenario, and the drama in every act depends on what went on in preceding acts.

The developmental approach is most notable in studies of immunity, cancer, metabolism, hormones, and the central nervous system. The ontogeny of such proteins as collagen, hemoglobin and immunoglobulins is being intensively investigated as the best known examples of switching on and off of genes according to a preordained schedule. Clinicians are becoming aware that accelerating or reversing the process may have great therapeutic value. For more than a decade we have watched cancer biologists wrestle with alpha-fetoprotein and have only recently glimpsed its possible function – to help maintain immunological tolerance necessary for mammalian gestation.

There have been several international workshops on 'onco-developmental proteins' and a concerted search may soon be made for a developmental role of C-type RNA viruses, seemingly universal in vertebrates. Predictable too is a push to delineate fetus- or embryo-specific proteins – enzymes, hormones, receptors, membrane antigens, carrier proteins – all presumably under genetic control and subject to mutation; deficiencies or delayed appearance of these may cause many birth defects of now unknown etiology. Future historians of birth defects may hail as the turning point in teratology the recent demonstration that mouse T-locus genes code for cell-surface antigens sequentially expressed during early embryonic development, and that T-locus mutations cause malformation in the heterozygote and embryo death in the homozygote.

All the areas mentioned have had a profound effect in shaping The National Foundation's scientific programs. In turn, these programs have contributed, sometimes decisively, to the advances recounted. The future is difficult to predict except that the unexpected is to be expected. At each international conference we have found that the preceding years have been rich in surprises. This is clear in even a cursory look at the program of the 5th International Conference, appropriately convened in Montreal, a city that has contributed so very much to our understanding of genetics and birth defects.

Foreword

It is quite possible that the major clinical reward from recombinant DNA technology, about which all of us have heard so much, will concern congenital malformations, rather than cancer, metabolic diseases, or 'genetic engineering'. This is because we cannot understand congenital malformations until we understand normal development, and here we have been blocked by an almost total lack of understanding of the structure and function of the human genome. Our ignorance of the chromosome has been reminiscent of our ignorance of DNA structure 'before Watson and Crick' 25 years ago, and perhaps even more of a bottleneck, considering the accumulated knowledge waiting to be applied to the study of development. Now, with rapid acceleration, studies with recombinant DNA and other techniques are beginning to provide a molecular model of the human chromosome, which will tell us how it stores and then progressively releases the incredibly complex information required to program development.

Due in part to our ignorance of the molecular mechanisms of development, the intellectual gap between the clinician interested in congenital malformations and the laboratory sciences which underly 'dysmorphology' is as great as that in any other specialty of pediatrics or medicine, if not greater. At the molecular level we simply cannot begin to consider ways in which development could go wrong! All the advances of molecular biology during the past 25 years are waiting to be applied to this problem. Yet presently the thoughts of the clinical dysmorphologist and of the scientist interested in development are far apart. Such an opportunity to bring the clinic and the laboratory together seems the sort of exciting long-term challenge which would provide a variety of satisfying careers.

As before, the goal of this Vth International Conference on Birth Defects was to cover broadly those advances in basic genetics, cell biology, and embryology relating to development; in biochemical genetics, somatic cell genetics, and cytogenetics; and in perinatology, clinical teratology, and clinical genetics. Although the Scientific Program Committee might be the last to learn otherwise, this meeting seemed to all of us particularly successful. The 'experts' who were present and have contributed to this volume were stellar. The afternoon sessions not included in this volume were limited to four each day, and were scheduled to avoid creating a 'conflict of interest' for the audience. The many free papers submitted were judged by a committee of experts; about 40% were considered appropriate for oral presentation, while the remainder were invited to submit posters. The workshops were chosen on the basis of interest in certain topics not represented in the morning sessions, and were more structured than before, with a number of invited speakers. A final innovation was two 'short courses' on Recombinant DNA Technology and the Cell Surface, designed to give especially interested individuals a detailed review of these rapidly evolving areas.

For all this, we are very grateful to the members of the Program Committee, who identified the fields where progress had been made, nominated potential speakers, suggested the improvements in the afternoon programs, and then participated individually in the Conference. To all of them, and to the many other chairpersons and speakers who helped to make this Conference unusually successful, many thanks indeed!

JOHN W. LITTLEFIELD
Chairman, Scientific Program Committee

List of authors

S. ABE
Laboratory of Developmental
  Biology and Anomalies
National Institute of Dental
  Research
National Institutes of Health
Building 30, Room 416
Bethesda, Maryland 20014
U.S.A.

V. G. ALLFREY
Department of Biochemistry
Rockefeller University
New York, New York 10021
U.S.A.

D. BENNETT
Sloan-Kettering Institute for
  Cancer Research
New York, New York 10021
U.S.A.

M. R. BERNFIELD
Department of Pediatrics
Stanford University
300 Pasteur Drive
Palo Alto, California 94304
U.S.A.

L. C. BOFFA
Department of Biochemistry
Rockefeller University
New York, New York 10021
U.S.A.

D. J. H. BROCK
Department of Human
  Genetics
University of Edinburgh
Western General Hospital
Edinburgh
United Kingdom

M. S. BROWN
Departments of Internal
  Medicine and Pathology
University of Texas Health
  Science Center at Dallas
Dallas, Texas 75235
U.S.A.

L. M. BUJA
Departments of Internal
  Medicine and Pathology
University of Texas Health
  Science Center at Dallas
Dallas, Texas 75235
U.S.A.

A. I. CAPLAN
Biology and Anatomy
  Departments
Developmental Biology Center
Case Western Reserve
  University
2119 Abington Road
Cleveland, Ohio 44106
U.S.A.

C. O. CARTER
MRC Clinical Genetics Unit
Institute of Child Health
30 Guilford Street
London WC1N 1EH
United Kingdom

B. CHILDS
Department of Pediatrics
The Johns Hopkins Hospital
601 North Broadway
Baltimore, Maryland 21205
U.S.A.

F. CLARKE FRASER
Department of Biology
McGill University
1205 McGregor Street
Montreal, Quebec H3A 1B1
Canada

J. E. CLEAVER
Laboratory of Radiobiology
University of California
School of Medicine
San Francisco, California
  94143
U.S.A.

M. D. COOPER
Department of Pediatrics and
  Microbiology and The Com-
  prehensive Cancer Center
University of Alabama in
  Birmingham
University Station
224 Tumor Institute
Birmingham, Alabama 35294
U.S.A.

B. DUTRILLAUX
Institut de Progénèse
Faculté de Médecine
15, rue de l'Ecole de
  Médecine-VIᵉ
Paris
France

Ch. J. EPSTEIN
Department of Pediatrics and
  Division of Genetics
Department of Biochemistry
  and Biophysics
University of California
San Francisco, California
  94143
U.S.A.

M. A. FERGUSON-SMITH
Department of Medical
  Genetics
Royal Hospital for Sick
  Children
University of Glasgow
Glasgow G3 8SJ
United Kingdom

List of authors

Ph. FIELDING
Cardiovascular Research
  Institute
University of California
  Medical Center
San Francisco, California
  94143
U.S.A.

R. L. GARDNER
Department of Zoology
University of Oxford
South Parks Road
Oxford OX1 3PS
United Kingdom

M. S. GOLBUS
Department of Obstetrics,
  Gynecology and Repro-
  ductive Sciences
University of California
  Medical Center
San Francisco, California
  94143
U.S.A.

J. L. GOLDSTEIN
Departments of Internal
  Medicine and Pathology
University of Texas Health
  Science Center at Dallas
Dallas, Texas 75235
U.S.A.

D. GOSPODAROWICZ
Cancer Research Institute
University of California
  Medical Center
San Francisco, California
  94143
U.S.A.

H. E. GREEN
The National Foundation–
  March of Dimes
79 West Monroe Street
Chicago, Illinois 60603
U.S.A.

H. HARRIS
Department of Human
  Genetics and U. of P.
  Human Genetics Center
Richards Building/G4
University of Pennsylvania
  School of Medicine
Philadelphia, Pennsylvania
  19174
U.S.A.

E. D. HAY
Harvard Medical School
Department of Anatomy
25 Shattuck Street
Boston, Massachusetts 02115
U.S.A.

R. M. HERNDON
The University of Rochester
  Medical Center
Center for Brain Research
601 Elmwood Avenue
Rochester, New York 14642
U.S.A.

E. M. JOHNSON
Department of Biochemistry
Rockefeller University
New York, New York 10021
U.S.A.

R. T. JOHNSON
Traylor Building, Room 709
The Johns Hopkins University
Baltimore, Maryland 21205
U.S.A.

J. F. KEARNEY
Departments of Pediatrics and
  Microbiology and The Com-
  prehensive Cancer Center
University of Alabama in
  Birmingham
University Station
224 Tumor Institute
Birmingham, Alabama 35294
U.S.A.

R. A. H. KINCH
Department of Obstetrics and
  Gynaecology
Montreal General Hospital
1650 Cedar Avenue
Montreal, Quebec H3G 1A4
Canada

H. K. KLEINMAN
Laboratory of Developmental
  Biology and Anomalies
National Institute of Dental
  Research
National Institutes of Health
Building 30, Room 416
Bethesda, Maryland 20014
U.S.A.

Cl. LABERGE
Centre Hospitalier
Université Laval
2705 Boulevard Laurier
Ste-Foy, Quebec
Canada

A. R. LAWTON III
Department of Pediatrics and
  Microbiology and The Com-
  prehensive Cancer Center
University of Alabama in
  Birmingham
University Station
224 Tumor Institute
Birmingham, Alabama 35294
U.S.A.

N. le DOUARIN
Institut d'Embryologie du
  C.N.R.S. et du Collège de
  France
49 bis, avenue de la Belle
  Gabrielle
94130 Nogent-sur-Marne
France

Chr. le LIEVRE
Institut d'Embryologie du
  C.N.R.S. et du Collège de
  France
49 bis, avenue de la Belle
  Gabrielle
94130 Nogent-sur-Marne
France

J. W. LITTLEFIELD
The Children's Medical and
  Surgical Center
The Johns Hopkins Hospital
Baltimore, Maryland 21205
U.S.A.

G. R. MARTIN
Laboratory of Developmental
  Biology and Anomalies
National Institute of Dental
  Research
National Institute of Health
Building 30, Room 416
Bethesda, Maryland 20014
U.S.A.

V. A. McKUSICK
Department of Medicine
The Johns Hopkins Hospital
Baltimore, Maryland 21205
U.S.A.

R. W. MILLER
Clinical Epidemiology Branch
A521 Landow Building
National Cancer Institute
National Institutes of Health
Bethesda, Maryland 20014
U.S.A.

M. MONGEAU
Rehabilitation Institute of
  Montreal
6300 Avenue Darlington
Montreal, Quebec H3S 2J4
Canada

A. G. MOTULSKY
Division of Medical Genetics
University of Washington
Seattle, Washington 98195
U.S.A.

D. E. OLINS
Biology Division
Graduate School of Biomedical
  Sciences
Oak Ridge National
  Laboratory
Oak Ridge, Tennessee 37830
U.S.A.

Th. PAPAYANNOPOULOU
Division of Medical Genetics
Department of Medicine
University of Washington
Seattle, Washington 98195
U.S.A.

P. E. POLANI
Paediatric Research Unit
Guy's Hospital Medical School
Guy's Tower
London Bridge
London SE1 9RT
United Kingdom

M.-O. RETHORE
Institute of Progenesis
15, rue de l'Ecole de Médecine
75006 Paris
France

L. E. ROSENBERG
Department of Human
  Genetics, Pediatrics and
  Medicine
Yale University School of
  Medicine
333 Cedar Street
New Haven, Connecticut
  06510
U.S.A.

S. ROTH
The Johns Hopkins University
Merganthaler Laboratory for
  Biology
Baltimore, Maryland 21218
U.S.A.

Ch. R. SCRIVER
McGill University
Montreal Children's Hospital
  Research Institute
2300 Tupper Street
Montreal, Quebec H3H 1P3
Canada

Th. B. SHOWS
Biochemical Genetics Section
Roswell Park Memorial
  Institute
New York State Department
  of Health
666 Elm Street
Buffalo, New York 14263
U.S.A.

R. W. SMITHELLS
Department of Paediatrics and
  Child Health
University of Leeds
27 Blundell Street
Leeds LS1 3ET
United Kingdom

G. STAMATOYANNO-
  POULOS
Division of Medical Genetics
Department of Medicine
University of Washington
Seattle, Washington 98195
U.S.A.

B. STEINMANN
Laboratory of Developmental
  Biology and Anomalies
National Institute of Dental
  Research
National Institutes of Health
Building 30, Room 416
Bethesda, Maryland 20014
U.S.A.

J. P. M. TIZARD
University Department of
  Paediatrics
John Radcliffe Hospital
Oxford OX3 9DU
United Kingdom

G. VIDALI
Department of Biochemistry
Rockefeller University
New York, New York 10021
U.S.A.

List of authors

I. VLODAVSKY
Cancer Research Institute
University of California
  Medical Center
San Francisco, California
  94143
U.S.A.

J. B. WARSHAW
Division of Perinatal Medicine
Department of Pediatrics and
  Obstetrics and Gynecology
Yale University School of
  Medicine
333 Cedar Street
New Haven, Connecticut
  06510
U.S.A.

J. A. C. WEATHERALL
Office of Population Censuses
  and Surveys
Medical Statistics Division
St Catherines House
10 Kingsway
London WC2B 6JP
United Kingdom

Contents

Contents

Mechanisms of disease

Prevention and diagnosis

Future prospects

WORKSHOP SUMMARIES

Opening ceremony

F. CLARKE FRASER

(Honorary President of the Conference)

The opening of a Conference of this kind is a very special moment. We can anticipate the excitement of learning new and stimulating facts about our own specialty, of mind-expanding overviews of other fields, of creative interactions with colleagues, of old friendships refreshed and new ones born. The National Foundation organized the First International Conference on Congenital Malformations in London, in 1960, and I have felt this expectation of an enriching experience, and its fulfilment, at each of the four previous meetings. It is particularly edifying, therefore, for me to be given, so early in my career, the honor of being the first to welcome you to this one. Welcome! I am glad you all got here, and I am sure you will not be disappointed.

Montreal is a wonderful city to live in and to work in. I hope you can sense while you are here, the vitality created by its multicultural nature, which makes this city one of Canada's outstanding national assets. Enjoy it.

Birth defects have been a focus of interest in Québec for many years, both with respect to the practical aspects of management, at the renowned Institut de Réhabilitation of Dr. Gingras and Dr. Mongeau, for example, and to research, at the Département de Génétique Médicale at Hôpital Sainte Justine and the Université de Montréal, at Université de Laval in Québec City, and at McGill and The Montreal Children's Hospital, among others.

The Provincial Government of Québec has played an enlightened and progressive role in developing research and screening programs for birth defects, as manifested by the Réseau Provincial de Médecine Génétique, for example. The current government was elected only last November, so it has not really had a good chance yet to introduce anything new into the Health Care Services with respect to birth defects, but I feel that the presence here, today, of the Ministre des Affaires Sociales (Minister of Health) demonstrates their interest and concern in this area.

Dr. Denis Lazure is a psychiatrist who has been working productively in the field of birth defects, and particularly mental retardation for many years, and has also had a great deal of administrative experience. He founded the department of child psychiatry at l'Hôpital Sainte Justine in 1957. He has been the Director-General of two major psychiatric hospitals and director of the first psychiatric hospital in Haiti, and he has organized the mental health services for the governments of Québec, Ontario and Manitoba. Last November he was elected to the Provincial Government and became Ministre des Affaires Sociales, and in this role he is here to speak to us today.

And so, may I say 'welcome' once again. May you work hard to increase your knowledge, but leave some time to enjoy the many pleasures of our city. May this meeting remain in your memories as the best yet. And may I now have the pleasure of introducing to you – Dr. Denis Lazure.

DENIS LAZURE

(Ministre des Affaires Sociales, Province de Québec)

I. RÉSEAU PROVINCIAL DE MÉDECINE GÉNÉTIQUE

Organisation, buts, fonctionnement et programmes

Organisation En 1969, en collaboration avec le ministère de la Santé, un groupe de représentants des départements universitaires de pédiatrie du Québec mettait sur pied un programme de dépistage de la phénylcétonurie. Un laboratoire central était créé en milieu hospitalier universitaire à Québec et commençait à dépister les nouveaux-nés par une méthode quantitative de dosage de la phénylalanine. Ce programme suivait alors la vague d'implantation de tels dépistages dans les pays développés.

En même temps, le dosage concommittant de la tyrosine était fait, répondant ainsi à un besoin épidémiologique de dépister la tyrosinémie héréditaire. Dès le début, l'organisation de ce programme était décentralisé du ministère. Elle reposait sur un comité interuniversitaire pédiatrique avec l'apport financier et administratif du ministère. Le financement venait du ministère sous forme de subventions et était alloué aux centres et laboratoires selon l'évaluation du comité. Ce type d'organisation était très simple et permettait de répondre rapidement aux besoins de la population.

Dès 1972, devant l'expansion des programmes et le développement des services génétiques régionaux, le programme de dépistage s'appela le Réseau provincial de médecine génétique pour bien démontrer la généralisation des services en terme de prévention, évaluation et traitement à toute la population.

Buts Les buts du Réseau sont: (a) De déceler le plus tôt possible et d'identifier les patients nouveaux-nés souffrant de phénylcétonurie, tyrosinémie héréditaire, d'erreurs innées du métabolisme décelables dans l'urine et récemment, d'hypothyroidie congénitale. (b) D'identifier les problèmes de la population susceptibles de prévention et de traitement par les services génétiques, et ce après des études-pilotes obligatoires. (c) De maintenir des communications étroites entre les laboratoires centraux d'analyse, les centres universitaires régionaux de traitement et les patients. (d) D'assumer la responsabilité de surveillance du traitement des patients identifiés et du conseil génétique aux familles.

Fonctionnement   Le Réseau fonctionne comme un organisme paragouvernemental ayant son budget du ministère et les mêmes normes administratives qu'un établissement de santé. Un comité exécutif composé de représentant de chaque centre universitaire de pédiatrie administre les programmes, alloue les ressources, évalue les budgets sectoriels et coordonne les programmes de dépistage, de traitement et de recherche épidemiologique.

Le dépistage n'étant pas un diagnostic et exigeant une confirmation, il est apparu que la personne ressource directement impliquée dans ce service de santé était le consommateur lui-même. Les parents sont donc mis à contribution directement pour la confirmation du diagnostic et par la suite, lorsque le diagnostic est positif, sont-ils référés à leurs médecins ou aux services hospitaliers régionaux. Cet aspect de communication avec les parents est original, est basé sur la philosophie même d'un système d'assurance-maladie où la prévention est la responsabilité finale du patient et permet aux services de distribution de soins d'être plus efficace au moment où le problème est identifié.

Programmes   Les services offerts à la population sont les dépistages de phénylcétonurie et ses variantes, de tyrosinémie héréditaire, d'hypothyroidie congénitale et d'erreurs innées des acides aminés urinaires.

La phénylcétonurie au Québec a une incidence de 1:35,000 alors que l'hyperphénylalaninémie est de 1:24,000. Le traitement pour le PCU est commencé dans les 4 premières semaines de vie.

La tyrosinémie héréditaire au Québec a une incidence de 1:8000 mais prend dans la région du nord-est un aspect presqu'épidémique avec une incidence de 1:800 naissances vivantes.

Le programme urinaire démontre encore le bien-fondé de l'approche individuelle au patient. En effet, la nouvelle mère est instruite à l'hôpital d'accouchement à recueillir de l'urine de son nouveau-né et de le faire parvenir par la poste à un laboratoire central à Sherbrooke. Cet échantillon est prélevé à 15 jours de vie sur papier filtre par la mère. Un taux de participation de 90% démontre bien que la population peut être sensibilisée à un programme de médecine préventive.

L'hypothyroidie congénitale étant plus spécifiquement du domaine des malformations, nous en traiterons plus loin séparément.

Collaboration inter-universitaire

L'aspect opérationnel le plus important du Réseau est la collaboration inter-universitaire. Comme presque partout ailleurs, les généticiens médicaux se retrouvent dans les milieux universitaires. Plutôt que de demeurer dans leurs tours d'ivoire et de se préoccuper essentiellement de recherche et d'enseignement, ces universitaires mus par un besoin d'appliquer les connaissances génétiques à la population se sont retrouvés au comité du Réseau.

Cette association d'intérêt, plutôt que formelle, a fait qu'un but commun a pu être poursuivi sans intégration officielle de structures (comité de doyens, etc...) universitaires tout en créant un réseau de services génétiques régionaux. Cette approche individuelle et d'intérêt empêche la formation de chasse-gardées, défendant un drapeau universitaire quelconque. L'autre avantage de cette association a été de normaliser la disparité existante entre les ressources des 'grandes' et 'petites' universités. L'obligation morale de chaque centre de surveiller la qualité du traitement et de s'assurer du conseil génétique aux familles à aider à créer et améliorer les ressources de ces centres pour dispenser les services génétiques.

Le comité du Réseau avait de plus la possibilité d'allouer les ressources nécessaires à l'implantation de nouveaux services, permettant ainsi un meilleur équilibre et faisant disparaître les disparités existantes. Si bien qu'actuellement, en partie par la politique du réseau, les centres universitaires de pédiatrie, ont les ressources nécessaires au diagnostic et traitement de leur clientèle en plus que celle générée par le Réseau. D'une certaine façon, toute la population peut maintenant avoir accès à ces services parce que le Réseau s'est développé d'une façon interuniversitaire. Les patients souffrants de maladies génétiques, par la complexité de leurs problèmes, seront admis dans ces hôpitaux, lesquels par ailleurs auront les ressources nécessaires en place grâce au Réseau. Cette planification de services aura donc dépassé les besoins immédiats des programmes de dépistage.

Assurance-maladie

La création de novo de services génétiques aurait été impossible, n'eut été l'arrivée de l'assurance-maladie universelle. Les services génétiques ne sont qu'un appendice à ce régime, appendice orienté vers une population de patients chroniques et répondant à un besoin particulier, même si ce besoin est important au niveau pédiatrique. Les coûts ont été marginaux pour son implantation. Il suffit de rappeler quelques chiffres connus. Des études à McGill et ailleurs ont démontré que 33 % des admissions d'un hôpital pédiatrique était relié à la génétique. Les études de Colombie-Britanique évaluent à 10 % le nombre de nouveaux-nés qui éventuellement manifesteront une maladie génétique au cours de leur vie. Si on se rappelle que la plupart de ces maladies sont chroniques, la prévention par les ressources appropriées et les traitements adéquats deviennent d'extrême importance.

En termes de coût, le Réseau a démontré que l'utilisation de personnel auxiliaire et des parents pour le traitement en externe de ces malades d'âge pédiatrique, permettait une économie très appréciable. Encore fallait-il que les ressources nécessaires soient en place pour permettre aux centres régionaux d'assumer leurs responsabilités de diagnostic et traitement.

Un des exemples souvent cité démontrant l'interaction assurance-maladie et génétique est l'efficacité de dépistage des leucinoses au Québec. Comparativement aux autres pays, le Québec est très efficace dans ce domaine. Cependant, il n'existe pas de programme spécifique de dépistage des leucinoses au Québec. Les nouveaux-nés souffrants de leucinose sont très malades, acidotiques et difficiles à traiter. Ils sont donc référés aux centres pédiatriques universitaires, ce que leur permet l'accessibilité aux soins du régime d'assurance-maladie.

Dans ces centres, les équipes médicales qui les reçoivent peuvent compter rapidement sur les services génétiques qui ont les ressources techniques nécessaires au diagnostic et qui en plus, grâce à la politique du Québec, peuvent obtenir les diètes nécessaires à leur traitement sans frais pour les parents. La création du Réseau favorise donc une intégration plus efficace des services de santé et ceci parce que les intérêts des universitaires sont coordonnés dans une organisation paragouvernementale. Nous sommes loin des services de laboratoire fournit par un laboratoire central et remis sans surveillance aux dispensateur de soins et sans contrôle sur la qualité du traitement.

Hypothyroidie congénitale

L'hypothyroidie congénitale n'est pas par définition une maladie génétique mais entre surtout dans le domaine des malformations congénitales. En effet, la plupart du temps, la cause est l'absence de thyroïde.

La possibilité d'utiliser le sang séché sur papier filtre pour doser l'hormone thyroidienne et le développement de micro-méthodes de dosage a permis au centre du réseau à Québec de mettre au point une méthode de dépistage. Après une étude pilote sur 50,000 naissances, Dussault et Laberge de Québec pouvaient recommander au réseau la mise en place de ce service. La méthodologie est différente de celle des programmes habituels de dépistage, utilisant des méthodes radio-immunologiques et des calculs sur ordinateurs. L'incidence d'hypothyroidie congénitale s'est avérée être de 1:6000 naissances vivantes, ce qui s'est avéré être la même dans des études d'autres populations qui ont suivi le Québec. Le traitement, après vérification du diagnostic, est commencé en moyenne vers la 4e semaine de vie, ce qui est dans les normes reconnues de début de traitement avant 3 mois pour prévenir l'arriération mentale et les troubles de croissance. Cette incidence a surpris tout le monde puisqu'on ne croyait pas ce problème aussi fréquent. De plus, il s'est avéré à l'étude prospective que plus de 50% des bébés ne montrait aucun signe clinique pouvant faire soupconner au clinicien averti la présence d'hypothyroidie.

Le programme est donc très efficace et offre les meilleures chances de succès thérapeutiques. En effet, des résultats préliminaires d'évaluation psychologique et du développement démontrent chez 14 patients sous traitement hormonal à l'âge d'un an, que leurs quotients de développement par le test de Griffith est égal à la population normale. L'évaluation prospective de ces patients est en cours dans une étude en collaboration nord-américaine et des résultats plus probants devraient sortir d'ici un an. Cette première québecoise a par la suite été reprise aux Etats-Unis et ailleurs et d'ici quelques années, on verra plusieurs populations avoir un tel programme. Un colloque international sous les auspices du Réseau aura lieu en 1979 et après l'évaluation des résultats des quelques programmes existants, dont le principal est au Québec, donnera probablement le feu vert final à l'implantation d'un tel programme. Ce dépistage de l'hypothyroidie congénitale est un évènement majeur dans la prévention de malformations congénitales et pourrait servir de modèle, la technologie aidant, dans d'autres syndromes.

Programmes divers du Réseau

En plus que des programmes de dépistage de masse, le Réseau participe à d'autres programmes. Ses centres sont occupées au dépistage de la maladie de Tay-Sachs dans la population juive de Montréal et certaines populations régionales canadienne-française, au dépistage de la thalassémie dans la population montréalaise d'origine méditerranéenne ainsi qu'une population canadienne-française de la région de Québec. Le Réseau participe à une banque de tissus permettant aux chercheurs l'accessibilité au matériel pathologique pour les travaux sur les mécanismes étiologiques de plusieurs maladies. Le Réseau a participé activement à la création d'une 'banque d'aliments' canadienne, en conjonction avec un mécène, permettant l'accessibilité des patients aux diètes spécifiques à leur maladie.

La coordination des membres du Réseau a permis la création à Montréal d'un centre d'amniocentèse pour fins génétiques où toutes les études sur liquide amniotique sont faites. Cette centralisation permet un meilleur contrôle de qualité, une évaluation génétique préalable et l'assurance d'un conseil génétique adéquat par la suite. Les patients des centres du Réseau sont donc référés à Montréal pour fin d'amniocentèse où les ressources existent dans les 2 universités pour faire les études de protéines fétales, l'analyse des chromosomes et les dosages biochimiques.

II. AUTRES PROGRAMMES DU QUÉBEC RELIÉS À LA PRÉVENTION DES MALFORMATIONS CONGÉNITALES

Centralisation des naissances

D'autres mesures de prévention que le Réseau existent au Québec. En terme purement préventif, la politique récente de centralisation des accouchements dans certains hôpitaux et surtout, la création d'unité néonatales régionales, permettent l'identification rapide et le traitement adéquat des malformations sur une base beaucoup plus efficace. Encore là, les membres du Réseau, sont appelés à aider dans l'identification, le traitement et le conseil génétique, les responsables de ces unités.

Banque de données

Les banques de données des régimes d'assurance hospitalisation et assurance-maladie, celle du comité néonatal et celle du Réseau pourraient éventuellement permettre la liaison de documents pour la surveillance des incidences de certaines malformations. Cette approche épidémiologique serait un grand pas dans l'identification de problèmes de santé et la prévention éventuelle.

Toxicologie

Un autre programme récemment développé au Québec en toxicologie pourrait aussi avoir un impact sur la prévention des malformations congénitales. Des programmes de pharmaco-vigilance et les études de tératogénicité des produits chimiques sont en train de s'implanter. Les programmes existants de toxicologie industrielle auront aussi possiblement un impact sur cette prévention.

III. CONCLUSION

Dans le domaine des malformations congénitales et plus spécifiquement celui des maladies génétiques le Québec s'est doté d'un programme intéressant de prévention, les programmes étant financés et approuvés par le ministère mais organisés et distribués par des universitaires, créant ainsi un réseau de centres régionaux. Ces centres en plus que d'offrir des services aux patients du Réseau, sont impliqués dans la distribution de soins génétiques à la population fréquentant ces institutions grâce au régime d'assurance-maladie.

Le réseau a développé un programme original et important démontrant l'efficacité de l'identification des hypothyroidiens congénitaux et de son traitement. Ce programme est maintenant suivi ailleurs dans le monde.

D'autres programmes en association avec celui du Réseau font du Québec une expérience intéressante dans le domaine de la prévention des maladies chroniques que sont les malformations congénitales.

DENIS LAZURE

(Minister of Health, Quebec Province)

I. PROVINCIAL NETWORK OF GENETIC MEDICINE

Organization, objectives, functioning and programs

Organization   In 1969, in collaboration with the Minister of Health, a group of representatives from university pediatric departments in Quebec launched a screening program for phenylketonuria. A central laboratory was set up within the environs of the Quebec University Hospital to screen the newborn by means of a quantitative assay method for phenylalanine. This program followed the wave of such screening activities embarked upon in the developed countries.

The assay of tyrosine was carried out at the same time, fulfilling the epidemiological need to screen for hereditary tyrosinemia. The organization of this program was from the start decentralized from the Ministry. It rested on an inter-university pediatric committee with the financial and administrative support of the Ministry. The financing was in the form of grants, which were allocated to the laboratories and centers according to the committee's evaluation. This simple organization allowed a rapid response to the needs of the population.

From 1972, with the expansion of the programs and the development of regional genetic services, the screening program was named the Provincial Network of Genetic Medicine in order to indicate clearly the generalization of its services to include prevention, evaluation and treatment in relation to the whole population.

Objectives   The objectives of the Network are: (a) The earliest possible detection and identification in the newborn of phenylketonuria, hereditary tyrosinemia, inborn metabolic defects detectable from the urine and, recently, hypothyroidism of a congenital nature. (b) After the necessary pilot studies the identification of problems susceptible to prevention or treatment by the genetic services. (c) To maintain direct communications between the central analytical laboratories, the regional university treatment centers and the patients. (d) To assume responsibility for the surveillance of the treatment given to identified patients, and to give genetic counselling to the families.

Functioning   The Network functions as a paragovernmental body receiving its budget from the Ministry and having the same administrative structure as a health establishment. An executive committee composed of representatives from each university pediatric center administers the programs, allocates the resources, evaluates the sector budgets and coordinates the screening, treatment and epidemiological research programs.

Since the detection is not a diagnosis and requires confirmation, it is clear that the responsible person directly involved in this health service is the consumer himself. The parents thus make a direct contribution to the confirmation of the diagnosis and, if the diagnosis is positive, are then referred to their doctor or to the regional hospital services. This aspect of communication with the parents is original, being based on the same philosophy as a health insurance scheme in which the aspect of prevention is the final responsibility of the patient, and this perhaps allows the services which provide the care to operate more effectively.

Programs The programs offered to the population are screening for phenylketonuria and its variants, for hereditary tyrosinemia, for congenital hypothyroidism and for inborn defects of urinary amino acids.

The incidence of phenylketonuria in Quebec is 1:35,000 while that of hyperphenylalaninemia is 1:24,000. Treatment for phenylketonuria is started during the first 4 weeks of life.

Hereditary tyrosinemia has an incidence of 1:8000 in Quebec, but has an almost epidemic aspect in the north-east region with an incidence of 1:800 amongst live newborn infants.

The urinary program again shows the effective basis of the individual approach to the patient. In fact the new mother is instructed in the maternity hospital to collect her newborn child's urine and to send it by post to the central laboratory at Sherbrooke. This sample is obtained by the mother on filter paper when the child is fifteen days old. The degree of participation of 90% clearly shows that the population can be made sensitive to a program of preventive medicine.

Since congenital hypothyroidism is more related to the field of malformations, it will be discussed separately later.

Inter-university collaboration

The most important operational aspect of the Network is the inter-university collaboration. As almost everywhere else, the medical geneticists are found within the university environment. Rather than stay in their ivory towers and become preoccupied with research and teaching, these university members are activated by a need to utilize their genetic knowledge for the population and are recruited by the Network committee.

This rather informal association of interests has a common objective and can be pursued without the official integration of university bodies (committee of deans, etc.). The individual approach and marriage of interests prevents the formation of exclusive groups defending any particular university flag. The other advantage has been to iron out the disparity between the resources of the 'big' and 'little' universities. The moral obligation of each center to monitor the quality of treatment and to ensure genetic counselling for families has helped to create and improve the resources of these centers.

The Network committee can also allocate the resources necessary for setting up new services, ensuring a better balance and reducing current disparities. Partly as a result, the university pediatric centers now have the resources necessary for diagnosing and treating their clientele over and above that generated by the Network, and to some extent the whole population now has access to these services. This service plan will thus exceed the immediate needs of the screening programs.

Health insurance

The creation of the genetic services from nothing would have been impossible if it had not been for the arrival of universal health insurance. The genetic services are only an appendage of this scheme, an appendage directed to a population of chronic patients and responding to a particular need, one which is of importance at the pediatric level. The costs of setting it up have been marginal. It is enough to note some well-known figures. From studies at McGill University and elsewhere it has been shown that 33 % of admissions to pediatric hospitals are related to genetic factors. Studies in British Columbia estimate that 10 % of the newborn will eventually show a genetic disease during the course of their lives. If it is recalled that the majority of these diseases are chronic, prevention by appropriate resources and adequate treatment take on a character of extreme importance.

In terms of cost the Network has shown that the use of auxiliary personnel and of parents for the out-patient treatment of these child patients has led to very appreciable economies. It has still been essential to make the necessary resources available to the regional centers.

One of the often quoted examples showing the interaction between health insurance and genetic services is the efficacy of leucinosis screening in Quebec, in comparison with other countries. However, there is no specific program for leucinosis screening in Quebec. Newborn infants suffering from leucinosis are very sick, acidotic and difficult to treat. They are thus referred to university pediatric centers, which allows them access to the care of the health insurance scheme.

The medical units which receive them can count on the rapid support of the genetic services, which have the technical resources for diagnosis and, due to the policies prevailing in Quebec, can also obtain the diets required for their treatment without cost to the parents. The creation of the Network thus promotes a more effective integration of the health services because the interests of the universities are coordinated within a paragovernmental organization. We have come a long way from central laboratory services provided to the physician but without surveillance or monitoring of the quality of the treatment.

Congenital hypothyroidism

Congenital hypothyroidism is not by definition a genetic disease but it is mainly placed within the field of congenital malformations. In fact, in most cases the cause is the absence of the thyroid gland.

The possibility of using blood dried on filter paper for thyroid hormone assay and the development of microassay methods have allowed the Quebec Network center to develop a screening method. After a pilot study on 50,000 newborn infants,

Dussault and Laberge in Quebec were able to recommend to the Network that this service should be set up. The methodology differs from that of traditional screening programs, using radioimmunological methods and computer calculations. The incidence of congenital hypothyroidism has been established as 1:6000 live births in Quebec, and proved the same in subsequent studies of other populations. After verification of the diagnosis, treatment is started on average towards the 4th week of life, which is within the recognized period for starting treatment before the age of 3 months so as to prevent mental retardation and disturbances of growth. This incidence surprised everybody since it had not been thought that the condition was so frequent. Moreover, prospective studies have established that more than 50% of the babies show no clinical sign to make the physician suspect the presence of hypothyroidism.

The program is thus very effective. In fact, the preliminary results of mental and developmental evaluation of 14 patients under hormonal treatment show that, at the age of 1 year, their development quotients in the Griffith test are equal to that in the normal population. The prospective evaluation of these patients is in progress as part of a North American collaborative study, and more searching results will become available in a year's time. This lead by Quebec has subsequently been taken up by the United States of America and elsewhere. An international colloquium under the auspices of the Network will take place in 1979, and in a few years from now there will be many populations with such a program.

Various programs of the Network

Apart from the mass screening, the Network participates in other programs. Its centers are involved in screening for Tay-Sachs' disease in the Jewish population of Montreal and in some regional French Canadian populations, as well as for thalassemia in the Montreal population of Mediterranean origins together with a French Canadian population of the Quebec region. The Network participates in a tissue bank allowing researchers access to pathological material for work on the etiological mechanisms of several diseases.

The Network, together with a patron, has actively participated in the creation of a Canadian 'food bank' providing patients access to diets specific for their disease.

The Network has promoted the creation in Montreal of an amniocentesis center for genetic purposes where all the studies on amniotic fluids are carried out. This centralization allows a better control of the quality of early genetic evaluation and an assurance of adequate genetic counselling afterwards. The resources of the 2 universities in Montreal are available for studies of fetal proteins, chromosome analysis and biochemical assays.

II. OTHER PROGRAMS IN QUEBEC RELATED TO THE PREVENTION OF CONGENITAL MALFORMATIONS

Centralization of births

Preventive measures other than the Network exist in Quebec. In purely preventive terms the recent policy of centralizing confinements in certain hospitals and, especially, the creation of regional neonatal units allows the rapid identification and adequate treatment of malformations on a much more effective basis. Apart from that, the Network members are called upon by those responsible for these units to aid in identification, treatment and genetic counselling.

Data bank

The data banks of the hospital insurance scheme, the health insurance scheme, the neonatal committee and the Network will eventually allow the combination of documents for monitoring the incidences of some malformations. This epidemiological approach will be a great step forward.

Toxicology

Other programs, in relation to drug vigilance and teratogenicity of chemical products, are currently being set up in Quebec and may also have an impact on the prevention of congenital malformations. Existing programs of industrial toxicology may be similarly relevant.

CONCLUSION

In the field of congenital malformations and, more specifically, that of genetic diseases, Quebec possesses a valuable overall preventive program in which the individual programs are financed and approved by the Minister of Health but are organized and distributed by the universities, thus creating a network of regional centers. Apart from offering services to the Network patients, these centers are involved in the provision of genetic care to the population consulting these centers as a result of the health insurance scheme.

The Network has developed an original and important program for efficaceous identification and treatment of congenital hypothyroidism.

Other programs associated with the Network give Quebec valuable experience in the field of preventing the chronic diseases which constitute congenital malformations.

VICTOR A. McKUSICK

(President, International Birth Defects Congress, Ltd.)

Dr. Lazure, thank you for that fine address. Dr. Fraser, fellow workers on birth defects, ladies and gentlemen.

To my knowledge the history of international congresses in science and medicine is yet to be written. Their impact on biomedical progress would be a useful matter for historical analysis. How has that usefulness changed over time? What, for example, is the relative value of congresses such as this one in 1977 and one in 1877, in view of the differences in communication and travel and in science itself?

Accounts are given of landmark medical congresses such as one held in London in 1881 at which Koch described solid media subsequently used in the discovery of the tuberculosis bacillus. Some of us here attended the First World Congress of Human Genetics in Copenhagen in 1956, a landmark meeting, and birth defects congresses beginning in 1960 have likewise been landmarks, starting with London and continuing with the congresses in New York, The Hague, Vienna and now Montreal.

In an age of increasing specialization the opportunity which a congress such as this provides for what Clarke Fraser has referred to as 'creative interaction' between diverse fields is one of its main objectives. This is particularly crucial in a field like birth defects which spans quite literally all of biology and medicine. Often in the past international congresses have served to delineate specialities, and in a sense this has occurred in these birth defects congresses, but I would say that more there has been a broad synthesis rather than the delineation of a narrow specialty. The basic sciences that have been brought together include genetics as a leading one, but also cell biology, molecular biology, embryology, teratology, and epidemiology to mention only a few, and in the clinical sphere, pediatrics, obstetrics, neonatology, orthopedics, neurology and, of course, clinical genetics.

I have spoken of a historical approach to the question 'How useful are these congresses?'. As you should have noted from the materials given you at the time of registration, a contemporary and prospective evaluation is being attempted at this meeting. I urge most strongly that each of you participating in this meeting give us the benefit of your experience by completing the evaluative questionnaire.

One can, furthermore, ask the relative value of congresses of broad scope such as this and of small, highly focused and specialized workshops, symposia and

14

conferences. You'll have noticed that the Program Committee for this meeting aims to have the best of both worlds by planning poster sessions, workshops and even short courses to supplement the plenary sessions that traditionally have characterized these birth defects conferences.

Science and certainly medicine are in the last analysis human activities. It is the people who do them that count. A main object of our getting together for a conference such as this, all said and done, is a social one. The informal and social aspects are as important as the formal plenary sessions, for example. In this connection I call your attention again to Dr. Fraser's useful term 'creative interaction'.

We are looking forward in this conference to an exciting mind-stretching, horizon-widening experience. The program has been laid on under the able leadership of my colleague at Johns Hopkins, Dr. John Littlefield, who has served as Chairman of the Program Committee. It is a special pleasure to be meeting in the hometown of my long-time friend Dr. Clarke Fraser and we all thank him for his warm welcome.

As President of the International Birth Defects Congress, which organizes these congresses, I'm delighted to welcome all of you to this fifth congress. International Birth Defects Congress, Ltd., was founded in the 1950's under the name International Medical Congress. It had, as its main objective at the outset, the organization of poliomyelitis congresses. It was founded by Mr. Basil O'Connor who was its first president and its president until his death in 1972. Because of the narrowed objectives of the organization we chose rather recently to change its name to International Birth Defects Congress.

It's next my pleasant task to introduce to you Mr. Harry Green who is Chairman of the Board of Trustees of the National Foundation–March of Dimes. As you know the March of Dimes is the 'angel' for these congresses. In the National Foundation and its predecessor in the field of poliomyelitis we have observed a marvelously effective alliance between dedicated laymen on the one hand and scientists and physicians on the other. This was illustrated by Franklin Delano Roosevelt, by Basil O'Connor and by the distinguished father of our next speaker, the late Mr. William Green who, in addition to being president of the American Federation of Labor, was a trustee of the National Foundation for Infantile Paralysis from its beginning in 1938. Mr. Harry Green, an honors graduate of Princeton University and of the Harvard Law School, has a distinguished record as a businessman. For us, however, the most important point is that he is a perceptive and supportive advocate to all who work in the field of birth defects.

HARRY E. GREEN

(Chairman, Board of Trustees, The National Foundation–March of Dimes)

Mr. President, distinguished participants in this Fifth International Conference on Birth Defects, and guests.

Ralph Waldo Emerson made this observation during the 19th century: 'Men love to wonder, and that is the seed of our science'. The timeless truth of this statement has even more validity today.

The National Foundation–March of Dimes invited scientists from all parts of the world to meet in London for the First International Conference on Congenital Malformations in 1960. The concept of such an assembly was a visionary one. Approaches to the age-old problem of birth defects would be seen from new points of view – multidisciplinary points of view – of genetics, anatomy, pathology, immunology, embryology, and other sciences.

Delegates came from 21 countries. They concentrated on the latest work in emerging fields such as cytogenetics, genetic variations in proteins, extrinsic factors in congenital malformations in man, and the management of human congenital defects. Never before had there been such an integrated presentation of the status of this complex problem. In the 17 years since that first international assembly, we have been able to share in the developments that hold such promise for our mutual quest: improving the quality of life at birth.

Basil O'Connor, president of The National Foundation, and president of the International Medical Congress, until his death in 1972, saw science as a struggle for truth – man's ageless war against his own ignorance, fiercely fought for his own improvement.

From its inception in 1938, The National Foundation–March of Dimes has acted upon the belief that answers can be achieved more readily when a voluntary health movement works with health professionals as an equal partner. We know what the association of laymen and scientists accomplished in the conquest of polio. This belief carries with it a responsibility to inform our constituents about advances in overcoming congenital disease and disability. We must communicate even the questions that you are asking. For it is these questions, directed as they are into your avenues of investigation, that offer so much hope to people throughout the world. In our fight against birth defects, rather than search for remedies, we seek, as you do, their ultimate prevention.

When this may be achieved is beyond prediction. But we have begun to see it happen. For example, 10 years ago, a pregnant woman and her unborn child were unprotected against congenital rubella or Rh blood disease. That is no longer true.

The world of science is contributing to an exciting tempo of progress in medical genetics. New techniques are at hand for studying the structure of chromosomes. New biochemical tests have been tried and made standard. New approaches for interpreting and understanding abnormalities have become indispensable in diagnosis. With each of these advances, a physician increases his ability to answer the questions: Why did it happen? Will it happen again?

By sharing these answers, the international community of scientists is bringing us closer to our cherished goal – that of protecting the unborn and the newborn from the incidence of birth defects.

Through such an exchange of expertise, The National Foundation has, this spring, published the 5th edition of the *International Directory of Genetic Services*. The most complete compilation of genetic study facilities in print, this new edition has been sent to geneticists, pediatricians, obstetricians, and other health professionals throughout the world.

When The National Foundation published the *Birth Defects Atlas and Compendium*, it represented information from 370 contributors from 22 countries. Each author was an expert in his particular field of birth defects. The *Atlas* was the first publication of its kind to give standard names, in 4 languages, and specific descriptions, treatment, and genetic background for some 850 congenital anomalies. An expanded second edition of the *Atlas* is being prepared.

Concurrently, the *Atlas and Compendium* is being updated by a computer memory bank. The system, now being tested, is a collaborative effort by The National Foundation, Tufts-New England Medical Center, and the Massachusetts Institute of Technology. When it is in full operation, the computer will provide physicians with rapid diagnostic information about any known birth defect that affects body structure or function. The system has the capacity to help doctors identify rare birth defects syndromes and alert them to unusual patterns in the occurrence of congenital disorders. Programmed for worldwide use, the computer may one day prevent another tragedy similar to the devastating one of thalidomide. This warning factor has the potential of giving professionals valuable extra time to trace the causes before many children are affected.

Protection of the unborn and the newborn is the mandate of The National Foundation–March of Dimes. 'Protection', to us, is not a passive word. Within our mandate, as a voluntary health organization, it calls for strongly positive action. Until recently, the world of fetal life, and how it is influenced, has been a neglected universe.

In the 17th century, Sir Thomas Browne wrote that man's life is encompassed by three worlds: this world in which we live; the world after death; and 'that other World, the truest microcosm, the Womb of our Mother', where we 'live, move, have being, and are subject to the actions of elements and malice of the disease'.

Little still is known about the adverse outside influences that affect the unborn child. We are aware of the classic cases of the afflicted fetus who survives, but is born with severe damage attributed to thalidomide or rubella.

But what of other possible sources of risks to the well-being of the fetus? Instead of causing obvious birth defects, does fetal malnutrition lead to a diminished quality of mind or behavior that the child will carry through life? An increasing number of investigators believe this, and there are reasons for their belief. But we don't know how one leads to the other, nor how frequently. If it is frequent, this will be one of the most challenging public health issues of the future.

While protection from outside agents will be a major aspect of future fetal medicine, the most important factor in fetal health undoubtedly will remain the mother's womb. Her hypertension and toxemia, her malnutrition or under-nutrition, her diabetes or metabolic disorders, some of the drugs she uses for these conditions, her chronic alcoholism, her cigarette consumption, all can have adverse effects on her unborn baby. And the fetus, just like the rest of us, can generate a disease of his own as a consequence of his genetic make-up that interacts with his environment in the womb.

'Fetal ecology', remarked the late Duncan Reid, '(is) the forerunner of the quality of life'. To master the ecology is the prime quest of fetal research. Implicit in its mastery is the promise of healthier babies rather than the tragedy of babies lost.

In a toast at a banquet attended by international scientists in Milan, Pasteur commented that 'Science knows no country because knowledge belongs to humanity, and it is the torch that illuminates the world'.

And, in that spirit, may I welcome you to the Fifth International Conference on Birth Defects. It will be a significant one, I am sure, to the well-being of generations who follow us.

A. G. MOTULSKY

(General Chairman of the Conference)

Ladies and Gentlemen

It gives me great pleasure to say a few words to introduce the 5th International Conference on Birth Defects. The birth defect congresses are somewhat different than most biological and medical meetings. Rather than focussing on a specific scientific discipline or medical specialty, the congresses have selected a single area of human suffering – birth defects – for their attention. With this focus, scientists and physicians from many fields are pooling their efforts and collective wisdom in these quadrennial exercises. This type of conference, therefore, deals with basic science, clinical investigation and clinical medicine in many different disciplines.

The primary goal of the congress is a consideration of a variety of scientific topics which bear upon etiology, mechanisms and management of the many different birth defects. This meeting is supported by public contributions to a private foundation – The March of Dimes–National Foundation – with the expectation that public philanthropy will speed the day when birth defects can be prevented or successfully managed. The example set by the conquest of a viral disease – poliomyelitis – largely through the efforts of the National Foundation is a 'hard act to follow'. We are dealing no longer with one illness but with many different congenital malformations and diseases. Their etiology is rarely unifactorial as it was with the viral cause of poliomyelitis. Complex multifactorial causations, often by subtle interaction of heredity and environment, largely occurring during inaccessible fetal development, are facing us in our task to understand and to prevent these human tragedies. We are beginning to develop some insights but should not mislead the public that prevention and cure for the majority of birth defects is 'just around the corner'. Much hard work in the basic sciences of molecular biology, immunology, membrane and cellular biology, genetics, developmental biology, pathology, virology and teratology is required to give us the understanding required for the conquest of birth defects. At the same time, clinical investigators in pediatrics, epidemiology, neonatology, medical genetics, dysmorphology and obstetrics/gynecology need to apply various basic concepts as well as methods unique to their disciplines to the study of birth defects in man. The past has shown that species differences may be considerable and that work on man, his cells and body fluids never can be entirely replaced by research work in lower species.

Despite these arduous tasks required for the future, considerable practical advances have already been taking place in prevention of Rh disease, in screening, in intrauterine diagnosis, in nosology and in surgical corrections of different birth defects. Prevention and cure requires recognition of the tremendous heterogeneity of birth defects. It is therefore likely that many different mechanisms apply in pathogenesis which require different strategies of research and management. No single panacea for prevention and treatment is likely. In fact, it may be that a certain fraction of birth defects may be the price the human species has to pay for biological variability. A search for better methods of intrauterine diagnosis to detect defects not otherwise preventable therefore remains an important area of our research strategy.

The conference will deal with many of these topics in plenary sessions, in workshops and contributed papers. I urge specialists to broaden their horizons and to attend meetings ordinarily outside of their interests and competence. Some of the most important contributions are likely to come by combining ideas and concepts of different fields into new insights. The conference is introducing a new kind of activity: courses in the important fields of cell surface biology and in 'recombinant DNA technology'. The latter field has suffered from exposure to mass hysteria in the recent past. Its scientific and practical potentials are enormous and the claimed dangers are hypothetical and highly unlikely.

It gives me great pleasure to welcome you to this congress. The intense biomedical research in the many areas touching on birth defects provides a solid opportunity for learning and discussions.

Priorities for research on birth defects *

BARTON CHILDS

Department of Pediatrics, Johns Hopkins University School of Medicine, Baltimore, Md., U.S.A.

It is a fundamental belief in medicine that knowledge of the cause of a disease is the key to its treatment and perhaps its cure.

Table 1, based on figures given by Wilson (1977), shows that although the causes of some developmental defects in human beings are known, the origins of the bulk of these conditions are not. In this, birth defects resemble other common disorders in which the causes of a few cases are assignable to genes or other well-defined influences, but the origins of the majority continue to defy attempts to discover them.

TABLE 1

Causes of developmental defects in man

Genetic transmission	20%
Chromosomal	3–5%
Environmental	
Radiation	< 1%
Infections	2–3%
Maternal metabolic	1–2%
Chemical	2–3%
Unknown	65–70%

After Wilson (1977).

Table 2, which summarizes the subjects of papers given in the plenary sessions of all 5 international conferences on birth defects, shows a heavy emphasis on the processes of normal embryogenesis and fetal development, as well as on disease mechanisms and other avenues to understanding which might lead to a reduction in the proportion of unknown causes (Birth Defects, Int. Conf., 1974, 1977; Congenital Malformations, Int. Congr., 1961, 1964, 1970). Indeed, only about 15% of these contributions were devoted to anything else. The idea embodied in these papers is that characterization of the molecular processes of normal embryogenesis, followed by discovery of the molecular mechanisms through which the defects are caused, will suggest some treatment or some intervention which might prevent the

* This work was supported in part by USPHS research grant HD 00486.

injury or malformation. This approach is perfectly compatible with the reductionist view which prevails in medicine in which it is presumed that the discovery of the causes of diseases and their consequences, preferably in molecular terms, must lead to some form of treatment, preferably a cure. No one can quarrel with this idea; it has brought some spectacular successes, most notably in the cure of infectious and nutritional diseases. But the causes of many other kinds of disease have eluded investigators and cures have not always followed even the most precise description of the molecular abnormality. In fact, much disease is chronic, much treatment only palliative, and many patients must endure physical and social handicaps which make life a trial rather than an adventure. Most birth defects fall into this category.

TABLE 2

Subjects of papers given in plenary sessions of 5 international conferences on birth defects

Basic aspects	Number	Clinical aspects	Number
Normal processes	56	Descriptive and taxonomic	10
Disease mechanisms	23	Causal factors	14
New techniques	16	Management	11
Epidemiology	17	Prevention	13
Total	112	Total	48

The conventional prescription for this deficiency is more of the same; more molecular elucidation, more search for mechanism and cure. That is an aim vigorously to pursue, but we should also consider alternatives, even ask whether the goal of mechanism and cure can soon be reached on any grand scale. It may turn out that the causes of many birth defects will be found to lie not proximally in the processes of generation, but distally in the social and evolutionary properties of the human race. And it may turn out that cures, and even prevention, will continue for some time to elude us.

This cause–cure paradigm is best exemplified in the conquest of infections (Thomas, 1974, 1976a). Here there is a clear-cut cause, in the form of a microbe that may be combatted by an antiserum or antibiotic or warded off by immunization. In this version, disease is the enemy, and we make war on it. Someone has pointed out how the language of warfare pervades our thinking and action. But is the mentality of warfare appropriate for all disease; should the cause of disease be seen invariably as something predatory and inimical to everyone? And can we count on devising some means of treatment for each case of each disease when we do discover its molecular properties? The answers to such questions, and the optimism with which one gives them, depend on definitions of causes and cures.

CAUSES AND CURES

Causes

If we think of disease as a state of homeostatic disharmony due to the intervention of some foreign or inappropriate substance, and if we are able to give a molecular description of both the immediate consequences of the intervening substance and all its ramifications, then we have the kind of insight into cause and mechanism of disease that may suggest a treatment with some chance of restoring homeostatic equilibrium. That is, we have a description of a disease, its cause, and its treatment, all at the molecular level.

In this version, the blame for the disease is implicit in the labels given; if the genotype is non-adaptive in all environments, the disease is said to be genetic; and if the adverse effects of an external agent are independent of the genotype, the disease is said to be environmental. When neither of these conditions obtains, the label 'multifactorial' is employed to give symmetry to the model and to suggest special combinations of genes and experiences. For each of these three kinds of disease, the aim is to hunt down the enemy, whether bad genes, microorganisms, or toxic substances, and to nullify their effects and to prevent recurrent attacks. All this focuses narrowly on the processes of the diseases themselves, visualizing each as a self-contained entity, as something alien which has the patient in its grip and from which he must be freed.

An alternative version avoids this typological rigidity and is wary of labels which suggest unitary causes. In this version, the cause of the disease is to be found in the complex relation between the individual qualities of the patient and his particular conditions of life. (Incidentally, this is not a modern idea, having been proposed in more or less this form by Virchow in the 19th century (Galdston, 1954)). The cause, then, is not expressed as the consequences of only one gene or one toxic substance, but lies, in addition, in a lifetime of experiences which have shaped a genetically unique person to respond non-adaptively in conditions which themselves have a cultural past, and the language of warfare is inappropriate here, since the only possible enemies in sight are one's self, one's species, and one's culture. This conception of cause also differs from the conventional one in its manifold nature. In the case of common diseases, the genes involved are the stuff of which most variation is made; and the non-genic elements involve not only drugs, diets, teratogens, carcinogens, and the like, but even the social and cultural conditions which predispose to their distribution and consumption. That is, in addition to these specific agents, unless one takes a parochial view of cause, there are the social and behavioral properties of a culture in which, in a clash of values, health sometimes loses out.

Cures

As to the need for some new thinking about the cure and prevention of birth defects (and chronic diseases), we have an eloquent witness in Lewis Thomas (1974, 1976a,b), who testifies to the inefficiency of palliative and expensive treatments which he describes as middle-level technology, and which he says must be replaced by a high-level technology through which diseases may be speedily, effectively, and simply resolved. Thomas' prescription for this deficiency is more research into mechanism, because with understanding will come the means to prevent irreversible damage; and he cites the conquest of infectious diseases as the example to follow. There is no doubt that this method will continue to pay off for a long time, but the problems will become more and more complex as the relatively simple cases are solved; and the remainder, which may well be a sizeable proportion, will turn out to be the result of the action of very particular, and often unpredictable, sets of polymorphic genes working under very particular and equally unpredictable conditions. The number of such gene sets, and genotype-environment combinations (which in birth defects must include both mother and fetus) could be very large, so that the precise description of cause of the same birth defect could differ from case to case and may be, in fact, unique in each. So the treatment, if any, would have to be tailored to each case, or at least to each of a number of types of case. In addition, the discovery of preventive measures could be made difficult because some of the environmental 'causes' might be substances in general use and so go unrecognized as harmful. For example, a drug in wide use shown not to be teratogenic in a large study might be strongly injurious to a few specially susceptible persons, a result which is diluted by the large number of non-susceptibles. This difficulty in distinguishing teratogenic properties of commonly used drugs was revealed in the Perinatal Collaboration Study (Heinonen et al., 1977). In short, there may be some irreducible minimum of birth defects, the result of both that genetic variability which is essential to the survival of the human species, and an environmental variability which technology causes to proliferate at a dizzying rate.

So, although the probes into molecular mechanism will continue to be rewarded, we might also search for new ways to detect causes in social organization. And because we are not going to have a disease-free society, we must devote more energy to dealing with those patients who will always be with us. I wish, therefore, to suggest some lines of research which will complement the work on mechanisms and which are not now being given the attention they deserve. These are: (1) a modification of the conventional epidemiological method to include some genetic considerations that may be helpful in the search for cause; (2) studies of attributes of personality and temperament which determine behaviors which on the one hand predispose to birth defects and on the other facilitate or preclude preventive actions; and (3) investigations into the attitudes of both public and patients which prevent, or promote, the development of self-sufficiency in people with birth defects and their incorporation into the polity as consequential citizens.

EPIDEMIOLOGICAL INVESTIGATIONS

Epidemiology offers a method for discovering relationships between variables; it is a means of studying distributions of conditions in populations and the factors which influence those distributions (Lilienfeld, 1976). It began as a study of the characteristics of infections and is now employed in the study of chronic diseases (Murphy, 1977). The similarity of aims between genetics and epidemiology is striking, but it is odd that although geneticists have been engaging in epidemiology since Penrose's Colchester study, the epidemiologists have seldom reciprocated. And it may be this lack of grasp of genetic variability which has caused epidemiologists, when looking for the causes of birth defects, to behave as if they see uniformity where the geneticist sees heterogeneity. For example, epidemiological methods have been used to show that the incidence of anencephaly varies geographically, with race, place and season of birth, SES, and maternal age, and that all of these relationships vary with time (Edwards, 1958; Leck and Record, 1966; Yen and MacMahon, 1967; Naggan,

1969; Fedrick, 1976; Anon, 1976; Sandahl, 1977). These and other observations have been taken to mean that there is some environmental agent which causes anencephaly, probably imposed on a genetic background, and that the secular variations mentioned are the result of variable exposure to it. Indeed, one such agent, potato blight, was recently proposed, but lost its glamour when various discordant observations were brought out (Renwick, 1972; Masterson et al., 1974). Now, while it would not have surprised the investigators if several agents had been discovered, in all these studies the methods used make an opposite impression: they do not accommodate to the idea of heterogeneity. That is, the distributions are treated as if they were characteristic of homogeneous populations. In contrast, it is the genetical view that no population may be assumed to be homogeneous, so the hypothesis of heterogeneity should be examined in anencephaly as in all else. The seasonal variations in birth, the maternal age effect, the geographical and ethnic differences, and the secular changes may all be manifestations of such heterogeneity. For example, the cases born during the winter months may differ in origin from those born in other parts of the year.

One way of deciding might be to divide the population into 2 parts according to season of birth and then to look at comparisons of variables between the 2 sets of individuals and at events in the families included in each. Leck and Record (1966) found that abortions in families of anencephalics were more frequent in the winter months, but did not say whether or not the anencephalic sibs of the abortuses born during the winter were themselves born in the winter. There are no data on season of birth of pairs of anencephalics; that is, whether or not season of birth of fetuses with this defect is a familial property. Stated more generally, one way to approach the possibility of heterogeneity is to break the distributions of traits found in epidemiological studies into at least 2 parts and then to study the 2 populations separately. This comes easily to the geneticist, who expects to find heterogeneity of cause at the extremes of distributions; the differences are revealed by the homogeneity of expression within the families and the differences between unrelated persons. The question to be tested in each study is whether the exceptional individuals, that is, those born of older mothers, or in some season of the year, or at one end of a spectrum of age of onset, or limited to some geographic, ethnic, or other group, are representative of a continuum or are causally distinct in some way. Study of the familial cases may be expected to help in this test.

STUDIES OF HEALTH BEHAVIOR

If we can accept that diseases have causes which reside in the organization of societies and in individual living habits, then the 'treatment' of such diseases should involve efforts to change the conditions which are involved in the network of cause (Galdston, 1954). Preventive agencies should try to accomplish these aims rather than to rely on homilies about healthful living or the after-the-event exhortations of physicians. Such changes will be slow in coming, requiring as they do such painful reordering of values as will put health above profits and before conventional standards of living. Perhaps the rising expressions of consumer resistance and the dawning recognition of the limits of the world's resources foreshadow such changes in values. Perhaps they are also precursors of some public awareness that diseases have ulterior causes and that good health requires self-protective actions. Physicians find it difficult to deal with these issues in office practice, but there are some ways medicine can participate in at least one aspect of this resolution of conflicting interests; namely, in helping to reorient public attitudes toward health and away from disease.

Students of health behavior are aware that good medical care depends upon an informed collaboration between patients and physicians (and their various agents) and that this collaboration depends upon more than formal knowledge. It depends upon psychological variables which may be summed up colloquially in saying that some people do what's good for them because they respond that way to authority in general, others because they see it as 'the thing to do' and because it gains them some social approbation, and others because the action is compatible with their own internal, sometimes quite irrational, scheme of things (Green, 1976). People must also have some grasp of what the disease or threat means to them, how serious it is, and how likely it is to involve themselves (Rosenstock, 1966). So, if preventive advice is to be accepted, it must be proffered through channels which meet each person's system of values and behavioral characteristics. For example, in an anti-smoking campaign, cognitive appeals alone may suffice for some of those who are internally directed, but others who take their cues from the actions of other people may not stop smoking even though they have understood the message perfectly. The origins of attitudes and beliefs about health and illness are not well understood; it is a field which has received little notice in medical circles despite abundant evidence that patients pay a good deal less attention to the doctor's 'orders' than the latter think (Sackett and Haynes, 1976). At the moment, ideas for changing attitudes having to do with the prevention of birth defects must be derivative of studies done in other fields, although since smoking, excessive drinking, and perhaps overuse of some drugs are habits which have been accused of causing some defects, results of research now in progress on these are directly applicable. One procedure, limited to the field of birth defects, which could be examined systematically in this way is antenatal diagnosis. We have little information about the psychological and social attributes of either the women who undergo it or of those who do not. The latter may have no knowledge of its existence or availability, perhaps because their doctors fail to mention it, or they may reject it because of inertia engendered by conflicts between advanced ideas and traditional beliefs, or perhaps they think it is riskier than we know it to be. Nor are there enough studies of the impact of the procedure on those parents who elected the abortion; are they advocates or antagonists? There is evidence that 'early adopters' of a procedure have a significant influence on followers (Green, 1975). In any case, this procedure represents a classical case of an innovation whose properties of diffusion and adoption could be studied. Adoption of preventive health measures has been shown to follow conventional S-shaped growth curves which are subject to the accelerating and decelerating effects of social pressures, including the compatibility of the procedure with existing values and past experiences, its complexity, and what others might think of one who falls in with the idea (Green, 1976). That is, there is an existing context in which to study the adoption of this practice; and since it can be regarded as an effective public health procedure only if it becomes a common and harmless medical practice available to all, the factors promoting or inhibiting its spread should be investigated.

Another aspect of health education of interest to students of birth defects is how people perceive general risks, as well as particular odds, say, for having another baby with a birth defect. In general, people guide risk-taking behavior by some subjective judgment of the utility of the action rather than by any objective valuation, and they often replace objective probabilities with subjective estimates of what the outcomes will be (Bem, 1971; Pearn, 1973). There are many studies of risk-taking behavior outlining the social settings and personality factors that determine who takes what risk under what circumstances, but few of these deal with peoples' own perceptions of the risks to their health of daily living or of reproductive decisions based on the odds for some genetic catastrophe. For example, I know of no studies of the perception of risk experienced by women who have or have not presented themselves for antenatal diagnosis. Further, the numerous papers and books on genetic counseling state the odds and allude to the relative importance in making decisions of burden and risk, but few report systematic efforts to discover the importance given these and other factors in individual cases, and I know of none which has reported a well-designed study of how these decisions are made (Murphy and Chase, 1975).

There is some evidence that subjective interpretation of odds may condition the behavior of physicians. In a study of physicians' attitudes to genetic screening, it was shown that doctors' perceptions of stated odds for common diseases varied from high to low; and if high, the doctor was much more likely to learn about the disease and to recommend action to his patients (Rosenstock et al., 1975). It would be useful to see if this subjective variation in the perception of risks operates in a sample of parents of offspring with birth defects and to test its relation to reproductive decisions. It would also be of interest to probe the social and psychological conditions which accompany, or predispose to, such subjective judgments with the idea of learning what to look for so as to bring the message of genetic counseling into consonance with the temperament, outlook and knowledge of those who need it. Such studies should be planned and carried out with the same scientific rigor as that demanded in laboratory research, and for this the collaboration of investigators of health behavior and health education are required.

SOCIAL ADAPTATION

People whose birth defects were not prevented and are not amenable to definitive treatment must become the object of the kind of care and support which will allow them to participate in life. Most of the care of patients with birth injuries, along with that of other chronic diseases, falls to agencies outside conventional medical practice. Research on the impact of such disabilities on the lives of patients, their families, and the community tends to take second place after investigations of cause or immediate treatment and is carried out by physicians, psychologists, special educators, and sociologists, again outside the usual medical channels. Table 3 shows the numerical relation of reports of such research to other kinds as it is tabulated in the *Index Medicus* for the years 1975–1976. There are, of course, other articles and books which are not listed in the *Index Medicus*, but that only reinforces the point these data make; namely the research is done outside the usual medical channels and its results are not likely to be seen by many physicians (Dybwad and Dybwad, 1977a). This separation of the handicapped from traditional medical practice is only the medical counterpart of a systematic isolation of such people, whether in custodial institutions, treatment centers, or special educational programs, and their exclusion from much daily life, not necessarily by virtue of their disability, but because the world is designed by, and operated for the benefit of those individuals who fit comfortably and inconspicuously within one or two standard deviations from the means of many distributions. But the outliers in the distributions stand apart and are seen to do so in stereotyped ways. They become 'funny looking kids', and they assume an identity which is determined by their most salient characteristic, their disability. And this disembodied view of the handicapped is translated into stereotyped social attitudes which lead to a developmental Catch 22; the handicapped are deprived of social stimulation because of their disabilities, which in turn leads to overprotective, non-stimulating treatment or custodial care, which, of course, alienates them the more from ordinary life.

TABLE 3

Subjects of papers listed in Index Medicus for the years 1975–1976 under several listing categories

Listing category	Subject of paper		Total
	Behavioral, social, and rehabilitation	Disease mechanism, diagnosis, treatment	
Congenital abnormality	21 (2%)	1067	1088
Spina bifida	27 (10%)	236	263
Cerebral palsy	45 (21%)	165	210
Mental retardation	298 (33%)	470	768
Diabetes mellitus	64 (3%)	2140	2204

Fortunately these restrictive attitudes are breaking up, due to the efforts of aroused relatives and citizens' groups as well as to those of enlightened physicians, sociologists, and other workers in the field (Dybwad and Dybwad, 1977b). These groups have recognized that bringing the handicapped into the community can promote their development and draw attention to their right to education, employment, and the enjoyment of life, and at the same time awaken the public to virtues, talents, and socially desirable attributes which go unnoticed and uncultivated in an institutional, or otherwise restricted, existence (Dybwad and Dybwad, 1977b). But to make this emergence successful, to reduce physical disability to mere variation in the public mind, and to readjust social institutions to accommodate disabled people as equals will require some massive tempering of traditional rigid attitudes on the part both of the public and the handicapped – clearly a state that calls for research.

Richardson (1976) has shown that it is the violation of the expectation of normal appearance and behavior by the handicapped which causes normal people to shy away from them. This aversion has powerful effects on the disabled, whose problems are derived less from the disability itself than from the reactions of other people, the inadequacy of public institutions to accommodate them, and the effects of these on their feelings about themselves (Anderson, 1976; Evans et al., 1974; Dorner,

1976). Both these actions and reactions are variable; some normal persons accept the handicapped easily and gracefully, while some disabled people surmount the most formidable obstacles with intact self-esteem; but the factors which contribute to this variability are unclear (Richardson, 1976). Here again we meet typological thinking in which 'the handicapped' are the object of study, observation, and conjecture as if all were the same. So the ranges of reaction for both normal and handicapped should be investigated, so that we may learn something about the responses of both disabled and normal individuals to each other. Then we may gain some insight into the factors that engender these behaviors. Without such insight it will be impossible to design educational programs capable of dissolving those prejudicial attitudes which deny the handicapped an atmosphere in which to thrive (Levin, 1976).

CONCLUSION

In conclusion, it is evident that we do not lack for attention to the molecular details of the mechanisms of differentiation and development. The techniques are there, or will be invented, and there is no lack of eager and talented investigators, and we may continue to expect rich dividends from their exertions. But medical practice is only partly involved with molecules, biochemistry, and physiology. Much of the biochemical and developmental configuration assumed by each human being originates in his social behavior; medical transactions are social, and the life of a patient with a disease is social. These aspects of health and disease have not been exactly neglected by investigators, but as subjects for research, they do not enjoy the attraction, not to say the glamour, of other more conventional scientific pursuits. Perhaps molecular biology is queen because the possibility to test hypotheses precisely and cleanly is at a maximum, while research into attitudes is beset by problems of definition, quantification, and research method. But thinking of the causes of birth defects as originating partly in the ways in which living is organized, that is, in the geographic, economic, and social elements which determine where and how we live, and learning something about how, or even whether, people perceive the connection between their everyday habits of living and their health; and learning about how to harmonize one's endowment with one's environment and how to accept people whose appearance and behavior is 'different'; are all as necessary to the solution of the problems posed by birth defects as learning about the molecular mechanisms. I think medicine is gradually being secularized, mainly as a result of public leverage; thoughtful people want to become collaborators in the protection of their health. Accordingly, in the field of birth defects, a greater priority should be given to investigation of ways in which social organization impinges on the preservation of health in all the senses of that word. New and rigorous research methods are needed, and so are more participants who know the problems of medicine at first hand. These issues, which lie at the heart of preventive medicine, are given too little weight by the medical establishment. Further, more opportunity for people working on apparently unrelated aspects of birth defects to meet, discuss, even to work together, would be salutary; a too restricted attention to each separate aspect of their problems is not in the interest of patients with birth defects. Perhaps future international conferences on birth defects will help in achieving these goals.

REFERENCES

Anderson, E. M. (1976): *Birth Defects: Orig. Art. Ser.*, *12/4*, 47.
Anon. (1976): *Brit. med. J.*, *2*, 1156.
Bem, D. J. (1971): In: *Risk Taking Behavior*, p. 4. Editor: R. E. Carney. Charles C Thomas, Springfield, Ill.
Birth Defects, IVth International Conference, Proceedings (1974): Editors: A. G. Motulsky, W. Levy and F. J. G. Ebling. Excerpta Medica, Amsterdam.
Birth Defects, Vth International Conference: Provisional Program (1977).
Congenital Malformations, Ist International Congress (1961): Editor: M. Fishbein. Lippincott, Philadelphia.
Congenital Malformations, IInd International Conference (1964): International Medical Congress, Ltd., New York.
Congenital Malformations, IIIrd International Conference (1970): Editors: C. F. Fraser and V. A. McKusick. Excerpta Medica, Amsterdam.
Dorner, S. (1976): *Arch. Dis. Childh.*, *51*, 439.
Dybwad, G. and Dybwad, R. (1977a): *Int. Child Welfare Rev.*, *32*, 63.
Dybwad, G. and Dybwad, R. (1977b): *Int. Child Welfare Rev.*, *32*, 55.
Edwards, J. H. (1958): *Brit. J. prev. soc. Med.*, *12*, 115.
Evans, K., Hickman, V. and Carter, C. O. (1974): *Brit. J. prev. soc. Med.*, *28*, 85.
Fedrick, J. (1976): *Brit. J. prev. soc. Med.*, *30*, 132.
Galdston, I. (1954): *The Meaning of Social Medicine*. Harvard Press, Cambridge.
Green, L. W. (1975): In: *Applying Behavioral Science to Cardiovascular Risk*, p. 84. Editors: A. J. Enelow and J. B. Henderson. American Heart Association, Inc., Seattle.
Green, L. W. (1976): *Publ. Hlth Rev.*, *5*, 5.
Heinonen, O. P., Slone, D. and Shapiro, S. (1977): *Birth Defects and Drugs in Pregnancy*. Publishing Sciences Group, Inc., Littleton, Mass.
Leck, I. and Record, R. G. (1966): *Brit. J. prev. soc. Med.*, *20*, 67.
Levin, L. S. (1976): *Birth Defects: Orig. Art. Ser.*, *12/4*, 171.
Lilienfeld, A. M. (1976): *Foundations of Epidemiology*. Oxford University Press, New York.
Masterson, J. G., Frost, C., Bourke, G. J., Joyce, N. A., Herity, B. and Wilson-Davis, K. (1974): *Brit. J. prev. soc. Med.*, *28*, 81.
Murphy, E. A. (1977): *Proceedings, VIIIth International Scientific Meeting of the International Epidemiological Association*. In press.
Murphy, E. A. and Chase, G. A. (1975): *Principles of Genetic Counseling*. Year Book Medical Publishers, Chicago.
Naggan, L. (1969): *Amer. J. Epidemiol.*, *89*, 154.
Pearn, J. H. (1973): *J. med. Genet.*, *10*, 129.
Renwick, J. H. (1972): *Brit. J. prev. soc. Med.*, *26*, 67.
Richardson, S. A. (1976): *Birth Defects: Orig. Art. Ser.*, *12/4*, 16.
Rosenstock, I. M. (1966): *Milbank mem. Fd Quart.*, *44*, 94.
Rosenstock, I. M., Childs, B. and Simopoulos, A. P. (1975): *Genetic Screening: A study of the knowledge and attitudes of physicians*. National Academy of Sciences, Washington, D.C.
Sackett, D. L. and Haynes, R. B. (1976): *Compliance with Therapeutic Regimens*: Johns Hopkins Press, Baltimore.
Sandahl, B. (1977): *Acta paediat. scand.*, *66*, 65.
Thomas, L. (1974): *Bioscience*, *24*, 99.
Thomas, L. (1976a): *J. med. Educ.*, *51*, 23.
Thomas, L. (1976b): *J. med. Philosophy*, *1*, 212.
Wilson, J. G. (1977): *Fed. Proc.*, *36*, 1698.
Yen, S. and MacMahon, B. (1967): *Lancet*, *2*, 623.

THE HUMAN GENOME

Chairman: Jean de Grouchy, Paris

Chromosome structure *

DONALD E. OLINS

The University of Tennessee Graduate School of Biomedical Sciences and the Biology Division, Oak Ridge National Laboratory, Oak Ridge, Tenn., U.S.A.

The last several years have witnessed a phenomenal growth in our knowledge and conceptions of eukaryotic chromatin structure. The most comprehensive and contemporary summary of the status of this field is the 1977 Cold Spring Harbor Symposium, entitled 'Chromatin'. Most of the references cited in this paper refer to that symposium. The purpose of this brief communication is 2-fold: (1) to assist the uninitiated reader in this burgeoning field by providing some overview; (2) to convey aspects of our laboratory's current and planned emphasis in the field of chromatin structure. Three general references are cited at the end of this paper – the results of three meetings largely devoted to chromatin structure, held in 1974, 1975 and 1977. The expansion and productivity of this field is readily conveyed by a comparison of these 3 symposia.

THE NUCLEOSOME CONCEPT

Early electron microscopic and biochemical studies, now amply confirmed, led to the concept of the repeating chromosomal subunit (the nucleosome or nu body). Spheroidal nucleohistone particles (*v* bodies), of approximately 10 nm diameter, connected by DNA strands were visualized from nuclei swollen and spread at low ionic strengths (see Olins et al., 1977. for earlier references). Figure 1 shows an example of this 'beads-on-a-string' appearance, and illustrates the bipartite internal structure, supported by more recent studies. The nucleolytic digestion studies (see Van Holde et al., 1977, for earlier references) suggested that the connecting DNA strands were readily digested with micrococcal nuclease to a core particle (v_1) consisting of ~ 140 nucleotide pairs (np) of DNA associated with an octamer of histones (i.e., 2 each of H4, H3, H2A and H2B).

More recent studies have refined our knowledge of the shape, dimensions and distribution of protein and DNA within the core particle. Neutron scattering studies (Pardon et al., 1977; Bradbury, 1977) and X-ray crystallographic analysis (Finch

*This research was sponsored by the Energy Research and Development Administration under contract with Union Carbide Corporation, and by a National Institute of Health research grant GM 19334 to DEO.

and Klug, 1977) of core particles have led to a bipartite model of v_1, i.e., 2 circular disks stacked into an oblate structure ~ 11 nm diameter and 5–6 nm thick. Each half-nucleosome would be associated with about 70 np DNA probably coiled on the outer perimeter of each disk. Evidence from DNase 1 digestion of chromatin (Noll, 1977) is also consistent with the view that the bulk of the DNA is on the outside of v_1. Many current models of DNA folding invoke the concept of DNA

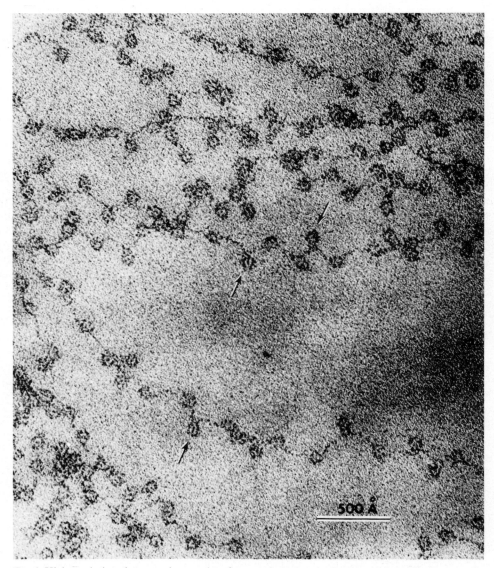

Fig. 1. High resolution electron micrography of a spread chicken erythrocyte nucleus. The arrows point to nu bodies with clear internal structure. Many chromatin fibers exhibit a zig-zag configuration with nu bodies lying on alternate sides of the connecting strand. Specimen swollen and fixed in 1 mM EDTA, pH 7.0, and dried on the grid in aqueous 5 mM uranyl acetate.

'kinking' (see e.g. Sobell et al., 1977), although calculations derived from the thermodynamics of DNA conformation in solution appear to make the concept of 'smooth' bending at least equally plausible (R. E. Harrington, manuscript in preparation). A core particle (v_1) normally includes a complete complement of 8 inner histones, but reconstructed particles consisting solely of H3 and H4 exhibit considerable resemblance to the native nucleosome (Camerini-Otero et al., 1977; Oudet et al., 1977a). Dissociation of a core particle in high salt buffer appears to liberate the inner histones as a heterotypic tetramer (Campbell and Cotter, 1976) or as an octamer (Thomas, 1977). The basis for this discrepancy between different laboratories remains to be resolved; either the preparation or the solvent conditions could account for this disagreement.

The NMR studies of isolated histones and of histone complexes (Bradbury, 1975, 1977; Bradbury et al., 1977) support the view that the N-terminal 40% of the inner histones (i.e., the most basic portions) are largely freely mobile; whereas, the apolar C-terminal regions are globular, and represent the regions of histone-histone interaction. Recent determinations of the secondary structure of the histones within purified nu bodies employing laser Raman spectroscopy (Thomas et al., 1977) yielded $\sim 50\%$ α-helix, $\sim 0\%$ β-sheet and $\sim 50\%$ 'random' structure. Assuming that essentially negligible secondary structure exists in the N-terminal portions of the histones, the C-terminal globular regions could consist of a high local density of α-helix (e.g., $\sim 80\%$ helix). These apolar regions would then resemble myoglobin or hemoglobin in α-helix density.

Our laboratory's interpretation of the conformational states of nu bodies (discussed below) is strongly dependent upon this emerging view of its internal structure: v_1 appears to consist of a DNA-rich outer shell associated with the irregularly folded N-terminal portions of the 8 inner histones; and of a protein-rich core composed of close-packed α-helix-rich histone globular regions, possibly arranged with point-group symmetry (Olins et al., 1977).

HIGHER-ORDER STRUCTURE OF NU BODIES

It has long been known that chromatin in situ or in the presence of sufficient divalent cations or ionic strength exists as an approximately 20 nm-wide fiber (see e.g. Ris, 1975). With the development of the nucleosome concept of chromatin, it was natural to suggest the possibility that the 20-nm fiber might represent some close-packed (e.g., helical) array of nu bodies (Olins et al., 1977). An alternative view of the 20-nm fibers, the solenoidal model (Finch and Klug, 1976), postulates that a continuous electron density 10 nm thick 'nucleofilament' is coiled into a helix with a pitch of ~ 10 nm and a channel down the middle of the fiber.

Current ultrastructural studies do not support simple continuous helical models. The solenoidal model claims that the nu bodies cannot be visualized in the 20-nm fibers (Davies, 1976). However, Figure 2 clearly shows that nu bodies can be visualized within close-packed structures. Figure 2 also illustrates that the 20-nm fibers frequantly fall apart into clusters of nu bodies (Olins, 1977; Renz et al., 1977; Franke et al., 1977). As a consequence of such micrographs, there remains the distinct possibility that the 20-nm chromatin fiber is a discontinuous structure composed of

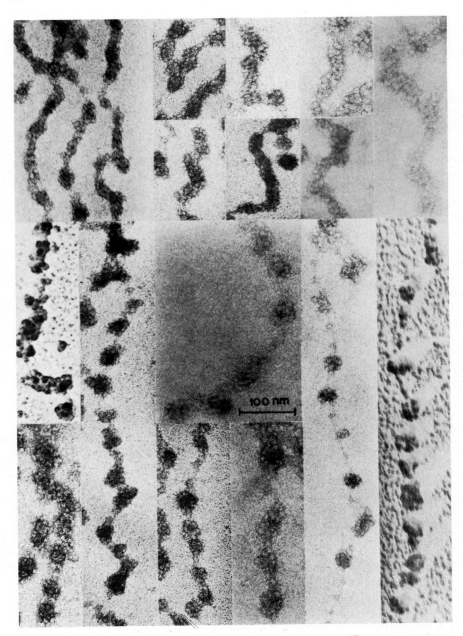

Fig. 2. A montage exhibiting samples of continuous and discontinuous nu body arrays. Electron micrographs of 20–30 nm chromatin fibers spilling out of chicken erythrocyte nuclei from many different preparations. Isolated nuclei were washed in 0.2 M KCl and diluted 1 : 150 in 0.02 M KCl, 0.5 mM MgCl$_2$. The slightly swollen nuclei were centrifuged onto freshly glowed carbon-coated grids, rinsed with Photo-Flo, dried and negatively stained with 5 mM uranyl acetate. The micrographs in the upper third of the figure illustrate continuous fibers; those on the bottom two-thirds of the figure discontinuous (clustered) nu body arrays.

close-packed clusters of nu bodies, rather than continuous helical arrangements of subunits.

Whatever the ultimate arrangement of the nucleosomes within the 20-nm fiber, there is strong circumstantial evidence that the H1 class of histones is responsible for its generation and/or stabilization (Bradbury, 1975, 1977; Cole et al., 1977). This importance of H1 for chromatin condensation is particularly well observed in the ultrastructural studies of SV-40 minichromosomes (Oudet et al., 1977b; Griffith and Christiansen, 1977; Keller et al., 1977).

The exact relationship of H1 histones to the nucleosomes core particles remains unclear. Most current models assume that H1 is primarily associated with the connecting DNA strands. The DNA between core particles can vary as much as 40–100 np in different tissues (see e.g. Morris, 1976), which may correlate with the size or basicity of the H1 proteins of that tissue.

When chromatin is condensed due to the presence of H1 and sufficient cations, treatment with DNase II results in cleavage of the DNA at the midpoint of the nucleosome (Zachau, 1977). This biochemical criteria suggests that during chromatin condensation (i.e., close-packing of nu bodies) conformational changes can also occur within the chromatin subunit.

CONFORMATIONAL STATES OF NU BODIES

Biochemical and ultrastructural studies of presumed transcriptionally active chromatin make it extremely likely that the native 'inactive' nucleosomal structure is conformationally altered. The most convincing biochemical studies derive from the demonstration of an enhanced sensitivity of 'active' chromatin to DNase I (for a summary of earlier results, see Garel and Axel, 1977). It is also apparent that although micrococcal nuclease cleaves active chromatin into the normal subunit DNA size, it is cleaved more rapidly than inactive chromatin (Bellard et al., 1977). Ultrastructural studies (Foe, 1977; McKnight et al., 1977; Franke et al., 1977) reveal that normal nu bodies are generally not observed in RNA polymerase-dense regions (i.e., sites of intense RNA synthesis), although they have been observed in regions of sparse transcription.

The view of this laboratory is that knowledge of the conformational states accessible to nu bodies is essential to understanding the probable structural transitions during activation of chromatin. Furthermore, we conceive the nu body as resembling other multisubunit enzymes and proteins (e.g., probably possessing internal symmetry and allosteric interactions). Because chromatin does not have a known catalytic or binding site (other than the internal histone-DNA and histone-histone interaction sites) it is not possible to search for effector molecules and allosteric transitions as with enzymes or hemoglobin. Instead we have chosen to employ biophysical techniques to define conformational states of nu bodies. Most of our studies have been on isolated chicken erythrocyte core particles (v_1), with some experiments on isolated chromatin (Zama et al., 1977).

We have examined the influence of increased urea concentration (0–10 M) on isolated v_1. Urea produces a diversity of structural transitions without dissociating the histone-DNA interactions. A model interpreting and summarizing these con-

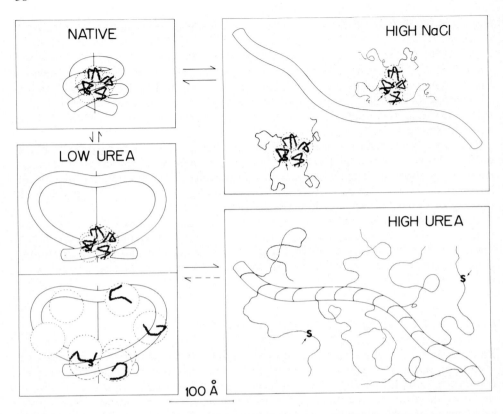

Fig. 3. Scheme of the effects of urea and of high NaCl on v_1. The postulated true dyad axis is represented as a vertical line penetrating the 'native' and 'low urea' structures. The equivalent single superhelical turn of DNA per v_1 is conceived of as being stabilized at the ends of the DNA fragment, presumably by interaction with H3 and H4. In the native v_1 model, additional folding of the DNA can be accomplished while the single equivalent superhelical turn is still maintained, by twisting the DNA clockwise or counter-clockwise around the particle dyad axis and binding to the histone core. α-Helical segments are represented in the globular domains of the histone molecules. Two different possible low urea states are represented with the DNA coil untwisting and expanding into a more asymmetric and open structure. In 'high urea', the histone globular regions have become random coils while the basic regions are still attached to the extended DNA rod. The H3 thiol groups are exposed and reactive ($\rightarrow$). In 'high NaCl' (pH 7.0), v_1 dissociates into the DNA fragment and 2 heterotypic tetramers.

formational perturbations is presented in Figure 3. To generalize these results, we believe that the disruptive effects of urea act differently upon the DNA-rich outer shell of v_1, than upon the protein-rich α-helical core of v_1. Urea appears to have progressive and non-cooperative effects on the DNA-rich shell and overall particle hydrodynamic properties: $S_{20,w}$ of v_1 decreases continuously with increased urea; the melting temperature (T_m) of most of the DNA decreases linearly with increased urea. Destabilizing effects on the close-packed apolar histone regions, however, appear to be highly cooperative. In low urea (0–3 M) the histone α-helix content (i.e., $[\theta]_{222\,nm}$) remains unchanged; the H3 thiol groups remain 'buried' to reaction with N-ethyl maleimide (NEM); the ultrastructure of v_1 remains essentially unchanged. Between 4–8 M urea dramatic and highly cooperative structural transitions are noted: α-helix is rapidly lost; H3 thiols are exposed; particle unravelling is observed by electron microscopy. Above 8 M urea, little biophysical changes are observed in v_1; the subunit appears to be completely unravelled, even though the histones remain bound to (and stabilize the melting of) the particle DNA. This differential response of the shell and core of v_1 to increased urea could furnish a model for possible structural transitions during chromatin activation. Perturbations of the DNA-rich shell adequate for transcription might occur with only minor structural effects upon the apolar core. The protein-rich core could then act as a restoring force to return the subunit to a compact inactive configuration.

Another type of perturbation of v_1 is observed during studies of the influence of ionic strength on hydrodynamic properties (see Zama et al., 1977). Oudet et al. (1977b) have observed v_1 splitting into half-nucleosomes at low ionic strength. Our hydrodynamic studies (V. Gordon, V. Schumaker, D. Olins and C. Knobler, manuscript in preparation) demonstrate 2 salt-dependent transitions at $\sim 10^{-3}$ and $\sim 10^{-2}$ M KCl. It is not yet clear whether either of these transitions would represent an 'opening up' of the bipartite structure of v_1. It is apparent, however, that these conformational transitions are readily reversible by changing the ionic strength, and they do not involve dissociation of histone and DNA. Further studies are in progress to ascertain the relative effects of ionic strength on the shell and core of v_1.

We have recently succeeded in incorporating a site-specific extrinsic fluorescent probe into nu bodies (Zama et al., 1977). N-pyrene maleimide (NPM) reacts with the exposed thiols of salt-dissociated v_1, and the particle can be reassociated by gradual removal of the high salt. These fluorescent-labelled v_1 exhibit both monomer NPM fluorescence and 'excimer' fluorescence. This latter emission indicates the possibility that the 2 pyrene rings are stacking with specific geometric constraints to permit coupling in the excited state. Changes in excimer and monomer fluorescence are being examined as a function of solvent conditions, and in the presence of possible conformational effector molecules. We have already observed that varying urea or KCl concentrations yield conformational transitions comparable to those observed by other biophysical techniques (see above). We believe that these NPM-labelled v_1 will permit us to rapidly search for conformational effector molecules, to identify stable states of v_1, and to examine the possibility of allosteric transitions within the chromatin subunit.

ACKNOWLEDGEMENTS

I wish to express my appreciation to my numerous colleagues and collaborators who have helped to develop many of the thoughts expressed in this brief communication. They include P. N. Bryan, R. E. Harrington, W. E. Hill, M. Hsie, B. Prescott, V. G. Schumaker, G. J. Thomas, E. B. Wright, M. Zama, and my principal collaborator, A. L. Olins.

REFERENCES

General references

The Structure and Function of Chromatin. The 1974 Ciba Foundation Symposium 28 (New Series) (1975). Editors: D. W. Fitzsimons and G. E. W. Wolstenholme. Elsevier – Excerpta Medica – North-Holland, Amsterdam – Oxford – New York.

The Molecular Biology of the Mammalian Genetic Apparatus. A 1975 international symposium held at the California Institute of Technology (1977). Editor: P. O. P. T'so. Elsevier–North-Holland, Amsterdam.

Chromatin. The 1977 Cold Spring Harbor Symposium on Quantitative Biology, XLII. Editors: M. Botchan and J. D. Watson. Cold Spring Harbor, New York.

Specific references

Bellard, M., Gannon, F. and Chambon, P. (1977): *Cold Spr. Harb. Symp. quant. Biol., 42.* In press.

Bradbury, E. M. (1975): In: *Ciba Foundation Symposium, 28 (New Series),* p. 131. Editors: D. W. Fitzsimons and G. E. W. Wolstenholme. Elsevier–Excerpta Medica–North-Holland, Amsterdam–Oxford–New York.

Bradbury, E. M. (1977): *Cold Spr. Harb. Symp. quant. Biol., 42.* In press.

Bradbury, E. M., Hjelm, R. P., Carpenter, B. G., Baldwin, J. P., Kneale, G. G. and Hancock, R. (1977): In: *The Molecular Biology of the Mammalian Genetic Apparatus,* Chapter 2, p. 53. Editor: P. O. P. Ts'o. Elsevier–North-Holland, Amsterdam.

Camerini-Otero, R. D., Sollner-Webb, B., Simon, R., Williamson, P., Zasloff, M. and Felsenfeld, G. (1977): *Cold Spr. Harb. Symp. quant. Biol., 42.* In press.

Campbell, A. M. and Cotter, R. I. (1976): *FEBS Letters, 70,* 1.

Cole, R. D., Lawson, G. M. and Hsiang, M. W. (1977): *Cold Spr. Harb. Symp. quant. Biol., 42.* In press.

Davies, H. G. (1976): *Nature (Lond.), 262,* 533.

Finch, J. T. and Klug, A. (1976): *Proc. nat. Acad. Sci. (Wash.), 73,* 1897.

Finch, J. T. and Klug, A. (1977): *Cold Spr. Harb. Symp. quant. Biol., 42.* In press.

Foe, V. E. (1977): *Cold Spr. Harb. Symp. quant. Biol., 42.* In press.

Franke, W. W., Scheer, V., Trendelenburg, M. F., Zentgraf, H. and Spring, H. (1977): *Cold Spr. Harb. Symp. quant. Biol., 42.* In press.

Garel, A. and Axel, R. (1977): *Cold Spr. Harb. Symp. quant. Biol., 42.* In press.

Griffith, J. and Christiansen, G. (1977): *Cold Spr. Harb. Symp. quant. Biol., 42.* In press.

Keller, W., Wendel, I., Eicken, I. and Zentgraf, H. (1977): *Cold Spr. Harb. Symp. quant. Biol., 42.* In press.

McKnight, S. L., Bustin, M. and Miller, O. L. (1977): *Cold Spr. Harb. Symp. quant. Biol., 42.* In press.

Morris, R. (1976): *Cell, 9,* 627.

Noll, M. (1977): *Cold Spr. Harb. Symp. quant. Biol., 42.* In press.

Olins, A. L. (1977): *Cold Spr. Harb. Symp. quant. Biol., 42.* In press.

Olins, A. L., Breillatt, J. P., Carlson, R. D., Senior, M. B., Wright, E. B. and Olins, D. E. (1977): In: *The Molecular Biology of the Mammalian Genetic Apparatus, Vol. 1,* Chapter 11, p. 211. Editor: P. O. P. T'so. Elsevier–North-Holland, Amsterdam.

Oudet, P., Germond, J. E., Bellard, M. and Chambon, P. (1977a): *Cold Spr. Harb. Symp. quant. Biol., 42.* In press.

Oudet, P., Spadafora, C. and Chambon, P. (1977b): *Cold Spr. Harb. Symp. quant. Biol., 42.* In press.

Pardon, J. F., Cotter, R. I., Lilley, D. M. J., Worcester, D. L., Campbell, A. M., Wolley, J. C. and Richards, B. M. (1977): *Cold Spr. Harb. Symp. quant. Biol., 42.* In press.

Renz, M. Nehls, P. and Hozier, J. (1977): *Cold Spr. Harb. Symp. quant. Biol., 42.* In press.

Ris, H. (1975): In: *Ciba Foundation Symposium, 28 (New Series),* p. 7. Editors: D. W. Fitzsimons and G. E. W. Wolstenholme. Elsevier–Excerpta Medica–North-Holland, Amsterdam–Oxford–New York.

Sobel, H. M., Jain, S. C., Tsai, C.-C., Sakore, T. D. and Gilbert, S. G. (1977): *Cold Spr. Harb. Symp. quant. Biol., 42.* In press.

Thomas Jr, G. J., Prescott, B. and Olins, D. E. (1977): *Science, 197,* 385.

Thomas, J. O. (1977): *Cold Spr. Harb. Symp. quant. Biol., 42.* In press.

Van Holde, K. E., Shaw, B. R., Tatchell, K., Pardon, J., Worcester, D., Wooley, J. and Richards, B. (1977): In: *The Molecular Biology of the Mammalian Genetic Apparatus, Vol. 1,* Chapter 12, p. 239. Editor: P. O. P. T'so. Elsevier–North-Holland, Amsterdam.

Zachau, H. G. (1977): *Cold Spr. Harb. Symp. quant. Biol., 42.* In press.

Zama, M., Bryan, P. N., Harrington, R. E., Olins, A. L. and Olins, D. E. (1977): *Cold Spr. Harb. Symp. quant. Biol., 42.* In press.

The role of DNA-associated proteins in the regulation of chromosome function *

VINCENT G. ALLFREY, GIORGIO VIDALI, LIDIA C. BOFFA and
EDWARD M. JOHNSON

The Rockefeller University, New York, N.Y., U.S.A.

Transcriptional control in differentiation – A brief overview

Of the many varied controls over cellular differentiation during embryonic development, those concerned with RNA synthesis, processing and utilization assume
paramount importance. Of these, the primary control mechanism is selective
transcription – the activation of a limited set of DNA sequences as templates for
RNA synthesis and suppression of the rest.

This type of control begins in oogenesis, when the changing transcriptional
activity of the developing oocyte is often directly evident in the changing morphology
and function of its chromosomes. The lampbrush chromosomes of amphibian
oocytes provide a particularly revealing model of the relationships between structure
and transcription. Ribonucleic acid synthesis in lampbrush chromosomes has been
shown to occur on DNA-containing 'loops' which project laterally from many
sites along the chromosome axis (Gall and Callan, 1962; Izawa et al., 1963; Miller
and Hamkalo, 1972; Malcolm and Sommerville, 1974; Mott and Callan, 1975;
Angelier and Lacroix, 1975). The complete chromosome complement contains at
least 10^4 loop-pairs containing nascent RNA chains. However, this represents
transcription of only about 4% of the total DNA; the great majority of the DNA
occurs in the dense chromomeres as tightly packed and transcriptionally inert
super-helical coils (Mott and Callan, 1975). Estimates of the proportion of DNA
present in the loops (5%) (Callan, 1963) are in good agreement with results showing
that somewhat over 4% of the non-repetitive DNA sequences hybridize with oocyte
nuclear RNA (Sommerville and Malcolm, 1976). The correlations between morphology and function in the lampbrush chromosome thus establish 2 main points about
transcription: (1) it is highly selective for particular DNA sequences, and, (2) transcriptionally active DNA exists in an extended configuration.

* This research was supported in part by grants from the National Foundation–March of Dimes (1–440),
the American Cancer Society (NP-228), the United States Public Health Service (GM 17383), and the
Rockefeller Foundation Program in Reproductive Biology.

41

An additional point is that the primary transcripts on the chromosome loops are generally much longer than the average-size messenger RNA in the cytoplasm (Miller and Hamkalo, 1972; Sommerville and Malcolm, 1976). In fact, some messenger-like sequences are apparently present in large primary transcripts up to 6×10^4 nucleotides long (Sommerville and Malcolm, 1976). This is in accord with the evidence that the sequence complexity of embryonic nuclear RNAs greatly exceeds that of cytoplasmic RNAs (Hough et al., 1975), and with the fact that globin mRNA sequences exist in the nucleus within much longer RNA molecules (Williamson et al., 1973; Ruiz-Carrillo et al., 1973; Macnaughton et al., 1974; Kwan et al., 1977). The nuclear transcripts also contain some repetitive sequences which may be involved in genetic control but do not appear in the final message (Smith et al., 1974).

The importance of post-transcriptional processing of nuclear RNA molecules is evident in the observations that only about 3% of the total RNA transcribed in the nucleus is destined to become cytoplasmic messenger RNA; mRNA sequences correspond to only about 1.2% of the non-repetitive DNA sequences (Davidson and Hough, 1971). This is equivalent to about 1.5×10^4 average-size messengers (Sommerville and Malcolm, 1976).

In addition to its enormously complex mRNA population, the oocyte contains even larger amounts of nucleic acid molecules necessary for ribosome structure and function. Most of the RNA synthesized during oogenesis is ribosomal RNA (Davidson et al., 1964) and 5S RNA (Brown and Sugimoto, 1973; Brownlee et al., 1974; Pukkila, 1975). In oocytes there is very little turnover of cytoplasmic RNAs; all types, including ribosomal (Davidson et al., 1964) and most messenger, 5S, and transfer RNAs (Rosbash and Ford, 1974; Ford et al., 1977), are stable for periods commensurate with the length of oogenesis (up to 2 years in *Xenopus*).

Among the approximately 20,000 different sequences of poly A-containing RNAs found in the mature oocyte many encode structural information for proteins destined to be synthesized after fertilization. For example, the *Xenopus* oocyte contains thousands of copies of mRNAs coding for histones (Levenson and Marcu, 1976) and for different hemoglobins (Perlman et al., 1977). The storage of so-called 'masked' messenger RNAs for long periods prior to their utilization is an important aspect of translational control in early embryogenesis (Gross, 1967; Gross et al., 1973). However, activation of cytoplasmic protein synthesis after fertilization may occur in the absence of a nucleus and thus, it does not appear to be under *immediate* genetic influence. This control mechanism will not be considered in the present analysis of transcriptional activity in the nucleus.

As maturation of the oocyte proceeds, the chromosome loops retract, and the incorporation of radioactive RNA precursors is drastically curtailed (Davidson et al., 1964). Suppression of RNA synthesis by actinomycin D also leads to retraction of the loops (Izawa et al., 1963), confirming the view that there is a close association between conformation of the DNA and its template activity.

After fertilization, the program of embryonic RNA synthesis is initiated. The patterns of RNA synthesis in early embryonic development include initiation of ribosomal RNA synthesis at the blastula stage (Emerson and Humphreys, 1970), and extensive activation of mRNA synthesis before the onset of gastrulation (Bachvarova et al., 1966; Davidson et al., 1968; Brandhorst and Humphreys, 1971; Galau et al.,

1977). The changing populations of mRNA during embryonic development indicate that each stage of differentiation involves the activation of different sets of structural genes, each set generally comprising several thousand specific sequences (Galau et al., 1976). The 'new' mRNAs are functional; the activation of 'new' genes at the onset of gastrulation is accompanied by the synthesis of 'new' protein species in the differentiating cell population (Brandhorst, 1976).

What controls the activation of specific genes during early embryonic development? Classical embryology has already established that morphogenetic substances synthesized during oogenesis and present in the egg cytoplasm determine the developmental pattern of the zygote. In *Ambystoma*, a genetic deficiency is known to lead to developmental arrest at gastrulation. The injection of nucleoplasm from a normal oocyte nucleus, or of cytoplasm from a normal mature egg, into a mutant egg corrects the deficiency (Briggs and Cassens, 1966). Gastrulation requires the presence of a nucleus (Gurdon, 1974). In the *Ambystoma* mutant the nucleus is functional, but proteins present in the normal egg cytoplasm appear to be essential for the activation of the nuclear genes required for gastrulation and organogenesis (Brothers, 1976).

A key inference from such experiments is that gene activity is subject to positive control. This fact has recently been made doubly clear by nuclear transplantation experiments in which nuclei from somatic cells were shown to change their patterns of mRNA synthesis after injection into oocytes. Analysis of the resulting proteins by 2-dimensional gel electrophoresis indicated that the transplanted nuclei were directing the synthesis of oocyte-type proteins. It follows that genes which became inactive during cell differentiation can be reactivated by substances present in the oocyte cytoplasm. Such reactivation does not require a new round of DNA synthesis (DeRobertis and Gurdon, 1977).

The selective activation of different gene sets in different tissues proceeds throughout development. It leads, for example, to the synthesis of over 140,000 copies of globin mRNA in the reticulocyte, as compared to only 70 copies in the adult hepatocyte (Humphries et al., 1976) – even though the number of globin genes does not differ in these cell types (Packman et al., 1972). Clearly, some mRNAs are highly characteristic of particular cell types, but many genes are expressed in common in different cell types (Axel et al., 1976; Hastie and Bishop, 1976). It has been suggested that the vast majority of the mRNAs may be required for the maintenance of cellular functions common to all tissues; others may play some regulatory role. It is significant that non-erythroid cells contain globin mRNA sequences largely restricted to the nucleus, while erythroid cells release almost all of their globin mRNAs to the cytoplasm (Humphries et al., 1976).

Apart from the differences in mRNA abundance in different tissues, it is also known that the concentration of a given mRNA in a particular tissue is subject to physiological control. Immature erythroblasts, for example, accumulate globin mRNAs in response to erythropoietin in vivo or in vitro (Conkie et al., 1975; Ramirez et al., 1975). The synthesis of ovalbumin mRNA in the oviduct is likewise responsive to hormonal stimulation, increasing from 0–10 molecules per tubular gland cell in estrogen-withdrawn animals to over 17,000 molecules per cell after estrogen treatment (Harris et al., 1975).

In the case of the globin genes, a defect in transcription appears to be the basis for some forms of β-thalassemia (Housman et al., 1973; Kacian et al., 1973; Benz et al., 1975; Tolstoshev et al., 1976). Whether the deficiency of the globin message reflects a reduced rate of synthesis of the high-molecular-weight globin mRNA precursor (Kwan et al., 1977) or deficiencies in its processing remains to be determined.

Differential expression of the globin gene in different cell types, as measured by hybridization-titration of the globin mRNAs to appropriate cDNA probes (Humphries et al., 1976), clearly establishes that differential gene activity is a major control mechanism in organogenesis. Given the fact that selective utilization of different DNA sequences takes place at successive stages in development, plus the evidence that gene activity is subject to control by factors originating in the cytoplasm, the question arises as to how DNA structure and function are regulated at the molecular level so that particular nucleotide sequences are active in one cell type but suppressed in another.

The experiments now to be described deal with some basic problems of DNA organization in active and inactive chromatin, and present some new approaches to the identification of DNA-associated proteins on active genes.

Active and inactive states of chromatin – The role of histone modification

The structural organization of the eukaryotic genome depends largely upon interactions between DNA and sets of small basic proteins called histones. In most cell types, histones may be grouped into 5 major classes differing in size, positive charge, and amino acid composition. The primary structures of the major histone classes have been determined, and numerous post-synthetic modifications of each polypeptide chain have been described. Much of this information is summarized in recent reviews (Elgin and Weintraub, 1975; Ruiz-Carrillo et al., 1975; Allfrey, 1977; Johnson and Allfrey, 1977). The structural function of histones is to organize the long, fibrillar molecules of DNA into a more compact form. This organization is achieved, in large part, by electrostatic interactions between the negatively charged phosphate groups of the DNA helix, and positively charged basic amino acids (lysine, arginine and histidine) in the histone polypeptide chain.

Current views of chromatin structure favor a model in which the DNA strand is periodically wrapped around clusters of histones, each cluster comprising an octamer made up of 2 each of the 4 histone classes – H2A, H2B, H3 and H4 (Kornberg, 1974; Olins and Olins, 1974; Thomas and Kornberg, 1975; Joffe et al., 1977). Coiling of the DNA strand around the histone core (Baldwin et al., 1975; Pardon et al., 1976; Hjelm et al., 1977) accounts for much of the compaction of the genetic material in interphase chromatin and in metaphase chromosomes.

In the assembly of such histone-DNA complexes, different regions of the histone polypeptide chains have different functions. Each of the 4 histone classes involved has a characteristic clustering of its basic amino acids in the NH_2-terminal region of the molecule. This positively charged region is most likely to interact with the negatively charged enveloping DNA helix (Bradbury and Crane-Robinson, 1971; Weintraub and Van Lente, 1974; Li, 1975), while the less polar and more hydrophobic regions of the histone molecule determine the selectivity of its interactions with other histones of the core complex (D'Anna and Isenberg, 1974; Martinson and McCarthy, 1975).

The resulting structures, generally referred to as 'nucleosomes' (Oudet et al., 1975) are arranged along the DNA like beads on a string. They are visible in the electron microscope as roughly spherical particles, about 100 Å in diameter, linked by interconnecting DNA strands (Olins and Olins, 1974; Woodcock, 1973; Oudet et al., 1975; Langmore and Wooley, 1975; Woodcock et al., 1976a; Olins et al., 1976). A typical electron micrograph – showing arrays of nucleosomes along DNA strands in avian erythrocyte chromatin – is presented in Figure 1.

In virtually all species examined, the nucleosome core particles contain a uniform length of DNA (140 nucleotide pairs) associated with the octameric histone complex $(H2A)_2$ $(H2B)_2$ $(H3)_2$ $(H4)_2$ (Axel, 1975; Sollner-Webb and Felsenfeld, 1975; Compton et al., 1976; Noll, 1976; Shaw et al., 1976). Histone H1 appears to be associated with DNA sequences adjoining the core particles (Baldwin et al., 1975; Shaw et al., 1976; Whitlock and Simpson, 1976; Varshavsky et al., 1976) about 20 nucleotide pairs long (Noll and Kornberg, 1977). There are indications that H1 may play a role in the control of higher orders of chromatin structure by cross-linking adjacent DNA strands in a superhelical array of nucleosomes.

Although the nucleosome 'cores' from diverse species contain a uniform length of DNA, the average lengths of DNA between the beads may vary from species to species (Compton et al., 1976; Johnson et al., 1976; Noll, 1976; Spadafora et al., 1976; Thomas and Furber, 1976; Lohr et al., 1977), from tissue to tissue (Morris, 1976), and in different cell types within a tissue (Thomas and Thompson, 1977; Todd and Garrard, 1977). The significance of the variability in spacer lengths remains unclear.

An important consequence of the bead-and-spacer organization of DNA in eukaryotic chromatin is that the DNA sequences in the interconnecting linker strands are more susceptible to nuclease attack than are DNA sequences in the nucleosome 'core particles'. Limited digestion with endogenous nucleases (Hewish and Burgoyne, 1973; Simpson and Whitlock, 1976) or with micrococcal (staphylo-coccal) nuclease (Rill and Van Holde, 1973; Noll, 1974; Axel, 1975; Sollner-Webb and Felsenfeld, 1975; Shaw et al., 1976) gives rise to an ordered series of chromatin fragments that can be separated by centrifugation in sucrose density gradients. This is shown for avian erythrocyte chromatin fragments in Figure 2. Electrophoretic sizing of the DNA in such digests shows a discrete series of fragments which are multiples of a fundamental unit corresponding to the DNA content of the core particle and its associated linker sequence. In avian erythrocytes and in many other species, the average repeat length is about 200 nucleotide pairs. The DNA lengths in erythrocyte mono-nucleosomes, di-nucleosomes, and higher oligomers are compared in Figure 3.

This new view of chromatin structure emphasizes the orderly array of nucleosomes in inactive chromatin (such as that of the mature avian erythrocyte), but leaves open the question of how such compact structures are modified to permit transcription in active regions of the chromatin. A clue to the problem is provided by observations indicating that the nucleosome 'core' possesses an axis of symmetry. This is suggested by cleavage at 100, rather than 200 nucleotide-pair intervals when chromatin is treated with DNase II (Altenburger et al., 1976), and by electron microscopic observations indicating that the nucleosomes of SV-40 mini-chromo-somes dissociate into half-nucleosomes at moderately high ionic strengths (Chambon, 1976).

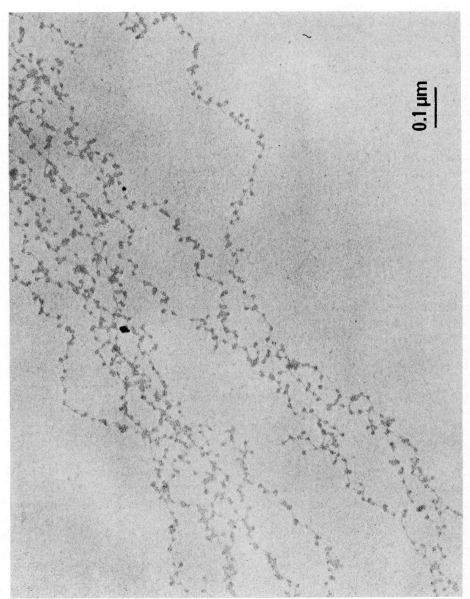

Fig. 1. Electron micrograph of avian erythrocyte chromatin spread and centrifuged onto carbon grids, and stained with phosphotungstic acid as described by Miller and Bakken (1972). Microscopy was performed using a Siemens 102 electron microscope.

0.1 μm

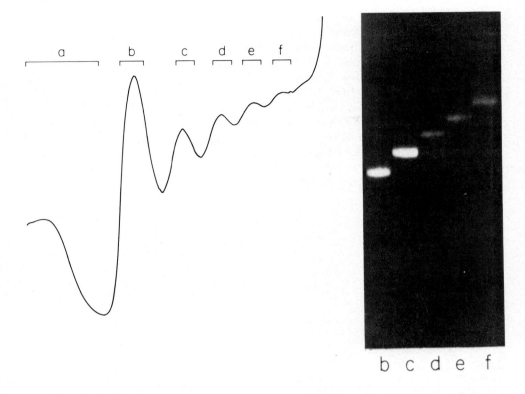

Fig. 2. Separation of chromatin fragments produced by limited digestion of avian erythrocyte chromatin with staphylococcal nuclease. The nucleosome monomers, dimers, and higher oligomers were separated by centrifugation on a 5–20% linear sucrose gradient. Peaks containing monomers (b), dimers (c), and higher oligomers (d–f) were collected as indicated by the lettered brackets and used for analysis of DNA length and protein composition.

Fig. 3. Electrophoretic sizing of the DNA fragments associated with the nucleosome peaks prepared by limited digestion with staphylococcal nuclease and separated as shown in Figure 2. The DNA associated with each peak was analyzed by electrophoresis in 2% agarose and localized by fluorescent staining with ethidium bromide. The average DNA repeat length in the avian erythrocyte is 196 nucleotide pairs (Compton et al., 1976; Lohr et al., 1977).

    The occurrence of 2 molecules of each histone (H2A, H2B, H3 and H4) in the octet comprising the nucleosome 'core', suggests the presence of heterotypic tetramers containing 1 molecule of each of the 4 histones; such tetramers have been detected in solution (Weintraub et al., 1975). A model has been proposed in which 2 heterotypic tetramers are organized about an axis of dyad symmetry (Weintraub et al., 1976). Opening of the compact structure to generate separate half-nucleosomes would facilitate access to the DNA by RNA polymerizing enzymes.

    In considering how the structure of the nucleosome could be reversibly unfolded, particular attention should be paid to the role of histone H3 and H4. It is now clear that many of the properties of the nucleosome, including the organization of discrete lengths of DNA into nuclease-resistant 'cores' depend mainly upon these 2 arginine-rich histone classes (Camerini-Otero et al., 1976; Sollner-Webb et al., 1976). Interaction between histones H3 and H4 and DNA depends upon the positive charges in the NH$_2$-terminal regions of the histone molecules. It is significant that both H3 and H4 are subject to a post-synthetic modification which neutralizes most of these positive charges (Allfrey, 1964, 1970, 1977; Allfrey et al., 1964; Gershey et al., 1968; DeLange et al., 1969, 1972; Candido and Dixon, 1971, 1972; Marzluff and McCarty, 1972; Hooper et al., 1973; Thwaits et al., 1976a, b). This is accomplished by enzymatic acetylation of the epsilon amino groups of specific lysine residues in the polypeptide chain. Histone H3 has sites of acetylation at positions 9, 14, 18 and 23 of the NH$_2$-terminal sequence. Histone H4 is subject to enzymatic acetylation at positions 5, 8, 12 and 16 of the polypeptide chain (Fig. 4).

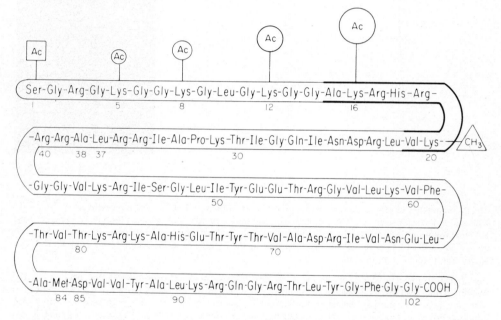

Fig. 4. Amino acid sequence of histone H4 (calf thymus), indicating the potential sites of acetylation of lysine residues at positions 5, 8, 12, and 16 in the amino-terminal region of the polypeptide chain. Histone H4 is also subject to acetylation at serine-1 and to methylation at lysine-20.

Since the original proposal that acetylation and deacetylation of the histones could provide a reversible mechanism for the control of chromatin structure (Allfrey, 1964; Allfrey et al., 1964), much evidence has accumulated relating the acetylation of histones to increased DNA reactivity and template function in RNA synthesis. This evidence has recently been reviewed in detail (Allfrey, 1977; Johnson and Allfrey, 1977), and only 6 key observations will be cited here:

1. Acetylation of histones in lymphocytes stimulated by mitogens (Pogo et al., 1966) follows a time course coincident with increasing accessibility of the DNA to intercalating dyes (Killander and Rigler, 1965, 1969). This is consistent with histone

acetylation as a mechanism for the release of DNA during unfolding of the nucleosomes (Allfrey, 1977).

2. Comparisons of cell types differing in their capacity for RNA synthesis show that histone acetylation is more pronounced in the more actively transcribing cells (Wangh et al., 1972; Sarkander et al., 1975). This is also true for erythroid cells at different stages in differentiation (Ruiz-Carrillo et al., 1975, 1976).

3. Measurements of the rates of histone acetylation in 'active' and 'inactive' subfractions of calf thymus chromatin (Frenster et al., 1963) have shown a direct proportionality with the activity of the fractions in RNA synthesis (Allfrey, 1964, 1970). Moreover, high resolution autoradiography of thymus nuclei after incubations with ^{3}H-acetate indicates that most of the acetylation occurs at the boundaries between the compact and diffuse regions of the chromatin, as expected if this modification of histones is related to changes in the physical state of the chromatin (Allfrey, 1970). The fractionation of *Drosophila melanogaster* chromatin also yields 'template-active' and 'template-inactive' regions. The acetylation of the histones is higher in the 'template-active' fraction (Levy-Wilson et al., 1977a).

4. The transcriptionally active maternal chromosome set of *Planococcus citrii* incorporates about 7 times more ^{3}H-acetate than does the heterochromatic and largely inactive paternal chromosome set (Berlowitz and Pallotta, 1972).

5. In multinucleated ciliates such as *Stylonychia mytilus* (Lipps, 1975) and *Tetrahymena pyriformis* (Gorovsky et al., 1973), the transcriptionally active macronucleus and the inactive micronucleus differ in their degree of histone acetylation; in both cases, the acetylation is greater in the macronucleus.

6. The extent to which the conformation of DNA is altered by added histone H4 depends upon the level of acetylation of the polypeptide chain (Adler et al., 1974).

In brief, histone acetylation involves histones which play a key role in chromatin organization, and it correlates both temporally and spatially with the activation of genes for RNA synthesis.

We have recently obtained new evidence in support of the view that such post-synthetic modifications of histone structure are related to the transcriptional activity of the associated DNA sequences. The evidence is based on experiments which exploit the differential sensitivity of 'active' and 'inactive' chromatin to pancreatic deoxyribonuclease I.

It has been shown that DNase I digestion of chromatin releases a large fraction of the newly synthesized RNA chains (Billing and Bonner, 1972) and that subfractions of transcriptionally active chromatin are more susceptible to DNase I attack than are transcriptionally inert fractions (Berkowitz and Doty, 1975). Of particular interest are recent observations showing that a limited digestion by DNase I preferentially removes the globin DNA sequences from nuclei isolated from chick red blood cells, but not from nuclei obtained from fibroblasts or brain (Weintraub and Groudine, 1976). Similarly, the ovalbumin genes are selectively degraded during DNase I digestion of nuclei from the oviduct, but not from the liver; over 70% of the ovalbumin sequences are digested when only 10% of the oviduct nuclear DNA has been solubilized (Garel and Axel, 1976). Moreover, it has been shown that the non-transcribed ovalbumin sequences in red cells and fibroblasts are relatively resistant to DNase I digestion (Weintraub and Groudine, 1976). In contrast, nucleolytic digestion of erythrocyte chromatin by staphylococcal nuclease does not result in preferential degradation of the active globin genes. Chromatin fragments produced by limited digestions with staphylococcal nuclease, when treated with DNase I, again show preferential hydrolysis of the globin sequences (Weintraub and Groudine, 1976). It follows that the genes that are active (or potentially active) in a given cell type exist in a subunit configuration which differs from that of genes which are inactive in that cell type.

We have employed limited digestions of chromatin with DNase I as a useful probe for the identification of proteins associated with the active genes. The first question considered was whether a limited DNase I digestion of erythrocyte chromatin releases acetylated histones from the susceptible DNA sequences. Erythrocytes were incubated in the presence of ^{3}H-acetate in order to label the acetylated forms of the histones prior to isolation of the nuclei. Aliquots of the nuclear suspension were then incubated with DNase I under conditions which release only about 12% of the DNA into the supernatant fraction (Vidali et al., 1977a). The histones remaining in the nuclei were then extracted, and histones H3 and H4 were purified by electrophoresis in SDS-polyacrylamide gels. The specific ^{3}H activities of the residual histones from DNase I-treated nuclei are compared with those of control nuclei (incubated in the absence of DNase I) in Figure 5. The specific ^{3}H activities of both H3 and H4 remaining after a brief DNase I treatment are appreciably

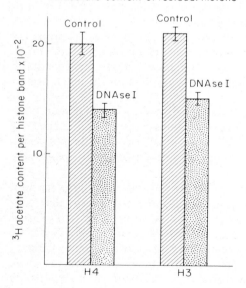

Fig. 5. Selective loss of acetylated histone H3 and H4 molecules from avian erythrocyte nuclei during limited digestion with DNase I. The erythrocyte histones were labeled with ^{3}H-acetate in intact cells; the nuclei were subsequently isolated and exposed to DNase I to release 11–12% of their total DNA content. The remaining histones were extracted and purified by electrophoresis in SDS-polyacrylamide gels. The specific ^{3}H activities of histones H3 and H4 in the DNase I-treated nuclei are significantly lower than the corresponding ^{3}H activities of the histones of control nuclei (incubated in the absence of DNase I). This is evidence for the preferential release of acetylated H3 and H4 under conditions known to selectively digest transcriptionally active regions of the chromatin.

lower than those of the corresponding histones in the control nuclei. It follows that the *acetylated forms* of H3 and H4 were selectively released during the digestion of the 'active' genes. Similar conclusions have been drawn from measurements of the rate of release of acetylated histones during DNase I digestions. The initial rate of release of chick erythrocyte histones previously labeled with ^{3}H-acetate is 3 times faster than the rate of DNA release (Wong and Alberts, 1977).

The results are consistent with a model in which histone acetylation in active regions of the chromatin has initiated an unfolding of nucleosomal DNA to a more extended configuration. This probably accounts for the increased DNase I sensitivity of the associated DNA sequences. A further implication is that 'active' and 'inactive' nucleosomes should differ in their physical properties. Evidence that the mono-nucleosome population is heterogeneous has been reported for mouse ascites tumor cells (Bakayev et al., 1975) and for *Physarum polycephalum* (Allfrey et al., 1977b). (The organization of the ribosomal genes in *Physarum* as a model for active genes will be considered later.)

Selective release of non-histone proteins associated with active genes

The technique of limited DNase I digestion has been employed for the identification and isolation of other proteins associated with active genetic loci. Erythrocyte nuclei were subjected to limited digestions with DNase I under conditions known to degrade most of the globin sequences while solubilizing only 12% of the total DNA. Proteins released into the supernatant (after low speed centrifugation of the nuclei) were analyzed by electrophoresis in SDS-polyacrylamide gels. For purposes of comparison, the effects of staphylococcal nuclease were also tested, since the latter enzyme does not show a preferential attack on the globin genes in erythrocyte chromatin (Weintraub and Groudine, 1976).

The supernatant fraction after DNase I treatment shows the presence of a characteristic subset of nuclear proteins (Fig. 6). Among these are 3 predominant bands in the molecular weight region 28,200–29,500 daltons; the corresponding bands in the residual chromatin after DNase I treatment are very faint (data not shown). These bands have been shown to correspond to the high-mobility group (HMG) proteins originally described by Johns and coworkers (Goodwin and Johns, 1973; Goodwin et al., 1973, 1975a,b; Johns et al., 1975; Walker et al., 1976; Vidali et al., 1977a). The HMG proteins appear to have a ubiquitous distribution in higher organisms (Vidali et al., 1977b; Levy-Wilson et al., 1977b; Watson et al., 1977) where they occur in concentrations exceeding 10^5 molecules per nucleus (Johns et al., 1975). Some of the HMG proteins have been shown to combine with DNA (Goodwin et al., 1975b) and to interact selectively with different subfractions of histone H1 (Smerdon and Isenberg, 1976).

Although the amount of HMG proteins is small relative to the histone or DNA content of the nucleus (about 3% by weight of the DNA of the calf thymus lymphocyte nucleus), the characteristic HMG bands are detectable in thymus nucleosomes isolated after limited digestions with staphylococcal nuclease (Goodwin et al., 1977). The presence of HMGs in avian erythrocyte nucleosomes has also been established (Vidali et al., 1977a). Figure 7 compares the protein compositions of the mono-, di-, tri-, tetra-, and penta-nucleosome peaks prepared by density gradient centrifugation of the staphylococcal nuclease digest described in Figures 2 and 3. The presence of 3 faint HMG bands is evident in the nucleosome monomers, dimers, and higher oligomers (Fig. 7,b–f), but no free HMGs are detected in the erythrocyte nuclear proteins at the top of the gradient (Fig. 7,a).

It is also of interest that the proportions of the core histones (H4, H2A, H2B,

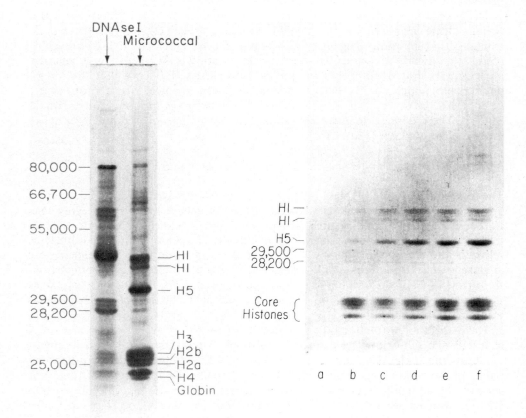

Fig. 6. Electrophoretic analysis of the proteins released during limited digestions of avian erythrocyte nuclei with DNase I (left-hand panel) and staphylococcal nuclease (termed 'micrococcal nuclease' in this figure) (right-hand panel). Note that 3 prominent protein bands in the molecular weight range 28,200–29,500 (HMG proteins) are present in the supernatant after centrifugation of the DNase I-treated nuclei. Only 11–12% of the DNA was solubilized under these conditions. In contrast, digestion of 24% of the nuclear DNA with staphylococcal nuclease did not result in an equivalent release of the HMG proteins, although a more extensive release of histones is evident, as expected for the greater degree of chromatin breakdown. DNase I attack on the transcriptionally active chromatin also releases a complex set of non-histone proteins showing prominent bands at 57–59,000 and at 80,000 daltons.

Fig. 7. Electrophoretic comparison of the protein compositions of nucleosome monomers (b), dimers (c) and higher oligomers (d–f) released by limited digestion of avian erythrocyte nuclei with staphylococcal nuclease and separated as described in Figure 2. Note the faint HMG bands (MW 28,200–29,500) in all nucleosome size classes. There is a progressive increase in the relative amounts of histones H1 and H5 with increasing size of the chromatin fragments, as expected if these histones are preferentially associated with DNA strands between the core particles.

and H3; in order of mobility) are invariant in all nucleosome fractions, while the histones associated with the interconnecting DNA strands (H1 and H5) become more prominent as the size of the chromatin fragments increases (Fig. 7,b–f).

When avian erythrocyte chromatin is treated with staphylococcal nuclease to release about 25% of the total DNA into the supernatant, one observes a proportionate release of histones and HMGs, but there is *no preferential release* of the HMG proteins (Fig. 6). In contrast, limited digestions with DNase I clearly release most of the HMG proteins (Fig. 6), even when only 12% of the DNA has been degraded. It follows that these proteins are not randomly distributed throughout the chromatin but are primarily associated with nucleosomes in a more DNase I-accessible state. Their presence on 'active' genes is consistent with an earlier report that HMG proteins stimulate transcription in vitro (Johns et al., 1975).

Other non-histone proteins are also released during limited DNase I digestions that are not released during comparable treatments with staphylococcal nuclease. Prominent among these are proteins of molecular weights 57–59,000 daltons and 80,000 daltons (Fig. 6). The functions of these proteins are not known, but in view of their likely association with transcriptionally active regions of the chromatin and their appreciable concentrations, it appears that such proteins must play a general, rather than a site-specific role in the synthesis or processing of nuclear RNAs.

A comparison of the electrophoretic banding patterns in Figure 6 shows that a broad molecular-weight spectrum of non-histone proteins is released differentially, depending upon the enzyme used to disrupt the chromatin, but many more proteins are released with DNase I. This is in agreement with earlier evidence that template-active subfractions of chromatin from many tissues are enriched in their non-histone protein complement (Frenster et al., 1963; Marushige and Bonner, 1971; Murphy et al., 1973; Simpson and Reeck, 1973; Doenecke and McCarthy, 1975; Gottesfeld et al., 1975). Some of the proteins associated with the DNase I-susceptible sequences are likely to be involved in transcriptional control mechanisms, and it would appear that this type of enzymatic release of a small fraction of the total nuclear proteins, combined with high-resolution DNA-affinity chromatography (Allfrey et al., 1974, 1977a) will provide a powerful and simplifying approach to the identification and purification of regulatory proteins in the eukaryotic genome.

Correlations between structure and function of ribosomal genes

The mechanisms of transcriptional control in eukaryotic cells, as in prokaryotes, involve the participation of proteins which interact directly with DNA to affect its conformation and influence its template function. The complexity of the eukaryotic genome and its differential expression in different cell types at different stages of development seriously complicate the analysis of genetic control at the molecular level. Somatic cell nuclei express thousands of genes, and their nuclei contain large numbers of non-histone proteins associated with their chromatin. For example, the number of electrophoretically distinct proteins in HeLa cell nuclei has been estimated at over 470 (Peterson and McConkey, 1976). Many of these proteins are structural components of the nucleus and the nuclear envelope; others are concerned with RNA and DNA synthesis and processing, with histone structural modifications, with the 'packaging' of nascent RNA chains, and with the assembly of ribosomal subunits in the nucleolus.

There is a large subset of chromosomal proteins, present in low concentrations, which appears to control both the rate (Teng et al., 1971; Kamiyama and Wang, 1971; Shea and Kleinsmith, 1973; Kostraba et al., 1976) and the specificity of transcription (Gilmour and Paul, 1969; Paul et al., 1975; Stein et al., 1974, 1977; Elgin and Weintraub, 1975; Tsai et al., 1976). The problem is to identify which of the nuclear proteins facilitate RNA chain initiation at specific gene loci and which proteins influence rates of RNA chain elongation or termination. It is also necessary to relate such proteins to the specificity of the different RNA polymerases, which are known to operate selectively on different gene sets (Roeder, 1976); polymerase I being selective for the ribosomal genes (Holland et al., 1977), polymerase II for mRNA coding sequences (Steggles et al., 1974), and polymerase III for the 5S genes (Parker and Roeder, 1977; Sklar and Roeder, 1977). On the premise that DNA sequence recognition is a prime prerequisite for selective gene readout, we have developed DNA-affinity chromatographic procedures for the fractionation of nuclear non-histone proteins (Allfrey et al., 1974, 1975). These methods have now been combined with nuclease digestion techniques to investigate the structure of a specific DNA sequence – that encoding the ribosomal RNAs of the myxomycete, *Physarum polycephalum*.

The genes for ribosomal RNA in this organism are extrachromosomal; they occur in the nucleolus in multiple copies (Zellweger et al., 1972; Ryser et al., 1973; Bradbury et al., 1973). Each of the diploid nuclei of the multinucleate syncytium contains about 1 pg of DNA, of which 0.2% is hybridizable to the 19S and 26S ribosomal RNA sequences of the organism (Newlon et al., 1973; Ryser and Braun, 1974; Bohnert et al., 1975). This corresponds to about 275 copies per nucleus of the sequences coding for 5.8S, 19S and 26S ribosomal RNAs (Hall and Braun, 1977). The reiteration of the ribosomal genes in *Physarum*, combined with the ease of growing the organism, its multinucleate structure, and rapid effective methods for preparing nucleoli on a large scale (Bradbury et al., 1973), permits the isolation of the ribosomal genes as a satellite DNA (rDNA) of characteristic density (Holt and Gurney, 1969; Zellweger et al., 1972; Bradbury et al., 1973; Newlon et al., 1973) in milligram amounts.

The deoxyribonucleotide sequences coding for *Physarum* ribosomal RNAs are localized in linear duplex DNA molecules of a uniform median length (18–20 μm; Vogt and Braun, 1976; R. M. Grainger, 1977, personal communication), and molecular weight 39×10^6 daltons (Molgaard et al., 1976). The sequence organization of the rDNA satellite has been analyzed by restriction nuclease cleavage, followed by sizing of the fragments (Molgaard et al., 1976; Vogt and Braun, 1976) and hybridization of the separate fragments to purified 19S and 26S ribosomal RNAs (Molgaard et al., 1976). The resulting 'map' shows that each rDNA molecule contains 2 genes for preribosomal RNA arranged at opposite ends of a long 'spacer' sequence in inverted polarity (Molgaard et al., 1976). The palindrome-like arrangement of the ribosomal genes can be directly visualized by electron microscopy of the transcription complexes (R. M. Grainger, 1977, personal communication). The long 'spacer' sequence between the ribosomal genes appears to be transcriptionally inert. Thus, the system offers the advantage of being able to compare regions on the same DNA molecule which differ markedly in transcriptional activity for a well-defined and easily characterized gene product.

An important basic problem is whether the actively transcribing ribosomal genes in rDNA are associated with histones to form nucleosomes, or whether they occur in a different structure or conformation. Electron microscopy of ribosomal RNA transcription complexes in *Notopthalmus* (Woodcock et al., 1976b), *Oncopeltus* (Foe et al., 1976), *Triturus* and other species (Franke et al., 1976a; Scheer et al., 1977) strongly suggest that the DNA of the actively transcribing regions occurs in an extended configuration. The nascent ribosomal RNP fibrils of *Oncopeltus* appear to be attached to an unbeaded chromatin strand (Foe et al., 1976). Similarly, the DNA strand within the transcribing matrix of ribosomal genes in *Notopthalmus* (Woodcock et al., 1976b) and *Xenopus* (Franke et al., 1976b) does not contain the 70–100 Å spherical particles seen in the non-transcribing spacer regions. The transcribed chromatin often appears thicker than a double-strand of free DNA, suggesting the presence of associated proteins (Foe et al., 1976; Woodcock et al., 1976b). Measurements of the DNA packing ratio in the ribosomal genes (1.2 μm of DNA per μm of chromatin; Foe et al., 1976) indicate that the DNA exists in a highly extended configuration, unlike that of the inactive strands of beaded chromatin.

Such observations confirm for ribosomal genes what has long been known about transcription in general; that RNA synthesis is much more active in the diffuse, euchromatic chromatin of mammalian (Littau et al., 1964; Granboulan and Granboulan, 1966), plant (Kemp, 1966) and insect (Lakhotia and Jacob, 1974) nuclei than in the highly condensed clumps of α-heterochromatin.

It is presumed that most of the spacer sequences in ribosomal DNA satellites are transcriptionally inert (but see Franke, 1976a), and the spacer regions have been reported to contain nucleosome-like particles (Woodcock et al., 1976b; McKnight and Miller, 1976), but the composition of such particles remains to be determined (Zentgraf et al., 1976).

An alternative approach to the analysis of the subunit organization of ribosomal DNA is to separate and analyze the fragments resulting from limited digestions with staphylococcal endonuclease. *Physarum* chromatin has been shown to yield a series of DNA fragments differing in length by 174–190 nucleotide pairs (Johnson et al., 1976). After more extensive nuclease digestion, the DNA is converted to a subunit monomer of average length 159 nucleotide pairs; this fragment is an intermediate in degradation to a core subunit containing 140 nucleotide pairs (Johnson et al., 1976). The lengths of the nuclease-accessible DNA sequences between the beads have been calculated as ranging from 13–31 nucleotide pairs. This estimate is in good agreement with the range of nucleosome spacings (14–30 nucleotide pairs) measured in electron micrographs of *Physarum* chromatin (Johnson et al., 1976).

The nucleosome monomers and oligomers produced by limited staphylococcal nuclease digestion of *Physarum* chromatin are separable by centrifugation in sucrose density gradients at moderate ionic strength (0.35 M NaCl), as shown in Figure 8. Of particular interest is the observation of a doublet in the monosome peak region (Fig. 8). The lighter component of the doublet (peak A) has been analyzed with respect to the length of its associated DNA sequences, and most of its DNA molecules were found to be 140 nucleotide pairs in length, i.e. not appreciably different in length than the DNA of the heavier monomer peak (Allfrey et al., 1977b). When peak A

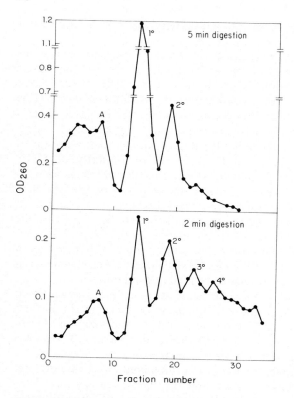

Fig. 8. Separation of chromatin fragments produced by limited digestions of *Physarum* nuclei with staphylococcal nuclease. After incubation for 2 minutes (lower panel) or 5 minutes (upper panel), the nucleosomes were fractionated in 5–20% linear sucrose gradients containing 0.35 M NaCl. The positions of the nucleosome monomers (1°), dimers (2°), trimers (3°), and tetramers (4°) are indicated. Particular attention is drawn to the peak A region of the gradient which, like the monomers, contains DNA approximately 140 nucleotide pairs in length. DNA from each peak was collected and tested for its content of sequences hybridizable to 19S and 26S ribosomal RNA as shown in Figure 9.

is further purified by recentrifugation in a shallower sucrose gradient, monomeric DNA lengths are still observed. The sedimentation coefficient of peak A has been estimated at 5.1S (H. R. Matthews and E. M. Bradbury, 1977, personal communication), well below that of the heavier monomer (11.5S).

The difference in sedimentation coefficient strongly suggests that the DNA in peak A exists in a highly extended configuration; this may reflect an altered protein complement of the more slowing sedimenting mononucleosome peak.

DNA fractions were prepared from each of the monomer peaks and from the larger chromatin digestion products and compared with respect to their content of ribosomal sequences by hybridization to ^{32}P-labeled 19S and 26S ribosomal RNAs. The results, showing the per cent DNA in each of the fractions hybridizable to increasing amounts of ^{32}P-labeled rRNAs, are summarized in Figure 9. By this test, the DNA in peak A is relatively enriched in sequences coding for ribosomal RNA as compared to the heavier monomer and larger chromatin fragments. It is significant that dimers and

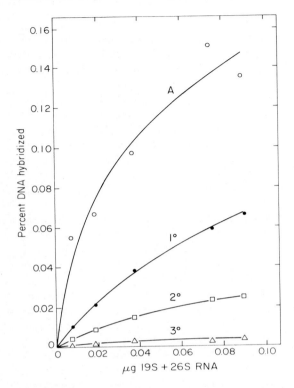

Fig. 9. Representation of 19S and 26S rDNA sequences in staphylococcal nuclease digestion products of *Physarum* chromatin. Chromatin fragments after 2 minutes digestion were isolated as shown in Figure 8, and DNA was purified from each peak. Each DNA sample was hybridized to increasing concentrations of ^{32}P-labeled 19S + 26S ribosomal RNA as described (Allfrey et al., 1977b). Note the relative enrichment of ribosomal genes in the peak A region.

larger oligomers obtained by limited digestions with staphylococcal nuclease are relatively deficient in their contents of hybridizable rDNA sequences; the higher the oligomer, the lower the per cent hybridization to ^{32}P-labeled 19S and 26S ribosomal RNA (Fig. 9). The reason for this unequal distribution of ribosomal genes in the various nucleosome classes has not yet been fully explained, but this result would be expected if the linker regions between histone-DNA complexes in the fully extended ribosomal genes were longer and more readily attacked by the staphylococcal nuclease. Changes in rDNA associated proteins might also influence spacer lability.

The recovery of rDNA sequences in nucleosome-size lengths of DNA in *Physarum* chromatin digests is in accord with similar findings for the ribosomal genes of *Xenopus* (Reeder, 1975; Reeves, 1976; Reeves and Jones, 1976) and *Tetrahymena* (Mathis and Gorovsky, 1976). However, the protection of rDNA sequences from random nuclease attack cannot be taken as proof that those sequences are entirely represented by a beaded chromatin structure. Such a conclusion would be inconsistent with the electron microscopic evidence for the absence of nucleosome beads in the transcription complex (Foe et al., 1976; Franke et al., 1976b) and with the low compaction ratio of rDNA. The presence of some rDNA sequences in beaded nucleosomes is, however, quite probable, as it is unlikely that all ribosomal genes are fully active at all times. This view is supported by data indicating that the ribosomal RNA cistrons in *Xenopus* are under-represented in nucleosomes from cells in which rRNA synthesis is particularly active (Reeves, 1976; Matthews, 1977). The percent of ribosomal genes actively transcribing in growing *Physarum* microplasmodia is not presently known, but may be presumed to be high at such a synthetically active stage of the life cycle. If the presence of ribosomal coding sequences in peak A is indicative of the active state, one would expect an association with nascent RNA chains. It is of interest in this regard that a major portion of rapidly labeled RNA appears in the corresponding zone of sucrose gradients of chromatin digests of *Physarum* labeled in vivo with ^{3}H-uridine (Staron et al., 1977).

As mentioned above, the large difference in sedimentation coefficient between peak A and the heavier monomer cannot be attributed to a major difference in the size of the DNA fragments in each peak, but may be a consequence of a change in DNA conformation and alterations in DNA-associated proteins. The proteins in each peak have been analyzed by electrophoresis in SDS-polyacrylamide gels (Allfrey et al., 1977b). The banding patterns showed a significant loss of the *Physarum* histones corresponding to mammalian H3 and H4 in the peak A region of the gradient. The selective loss of these histones is not likely to be an artefact of proteolysis, since all operations were carried out in the presence of the protease inhibitor, phenylmethylsulfonyl fluoride. The apparent deficiency of H3 and H4 in peak A may indicate selective detachment of those proteins from actively transcribing DNA, either in situ, or during the centrifugation of chromatin fragments at moderately high ionic strengths (0.35 M NaCl). This salt concentration would not displace unmodified H3 and H4 molecules from DNA, but might be sufficient to disrupt the much weaker interactions between DNA and highly acetylated H3 and H4 chains. An unfolding of the nucleosome as a result of modification or loss of histones H3 and H4 would account for the absence of a beaded structure in the transcription complex of *Physarum*, as visualized by electron microscopy.

The nucleoprotein complexes in the peak A region of the gradient also differ from the heavier monosomes and higher oligomers in their higher content of non-histone proteins. These proteins remain with peak A when it is purified by recentrifugation through a shallower sucrose density gradient. Which of the non-histone proteins associated with peak A take part in transcriptional control is not presently known, but in view of their association with the presumably active DNA sequences, an enrichment of regulatory proteins may have been achieved.

On the premise that proteins involved in the control of ribosomal RNA synthesis will be localized in the nucleolus and interact with rDNA sequences, we have also begun to study the DNA-binding properties of *Physarum* nucleolar proteins. The proteins were extracted from purified nucleoli (Bradbury et al., 1973) under nondenaturing conditions in 0.5 M $(NH_4)_2SO_4$. The proteins in the extract were fractionated by affinity chromatography on *Physarum* DNA covalently attached to Sephadex G-25 (Allfrey et al., 1974, 1975). The affinity chromatography of nuclear proteins under these conditions has been shown to be highly reproducible. The columns fractionate nuclear proteins into subsets of characteristic DNA-binding and electrophoretic properties. The elution procedure, involving the displacement of different sets of proteins by successive increments in salt concentration of the eluting buffer, has been shown to preserve both enzyme activity (Johnson et al., 1975) and hormone-receptor function (Inoue et al., 1977) of the DNA-binding proteins. The sensitivity of the method is indicated by its capacity to detect which proteins differ in their affinities for repeated and unique DNA sequences from the same species (Allfrey et al., 1974, 1975).

A fractionation of *Physarum* nucleolar proteins on *Physarum* DNA linked to Sephadex G-25 separates the majority of the proteins (more than 70% have little or no DNA affinity) from a DNA-binding set. The latter were fractionated by elution in a stepwise salt gradient. Protein fractions eluted at different ionic strengths were compared with respect to their capacity to bind preferentially to the rDNA satellite, as compared to main-band DNA. Binding was measured by retention of ^{125}I-labeled rDNA or ^{125}I-labeled main-band DNA on nitrocellulose filters (Riggs et al., 1970; Johnson et al., 1975; Allfrey et al., 1977a), both types of DNA being sheared to equal lengths. The results shown in Figure 10 show that protein fraction IV (a fraction eluting from the DNA column at high ionic strength (1 M KCl) has a higher affinity for rDNA than for main-band DNA. Such a preferential binding to the rDNA satellite was not seen in another fraction of nucleolar proteins (fraction I) which eluted from the DNA column at low ionic strength (0.05 M KCl) (Fig. 10). This preliminary indication that *Physarum* nucleoli contain proteins which preferentially combine with ribosomal DNA sequences is supported by competition-binding studies in which the same nucleolar protein fraction (fraction IV) was allowed to interact with ^{125}I-rDNA in the presence of increasing amounts of either unlabeled rDNA or unlabeled main-band DNA. It was found that excess rDNA could completely displace the ^{125}I-rDNA in the complex; excess main-band DNA was less effective in displacing the ^{125}I-rDNA from its associated proteins (Allfrey et al., 1977a). These experiments provide the first direct evidence for the presence in the nucleolus of non-histone proteins with a preferential affinity for ribosomal DNA. A distinctive

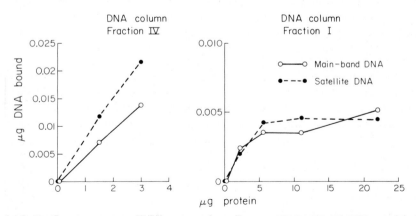

Fig. 10. Differential DNA binding by nucleolar protein fractions eluted at different ionic strengths from a column of *Physarum* DNA covalently linked to Sephadex G-25. The binding of the protein fractions to ^{125}I-labeled rDNA or ^{125}I-labeled main-band DNA is compared. Note that protein fraction IV has a preferential affinity for the rDNA satellite; fraction I does not.

set of non-histone proteins associated with ribosomal chromatin has also been reported in *Xenopus* (Higashinakagawa et al., 1977) and in the nucleoli of tumor cells (Soiero and Basile, 1973; Olson et al., 1974). As yet, the functional role of any of these proteins has not been determined, but in view of the evidence that fidelity of transcription of the ribosomal genes requires the presence of nucleolar proteins (Roeder et al., 1976; Reeder and Roeder, 1972; Honjo and Reeder, 1974; Grummt, 1975; Matsui et al., 1977; Ballal et al., 1977), as well as the appropriate RNA polymerase (Roeder, 1976; Holland et al., 1977), one may surmise that some of the rDNA-binding proteins of the *Physarum* nucleolus direct the binding of polymerase I to promotor or initiation sites in the rDNA molecule.

The eventual aim of our studies is to identify which of the rDNA-binding proteins influence the transcription of ribosomal RNA. We have begun by developing a cell-free system capable of ribosomal RNA synthesis. Isolated *Physarum* nuclei have been found to synthesize RNA in the presence of α-amanitin (to inhibit RNA polymerase II activity), and the newly synthesized polyribonucleotides hybridize to the purified rDNA satellite (Allfrey et al., 1977a). Isotopic labeling experiments indicate that isolated nuclei produce a high-molecular-weight precursor of the 19S and 26S ribosomal RNAs (Sun et al., 1977). The effects of purified rDNA-binding proteins upon rRNA initiation, elongation and termination are currently being investigated.

Chromosomal proteins and transcriptional control during differentiation

Both structure and function of the eukaryotic chromosome are altered during embryogenesis and post-natal development. The changes are known to involve qualitative alterations in the histones (Seale and Aronson, 1973b; Ruderman et al., 1974; Cohen et al., 1975) and quantitative and qualitative changes in the non-histone protein complement (Hill et al., 1971; Cognetti et al., 1972; Seale and Aronson, 1973a; Chytil et al., 1974; Platz et al., 1975). Changes in the patterns of RNA synthesis at successive stages in sea urchin development have been correlated with altered proportions of RNA polymerases I, II and III, but there are numerous indications that other factors modulate the activity of the polymerases and the accessibility of the DNA template (Roeder and Rutter, 1970).

Much of the evidence that differential gene activity is controlled by characteristic sets of non-histone nuclear proteins has been reviewed recently (Stein et al., 1977). DNA-binding proteins of nuclear origin have been shown to stimulate RNA synthesis in vitro (Teng et al., 1971) by a mechanism which probably involves an enhancement of RNA chain initiation (Kostraba et al., 1976); but other non-histone chromosomal proteins are known to inhibit transcription (Kostraba and Wang, 1975). Thus, both positive and negative control mechanisms may require interactions between specific sets of non-histone chromosomal proteins and DNA templates.

Considering the enormous complexity of the mammalian genome and the range of gene expression in different cell types during embryogenesis, one may anticipate that the nuclear non-histone protein complement must vary in a very complex way as cell differentiation proceeds. Variations have been observed during embryonic development of mammalian liver (Chytil et al., 1974) and in avian erythroid cells at different stages of differentiation (Gershey and Kleinsmith, 1969; Shelton and

Neelin, 1971; Vidali et al., 1973; Ruiz-Carrillo et al., 1974), as well as in other cell types. The problem is to identify the proteins involved in the regulation of a specific gene. Progress in this area is now likely to be rapid, because of new techniques which permit the localization by immunofluorescence of specific proteins at specific bands in Dipteran chromosomes (Silver and Elgin, 1976; Alfageme et al., 1976), with the availability of reiterated or cloned DNA sequences for studies of DNA sequence recognition by nuclear protein fractions, and with sensitive hybridization techniques for assessment of the fidelity of transcription in reconstituted chromatin fractions. The study of ribosomal gene control in *Physarum* provides a useful paradigm of transcriptional control in eukaryotes. The system has great potential for detailed chemical analysis of how the structure and organization of the transcription complex are modified to regulate gene function during differentiation.

ACKNOWLEDGEMENT

We are greatly indebted to Dr. Hans-Peter Hoffmann of the Rockefeller University for the electron micrograph of avian erythrocyte chromatin shown in Figure 1.

REFERENCES

Adler, A. J., Fasman, G. D., Wangh, L. J. and Allfrey, V. G. (1974): *J. biol. Chem.*, *249*, 2911.
Alfageme, C. R., Rudkin, G. T. and Cohen, L. H. (1976): *Proc. nat. Acad. Sci. (Wash.)*, *73*, 2038.
Allfrey, V. G. (1964): *Canad. Cancer Conf.*, *6*, 313.
Allfrey, V. G. (1970): *Fed. Proc.*, *29*, 1447.
Allfrey, V. G. (1977): In: *Chromatin and Chromosome Structure*, p. 167. Editors: H. J. Li and R. A. Eckhardt. Academic Press, New York.
Allfrey, V. G., Faulkner, R. and Mirsky, A. E. (1964): *Proc. nat. Acad. Sci. (Wash.)*, *51*, 786.
Allfrey, V. G., Inoue, A., Karn, J., Johnson, E. M. and Vidali, G. (1974): *Cold Spr. Harb. Symp. quant. Biol.*, *38*, 785.
Allfrey, V. G., Inoue, A. and Johnson, E. M. (1975): In: *Chromosomal Proteins and their Role in the Regulation of Gene Expression*, p. 265. Editors: G. S. Stein and L. J. Kleinsmith. Academic Press, New York.
Allfrey, V. G., Johnson, E. M., Sun, I. Y-C., Littau, V. C., Matthews, H. R. and Bradbury, E. M. (1977a): In: *Human-Molecular Cytogenetics–ICN-UCLA Symposia on Molecular and Cellular Biology*, *Vol. VII*, pp. 159–177. Editors: R. S. Sparkes, D. Comings and C. F. Fox. Academic Press, New York.
Allfrey, V. G., Johnson, E. M., Sun, I. Y-C., Littau, V. C., Matthews, H. R. and Bradbury, E. M. (1977b): *Cold Spr. Harb. Symp. quant. Biol.*, *42*, in press.
Angelier, N. and Lacroix, J. C. (1975): *Chromosoma (Berl.)*, *51*, 323.
Altenburger, W., Hörz, W. and Zachau, H. G. (1976): *Nature (Lond.)*, *264*, 517.
Axel, R. (1975): *Biochemistry*, *14*, 2921.
Axel, R., Feigelson, P. and Schutz, G. (1976): *Cell*, *7*, 247.
Bachvarova, R., Davidson, E. H., Allfrey, V. G. and Mirsky, A. E. (1966): *Proc. nat. Acad. Sci. (Wash.)*, *55*, 358.
Bakayev, V. V., Melnickov, A. A., Osicka, V. D. and Varshavsky, A. J. (1975): *Nucl. Acids Res.*, *2*, 1401.
Baldwin, J. P., Boseley, P. G., Bradbury, E. M. and Ibel, K. (1975): *Nature (Lond)*, *253*, 245.
Ballal, N. R., Choi, Y. C., Mouche, R. and Busch, H. (1977): *Proc. nat. Acad. Sci. (Wash.)*, *74*, 2446.
Benz, E. J., Swerdlow, P. S. and Forget, B. G. (1975): *Blood*, *45*, 1.
Berkowitz, C. and Doty, P. (1975): *Proc. nat. Acad. Sci. (Wash.)*, *72*, 3328.
Berlowitz, L. and Pallotta, D. (1972): *Exp. Cell Res.*, *71*, 45.
Billing, R. J. and Bonner, J. (1972): *Biochim. biophys. Acta (Amst.)*, *281*, 453.
Bohnert, H. J., Schiller, B., Bohme, R. and Sauer, W. (1975): *Europ. J. Biochem.*, *57*, 361.

Bradbury, E. M. and Crane-Robinson, C. (1971). In: *Histones and Nucleohistones*, p. 85. Editor: D. M. P. Phillips, Plenum Press, London.

Bradbury, E. M., Matthews, H. R., MacNaughton, J. and Molgaard, H. V. (1973): *Biochim. biophys. Acta (Amst.)*, *335*, 19.

Brandhorst, B. P. (1976): *Develop. Biol.*, *52*, 310.

Brandhorst, B. P. and Humphreys, T. (1971): *Biochemistry*, *10*, 877.

Briggs, R. and Cassens, G. (1966): *Proc. nat. Acad. Sci. (Wash.)*, *55*, 1103.

Brothers, A. J. (1976): *Nature (Lond.)*, *260*, 112.

Brown, D. D. and Sugimoto, K. (1973): *J. molec. Biol.*, *78*, 397.

Brownlee, G. G., Cartwright, E. M. and Brown, D. D. (1974): *J. molec. Biol.*, *89*, 703.

Callan, H. G. (1963): *Int. Rev. Cytol.*, *15*, 1.

Camerini-Otero, R. D., Sollner-Webb, B. and Felsenfeld, G. (1976): *Cell*, *8*, 333.

Candido, E. P. M. and Dixon, G. H. (1971): *J. biol. Chem.*, *246*, 3182.

Candido, E. P. M. and Dixon, G. H. (1972): *Proc. nat. Acad. Sci. (Wash.)*, *69*, 2015.

Chambon, P. (1976): In: *Organization and Expression of Chromosomes*, p. 24. Editors: V. G. Allfrey, E. K. F. Bautz, B. J. McCarthy, R. T. Schimke and A. Tissieres. Life Sciences Research Report 4, Dahlem Konferenzen, Berlin.

Chytil, F., Glasser, S. R. and Spelsberg, T. C. (1974): *Develop. Biol.*, *37*, 295.

Cognetti, G., Settineri, D. and Spinelli, G. (1972): *Exp. Cell Res.*, *71*, 465.

Cohen, L. H., Newrock, K. M. and Zweidler, A. (1975): *Science*, *190*, 994.

Compton, J. L., Bellard, M. and Chambon, P. (1976): *Proc. nat. Acad. Sci. (Wash.)*, *73*, 4382.

Conkie, D., Kleiman, L., Harrison, P. R. and Paul, J. (1975): *Exp. Cell Res.*, *93*, 315.

D'Anna, J. A. and Isenberg, I. (1974): *Biochemistry*, *13*, 4992.

Davidson, E. H., Allfrey, V. G. and Mirsky, A. E. (1964): *Proc. nat. Acad. Sci. (Wash.)*, *52*, 501.

Davidson, E. H., Crippa, M. and Mirsky, A. E. (1968): *Proc. nat. Acad. Sci. (Wash.)*, *60*, 152.

Davidson, E. H. and Hough, B. R. (1971): *J. molec. Biol.*, *56*, 491.

DeLange, R. J., Fambrough, D. M., Smith, E. L. and Bonner, J. (1969): *J. biol. Chem.*, *244*, 319.

DeLange, R. J., Hooper, J. A. and Smith, E. L. (1972): *Proc. nat. Acad. Sci. (Wash.)*, *69*, 882.

DeRobertis, E. M. and Gurdon, J. B. (1977): *Proc. nat. Acad. Sci. (Wash.)*, *74*, 2470.

Doenecke, D. and McCarthy, B. J. (1975): *Biochemistry*, *14*, 1366.

Elgin, S. C. R. and Weintraub, H. (1975): *Ann. Rev. Biochem.*, *44*, 725.

Emerson, C. P. and Humphreys, T. (1970): *Develop. Biol.*, *23*, 86.

Foe, V. E., Wilkinson, L. E. and Laird, C. D. (1976): *Cell*, *9*, 131.

Ford, P. J., Mathieson, T. and Rosbash, M. M. (1977): *Develop. Biol.*, in press.

Franke, W. W., Scheer, U., Spring, H., Trendelenburg, M. F. and Krohne, G. (1976a): *Exp. Cell Res.*, *100*, 233.

Franke, W. W., Scheer, U., Trendelenburg, M. F., Spring, H. and Zentgraf, H. W. (1976b): *Cytobiologie*, *13*, 401.

Frenster, J. H., Allfrey, V. G. and Mirsky, A. E. (1963): *Proc. nat. Acad. Sci. (Wash.)*, *50*, 1026.

Galau, G. A., Klein, W. H., Davis, M. M., Wold, B. J., Britten, R. J. and Davidson, E. H. (1976): *Cell*, *7*, 487.

Galau, G. A., Lipson, E. D., Britten, R. J. and Davidson, E. H. (1977): *Cell*, *10*, 415.

Gall, J. G. and Callan, H. G. (1962): *Proc. nat. Acad. Sci. (Wash.)*, *48*, 562.

Garel, A. and Axel, R. (1976): *Proc. nat. Acad. Sci. (Wash.)*, *73*, 3966.

Gershey, E. L. and Kleinsmith, L. J. (1969): *Biochim. biophys. Acta (Amst.)*, *194*, 519.

Gershey, E. L., Vidali, G. and Allfrey, V. G. (1968): *J. biol. Chem.*, *243*, 5018.

Gilmour, R. S. and Paul, J. (1969): *J. molec. Biol.*, *40*, 137.

Goodwin, G. H. and Johns, E. W. (1973): *Europ. J. Biochem.*, *40*, 215.

Goodwin, G. H., Nicholas, R. H. and Johns, E. W. (1975a): *Biochim. biophys. Acta (Amst.)*, *405*, 280.

Goodwin, G. H., Sanders, C. and Johns, E. W. (1973): *Europ. J. Biochem.*, *38*, 14.

Goodwin, G. H., Shooter, K. V. and Johns, E. W. (1975b): *Europ. J. Biochem.*, *54*, 427.

Goodwin, G. H., Woodhead, L. and Johns, E. W. (1977): *FEBS Letters*, *73*, 85.

Gorovsky, M. A., Pleger, G. L., Keevert, J. B. and Johmann, C. A. (1973): *J. Cell Biol.*, *57*, 773.

Gottesfeld, J. M., Murphy, R. F. and Bonner, J. (1975): *Proc. nat. Acad. Sci. (Wash.)*, *72*, 4404.

Granboulan, N. and Granboulan, P. (1966): *Exp. Cell Res.*, *38*, 604.

Gross, P. R. (1967): In: *Current Topics in Developmental Biology*, Vol. 2, p. 1. Editors: A. Monroy and A. A. Moscona. Academic Press, New York.

Gross, K. W., Lorena, J. M., Baglioni, C. and Gross, P. R. (1973): *Proc. nat. Acad. Sci. (Wash.)*, 70, 2614.
Grummt, I. (1975): *Europ. J. Biochem.*, 57, 159.
Gurdon, J. B. (1974): *The Control of Gene Expression in Animal Development*. Harvard University Press, Cambridge.
Hall, L. and Braun, R. (1977): *Experientia (Basel)*, 33, 829.
Harris, S. E., Rosen, J. M., Means, A. R. and O'Malley, B. W. (1975): *Biochemistry*, 14, 2072.
Hastie, N. D. and Bishop, J. O. (1976): *Cell*, 9, 761.
Hewish, D. R. and Burgoyne, L. A. (1973): *Biochem. biophys. Res. Commun.*, 52, 504.
Higashinakagawa, T., Wahn, H. and Reeder, R. H. (1977): *Develop. Biol.*, 55, 375.
Hill, R. J., Poccia, D. L. and Doty, P. (1971): *J. molec. Biol.*, 61, 445.
Hjelm, R. P., Kneale, G. G., Suau, P., Baldwin, J. P., Bradbury, E. M. and Ibel, K. (1977): *Cell*, 10, 139.
Holland, M. J., Hager, G. L. and Rutter, W. J. (1977): *Biochemistry*, 16, 16.
Holt, C. E. and Gurney, E. G. (1969): *J. Cell Biol.*, 40, 484.
Honjo, T. and Reeder, R. H. (1974): *Biochemistry*, 13, 1896.
Hooper, J. A., Smith, E. L., Summer, K. R. and Chalkley, R. (1973): *J. biol. Chem.*, 248, 3275.
Hough, B. R., Smith, M. J., Britten, R. J. and Davidson, E. H. (1975): *Cell*, 5, 291.
Housman, D., Forget, B. G., Skoultchi, A. and Benz, E. J. (1973): *Proc. nat. Acad. Sci. (Wash.)*, 70, 1809.
Humphries, S., Windass, J. and Williamson, R. (1976): *Cell*, 7, 267.
Inoue, A., Silva, E., Oppenheimer, J. and Allfrey, V. G. (1977): Manuscript in preparation.
Izawa, M., Allfrey, V. G. and Mirsky, A. E. (1963): *Proc. nat. Acad. Sci. (Wash.)*, 49, 544.
Joffe, J., Keene, M. and Weintraub, H. (1977): *Biochemistry*, 16, 1236.
Johns, E. W., Goodwin, G. H., Walker, J. M. and Sanders, C. (1975): In: *Ciba Foundation Symposium 28, (New Series)*, p. 95. Editors: David W. Fitzsimons and G. E. W. Wolstenholme. Elsevier–Excerpta Medica–North-Holland, Amsterdam–Oxford–New York.
Johnson, E. M. and Allfrey, V. G. (1977): In: *Biochemical Actions of Hormones, Vol. 5*, pp. 1–56. Editor: G. Litwack. Academic Press, New York.
Johnson, E. M., Hadden, J. W., Inoue, A. and Allfrey, V. G. (1975): *Biochemistry*, 14, 3873.
Johnson, E. M., Littau, V. C., Allfrey, V. G., Bradbury, E. M. and Matthews, H. R. (1976): *Nucl. Acids Res.*, 3, 3313.
Kacian, D. L., Gambino, R., Dow, L. W., Grossbard, E., Natta, C., Ramirez, F., Spiegelman, S., Marks, P. A. and Bank, A. (1973): *Proc. nat. Acad. Sci. (Wash.)*, 70, 1886.
Kamiyama, M. and Wang, T. Y. (1971): *Biochim. biophys. Acta (Amst.)*, 228, 563.
Kemp, C. L. (1966): *Chromosoma (Berl.)*, 19, 137.
Killander, D. and Rigler, R. (1965): *Exp. Cell Res.*, 39, 710.
Killander, D. and Rigler, R. (1969): *Exp. Cell Res.*, 54, 163.
Kornberg, R. D. (1974): *Science*, 184, 868.
Kostraba, N. C., Montagna, R. A. and Wang, T. Y. (1976): *Biochem. biophys. Res. Commun.*, 72, 334.
Kostraba, N. C. and Wang, T. Y. (1975): *J. biol. Chem.*, 250, 8938.
Kwan, S. P., Wood, T. G. and Lingrel, J. B. (1977): *Proc. nat. Acad. Sci. (Wash.)*, 74, 178.
Lakhotia, S. C. and Jacob, J. (1974): *Exp. Cell Res.*, 86, 253.
Langmore, J. P. and Wooley, J. C. (1975): *Proc. nat. Acad. Sci. (Wash.)*, 72, 2691.
Levenson, R. G. and Marcu, K. B. (1976): *Cell*, 9, 311.
Levy-Wilson, B., Gjerset, R. and McCarthy, B. J. (1977a): *Biochim. biophys. Acta (Amst.)*, 475, 168.
Levy-Wilson, B., Wong, N. C. W. and Dixon, G. H. (1977b): *Proc. nat. Acad. Sci. (Wash.)*, 74, 2810.
Li, H. J. (1975): *Nucl. Acids Res.*, 2, 1275.
Lipps, H. J. (1975): *Cell Differentiation*, 4, 123.
Littau, V. C., Allfrey, V. G., Frenster, J. H. and Mirsky, A. E. (1964): *Proc. nat. Acad. Sci. (Wash.)*, 52, 93.
Lohr, D., Corden, J., Tatchell, K., Kovacic, R. T. and Van Holde, K. E. (1977): *Proc. nat. Acad. Sci. (Wash.)*, 74, 79.
MacNaughton, M., Freeman, K. B. and Bishop, J. O. (1974): *Cell*, 1, 117.
Malcolm, D. B. and Sommerville, J. (1974): *Chromosoma (Berl.)*, 48, 137.
Martinson, H. G. and McCarthy, B. J. (1975): *Biochemistry*, 14, 1073.
Marushige, K. and Bonner, J. (1971): *Proc. nat. Acad. Sci. (Wash.)*, 68, 2941.
Marzluff Jr, W. F. and McCarty, K. S. (1972): *Biochemistry*, 11, 2677.
Mathis, D. and Gorovsky, M. A. (1976): *Biochemistry*, 15, 750.
Matsui, S., Fuke, M. and Busch, H. (1977): *Biochemistry*, 16, 39.

Matthews, H. R. (1977): *Nature (Lond.)*, *267*, 203.
McKnight, S. L. and Miller Jr, O. L. (1976): *Cell*, *8*, 305.
Miller Jr, O. L. and Bakken, A. H. (1972): *Acta endocr., Suppl.*, *168*, 155.
Miller Jr, O. L. and Hamkalo, B. A. (1972): *Int. Rev. Cytol.*, *33*, 1.
Molgaard, H. V., Matthews, H. R. and Bradbury, E. M. (1976): *Europ. J. Biochem.*, *68*, 541.
Morris, N. R. (1976): *Cell*, *9*, 627.
Mott, M. R. and Callan, H. G. (1975): *J. Cell Sci.*, *17*, 241.
Murphy, E. C., Hall, S. H., Sheperd, J. H. and Weiser, R. S. (1973): *Biochemistry*, *12*, 3843.
Newlon, C. S., Sonenshein, G. E. and Holt, C. E. (1973): *Biochemistry*, *12*, 2338.
Noll, M. (1974): *Nature (Lond.)*, *251*, 249.
Noll, M. (1976): *Cell*, *8*, 349.
Noll, M. and Kornberg, R. D. (1977): *J. molec. Biol.*, *109*, 393.
Olins, A. L. and Olins, D. E. (1974): *Science*, *183*, 330.
Olins, A. L., Senior, M. B. and Olins, D. E. (1976): *J. Cell Biol.*, *68*, 787.
Olson, M. O. J., Prestayko, A. W., Jones, C. W. and Busch, H. (1974): *J. molec. Biol.*, *90*, 161.
Oudet, P., Gross-Bellard, M. and Chambon, P. (1975): *Cell*, *4*, 281.
Packman, S., Aviv, H., Ross, J. and Leder, P. (1972): *Biochem. biophys. Res. Commun.*, *49*, 813.
Pardon, J. F., Worcester, D. L., Wooley, J. C., Tatchell, K., Van Holde, K. and Richards, B. (1976): *Nucl. Acids Res.*, *2*, 2163.
Parker, C. S. and Roeder, R. G. (1977): *Proc. nat. Acad. Sci. (Wash.)*, *74*, 44.
Paul, J., Gilmour, R. S., More, I., MacGillivray, A. J. and Rickwood, D. (1975): In: *Regulation of Transcription and Translation in Eukaryotes*, p. 143. Editors: E. K. F. Bautz, P. Karlson and H. Kersten. Springer-Verlag, New York.
Perlman, S. M., Ford, P. J. and Rosbash, M. M. (1977): *Proc. nat. Acad. Sci. (Wash.)*, *74*, 3835.
Peterson, J. L. and McConkey, E. H. (1976): *J. biol. Chem.*, *251*, 548.
Platz, R. D., Grimes, S. R., Hard, G., Meistrich, M. L. and Hnilica, L. S. (1975): In: *Chromosomal Proteins and their Role in the Regulation of Gene Expression*, p. 67. Editors: G. S. Stein and L. J. Kleinsmith. Academic Press, New York.
Pogo, B. G. T., Allfrey, V. G. and Mirsky, A. E. (1966): *Proc. nat. Acad. Sci. (Wash.)*, *55*, 805.
Pukkila, P. J. (1975): *Chromosoma (Berl.)*, *53*, 71.
Ramirez, F., Gambino, R., Maniatis, G. M., Rifkind, R. A., Marks, P. A. and Bank, A. (1975): *J. biol. Chem.*, *250*, 6054.
Reeder, R. H. (1975): *J. Cell Biol.*, *67*, 357a.
Reeder, R. H. and Roeder, R. G. (1972): *J. molec. Biol.*, *67*, 433.
Reeves, R. (1976): *Science*, *194*, 529.
Reeves, R. and Jones, A. (1976): *Nature (Lond.)*, *260*, 495.
Riggs, A. D., Suzuki, H. and Bourgeois, S. (1970): *J. molec. Biol.*, *48*, 67.
Rill, R. and Van Holde, K. E. (1973): *J. biol. Chem.*, *248*, 1080.
Roeder, R. G. (1976): In: *RNA Polymerases*, p. 285. Editors: R. Losick and M. Chamberlin, Cold Spring Harbor Press, New York.
Roeder, R. G., Reeder, R. H. and Brown, D. D. (1976): *Cold Spr. Harb. Symp. quant. Biol.*, *35*, 727.
Roeder, R. G. and Rutter, W. J. (1970): *Biochemistry*, *9*, 2543.
Rosbash, M. M. and Ford, P. J. (1974): *J. molec. Biol.*, *85*, 87.
Ruderman, J. V., Baglioni, C. and Gross, P. R. (1974): *Nature (Lond.)*, *247*, 36.
Ruiz-Carrillo, A., Beato, M., Schutz, G., Feigelson, P. and Allfrey, V. G. (1973): *Proc. nat. Acad. Sci., (Wash.)*, *70*, 3641.
Ruiz-Carrillo, A., Wangh, L. J. and Allfrey, V. G. (1975): *Science*, *190*, 117.
Ruiz-Carrillo, A., Wangh, L. J. and Allfrey, V. G. (1976): *Arch. Biochem.*, *174*, 273.
Ruiz-Carrillo, A., Wangh, L. J., Littau, V. C. and Allfrey, V. G. (1974): *J. biol. Chem.*, *249*, 7358.
Ryser, U. and Braun, R. (1974): *Biochim. biophys. Acta (Amst.)*, *361*, 33.
Ryser, U., Fakan, S. and Braun, R. (1973): *Exp. Cell Res.*, *78*, 89.
Sarkander, H. J., Fleischer-Lambropoulos, H. and Brade, W. P. (1975): *FEBS Letters*, *52*, 40.
Scheer, U., Trendelenburg, M. F., Krohne, G. and Franke, W. W. (1977): *Chromosoma (Berl.)*, *60*, 147.
Scott, S. E. M. and Sommerville, J. (1974): *Nature (Lond.)*, *250*, 680.
Seale, R. L. and Aronson, A. I. (1973a): *J. molec. Biol.*, *75*, 633.
Seale, R. L. and Aronson, A. I. (1973b): *J. molec. Biol.*, *75*, 647.
Shaw, B. R., Herman, T. M., Kovacic, R. T., Beaudreau, G. S. and Van Holde, K. E. (1976): *Proc. nat.*

Acad. Sci. (Wash.), 73, 505.

Shea, M. and Kleinsmith, L. J. (1973): *Biochem. biophys. Res. Commun., 50,* 473.

Shelton, K. M. and Neelin, J. M. (1971): *Biochemistry, 10,* 2342.

Silver, L. M. and Elgin, S. C. R. (1976): *Proc. nat. Acad. Sci. (Wash.), 73,* 423.

Simpson, R. T. and Reeck, G. R. (1973): *Biochemistry, 12,* 3853.

Simpson, R. T. and Whitlock, J. (1976): *Nucl. Acids Res., 3,* 117.

Sklar, V. E. F. and Roeder, R. G. (1977): *Cell, 10,* 405.

Smerdon, M. J. and Isenberg, I. (1976): *Biochemistry, 15,* 4242.

Smith, M. J., Hough, B. R., Chamberlin, M. E. and Davidson, E. H. (1974): *J. molec. Biol., 85,* 103.

Soiero, R. and Basile, C. (1973): *J. molec. Biol., 79,* 507.

Sollner-Webb, B., Camerini-Otero, R. D. and Felsenfeld, G. (1976): *Cell, 9,* 179.

Sollner-Webb, B. and Felsenfeld, G. (1975): *Biochemistry, 14,* 2915.

Sommerville, J. and Malcolm, D. B. (1976): *Chromosoma (Berl.), 55,* 183.

Spadafora, C., Bellard, M., Compton, J. L. and Chambon, P. (1976): *FEBS Letters, 69,* 281.

Staron, K., Jerzmanowski, A., Tyniec, B., Urbanska, A. and Toczko, K. (1977): *Biochim. biophys. Acta (Amst.), 475,* 131.

Steggles, A. W., Wilson, G. N., Kantor, J. A., Picciano, D. J., Falvey, A. K. and Anderson, W. F. (1974): *Proc. nat. Acad. Sci. (Wash.), 71,* 1219.

Stein, G. S., Spelsberg, T. C. and Kleinsmith, L. J. (1974): *Science, 183,* 817.

Stein, G. S., Stein, J. L., Kleinsmith, L. J., Jansing, R. L., Park, W. D. and Thomson, J. A. (1977): *Biochem. Soc. Symp. (Lond.), 42,* 137.

Sun, I. Y-C., Johnson, E. M., Matthews, H. R. and Allfrey, V. G. (1977): Manuscript in preparation.

Teng, C. S., Teng, C. T. and Allfrey, V. G. (1971): *J. biol. Chem., 246,* 3597.

Thomas, J. O. and Furber, V. (1976): *FEBS Letters, 66,* 274.

Thomas, J. O. and Kornberg, R. D. (1975): *FEBS Letters, 58,* 353.

Thomas, J. O. and Thompson, R. J. (1977): *Cell, 10,* 633.

Thwaits, B. H., Brandt, W. F. and Von Holt, C. (1976a): *FEBS Letters, 71,* 193.

Thwaits, B. H., Brandt, W. F. and Von Holt, C. (1976b): *FEBS Letters, 71,* 197.

Todd, R. D. and Garrard, W. T. (1977): *J. biol. Chem., 252,* 4729.

Tolstoshev, P., Mitchell, J., Lanyon, G., Williamson, R., Ottolenghi, S., Comi, P., Giglioni, B., Masera, G., Modell, B., Weatherall, D. J. and Clegg, J. B. (1976): *Nature (Lond.), 259,* 95.

Tsai, S. Y., Harris, S. E., Tsai, M. J. and O'Malley, B. W. (1976): *J. biol. Chem., 251,* 4713.

Varshavsky, A. J., Bakayev, V. V. and Georgiev, G. P. (1976): *Nucl. Acids Res., 3,* 477.

Vidali, G., Boffa, L. C. and Allfrey, V. G. (1977a): *Cell, 12,* 409.

Vidali, G., Boffa, L. C., Littau, V. C., Allfrey, K. M. and Allfrey, V. G. (1973): *J. biol. Chem., 248,* 4065.

Vidali, G., Boffa, L. C., Sterner, R. and Allfrey, V. G. (1977b): Manuscript in preparation.

Vogt, V. M. and Braun, R. (1976): *J. molec. Biol., 106,* 567.

Walker, J. M., Goodwin, G. H. and Johns, E. W. (1976): *Europ. J. Biochem., 62,* 461.

Wangh, L. J., Ruiz-Carrillo, A. and Allfrey, V. G. (1972): *Arch. Biochem., 150,* 44.

Watson, D. C., Peters, E. H. and Dixon, G. H. (1977): *Europ. J. Biochem., 74,* 53.

Weintraub, H. and Groudine, M. (1976): *Science, 193,* 848.

Weintraub, H., Palter, K. and Van Lente, F. (1975): *Cell, 6,* 85.

Weintraub, H. and Van Lente, F. (1974): *Proc. nat. Acad. Sci. (Wash.), 71,* 4249.

Weintraub, H., Worcel, A. and Alberts, B. (1976): *Cell, 9,* 409.

Whitlock, J. P. and Simpson, R. T. (1976): *Biochemistry, 15,* 3307.

Williamson, R., Drewienkiewicz, C. and Paul, J. (1973): *Nature New Biol., 241,* 66.

Wong, L. J. C. and Alberts, B. M. (1977): *Fed. Proc., 36,* 784a.

Woodcock, C. L. F. (1973): *J. Cell Biol., 59,* 368a.

Woodcock, C. L. F., Frado, L. L. Y., Hatch, C. L. and Ricciardiello, L. (1976b): *Chromosoma (Berl.), 58,* 33.

Woodcock, C. L. F., Safer, J. P. and Stanchfield, J. E. (1976a): *Exp. Cell Res., 97,* 101.

Zellweger, A., Ryser, U. and Braun, R. (1972): *J. molec. Biol., 64,* 681.

Zentgraf, H., Scheer, U., Franke, W. W. and Trendelenburg, M. F. (1976): *J. Cell Biol., 70,* 390a.

Mapping the human genome and metabolic diseases *

THOMAS B. SHOWS

Biochemical Genetics Section, Roswell Park Memorial Institute, New York State Department of Health, Buffalo, N.Y., U.S.A.

It is reasoned from successful gene mapping studies in experimental organisms that a detailed knowledge of the specific location of individual human genes on chromosomes is basic for understanding the organization of the human genome; the function of genes individually and as a total genome; and the regulation of gene expression. Understanding these principles individually should promote a genetic knowledge of how they function together in man. Such information on organization, function, and expression of the human genome is essential for understanding all stages of normal and abnormal human development and physiology. Furthermore, a knowledge of the gene map of each human chromosome will be useful in prenatal diagnosis and genetic dissection of metabolic diseases as well as in understanding the evolution of man through comparative gene mapping. Comparative mapping studies are becoming increasingly important in choosing laboratory animals with a homologous or suitable arrangement of genes for experimental studies and possible gene therapy.

It has been estimated that there are in the order of 50,000 structural genes coding for proteins in man (Ohta and Kimura, 1971; Bishop, 1974; Judd et al., 1972; Searle et al., 1970). This is an estimated number derived from Mendelian genetic and molecular studies of microorganisms, Drosophila, and the mouse. It is of considerable importance for understanding the biology and evolution of man to assign these genes to specific locations on human chromosomes. The gene map as of September, 1977, will be presented here with a discussion on the organization of the map; regional assignment of genes on specific chromosome regions; usefulness of the human gene map; and the genetics of fatal childhood diseases.

MAPPING THE HUMAN GENOME

The human genome is divided into 24 gene maps representing the 24 different human chromosomes. Some 1200 inherited traits have been reported in man, but most are rare and are not useful in classical gene mapping studies (McKusick, 1975). There

* Supported in part by NIH grants HD 05196 and GM 20454, and by a National Foundation–March of Dimes grant 1–485.

have been over 100 X-linked traits and a few Y traits described (McKusick, 1975) but only a few are frequent enough in the population to be useful for pedigree analysis. A detailed gene map in man determined by classical Mendelian genetics has been prevented because of a paucity of common variants at each locus, restrictions on controlled matings, small numbers of progeny, long generation times, suitable methodology to program chromosome variations for localization of genes, and a methodology to acquire and test mutants affecting all stages of human biology. Requirements essential for a detailed Mendelian mapping of the human genome include being able to identify common genetic variants at all loci; having unrestricted matings for test crosses; a reduction of the generation time from 20–25 years to weeks, days, or even hours; the meiotic segregation and recombination of chromosomes; an unlimited number of progeny; the methods to identify each chromosome and to obtain unlimited chromosome variants for gene assignments; and experimental procedures to acquire mutants at all stages of development. Clearly, the majority of these requirements cannot be met for a classical genetic examination of man.

To bypass these difficulties, alternative strategies have been developed to map the human genome. For example, the development of parasexual systems such as somatic cell hybridization (see Ruddle, 1972); molecular procedures to identify gene location by annealing complementary nucleic acid to specific chromosome sites (Evans et al., 1974); gene dosage methods (Ferguson-Smith et al., 1976); comparative gene mapping (Minna et al., 1976); and a combination of these alternative procedures with pedigree analyses have all become suitable alternatives and quite essential for arriving at a detailed gene map of each human chromosome.

The alternative system that has contributed most significantly to developing the human gene map has been the use of interspecific somatic cell hybridization. The advantages of the man–rodent cell hybridization strategy are that a large number of genetic variants are available as a result of the more than 80 million years of evolutionary divergence between man and rodents; employing man–rodent cell fusions the genetic crosses that are necessary are practically unrestricted; there is a loss of human chromosomes similar to that of meiotic segregation; each human chromosome and specific regions can be identified; a generation time of about 20 hours exists for cell hybrids; there is an unlimited number of progeny and lifespan; cell hybrids are amenable to gene transfer techniques; and cell hybrid characteristics lend themselves to combining data from parasexual, Mendelian, and molecular methodologies which are all necessary for developing a detailed gene map of man.

Somatic cell hybridization and gene mapping

Procedures for obtaining man–rodent cell hybrids and mapping human genes in a parasexual way are illustrated in Figure 1. Human cells in monolayer culture or as cell suspensions are fused to rodent cells, either mouse or Chinese hamster, which possess enzyme deficiencies or other characteristics which can be selected against. Human and rodent cells are fused using inactivated Sendai virus or polyethylene glycol (PEG) fusing agents (Klebe et al., 1970; Pontecorvo, 1975) and are plated for monolayer cell culture. The fused cells, termed heterokaryons, are subjected to a selection medium that prevents the growth of rodent cells. If the rodent parental cells,

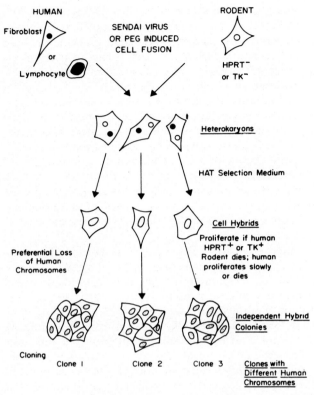

Fig. 1. Somatic cell hybridization scheme featuring gene mapping strategy. Development of these methodologies has been reviewed (see Ruddle, 1972).

for example, are deficient for thymidine kinase (TK) or hypoxanthine phosphoribosyl transferase (HPRT) which function in DNA-RNA salvage pathways, they will not grow in HAT (hypoxanthine-aminopterin-thymidine) medium (Szybalski et al., 1962; Littlefield, 1964). Human cells are selected against since human leukocytes are removed with media changes and human fibroblasts replicate slowly in low dilution. Hybrid cells are able to proliferate if nuclear fusion occurs and the genes for human HPRT or TK are retained to compensate for the enzyme deficiencies of the rodent cells. Hybrid colonies derived from independent fusions proliferate and are cloned and expanded for analysis. The important characteristic of man–rodent cell hybrids is that human but not rodent chromosomes are lost, which results in hybrid clones that retain different numbers and combinations of functioning human chromosomes. When the cells of an individual are investigated by hybridization studies and several independent clones are isolated, it is possible to obtain a population of primary hybrid clones in which the total human chromosome complement of an individual is represented but distributed in reduced numbers of chromosomes in the hybrid clones. These characteristics present a methodology to genetically analyze the somatic cells of an individual and dissect the human genome chromosome-by-chromosome. Detailed accounts of the somatic cell hybridization methodology and strategies have been reviewed (Ruddle, 1972; Ruddle and Creagan, 1975; Shows, 1978).

Chromosomes and enzymes representative of a man–mouse hybrid cell are illustrated in Figure 2. Only human chromosomes 7 and 10 are retained in this cell hybrid. All other human chromosomes have been lost and the remaining chromosomes are of mouse origin. Since the other human chromosomes and genes have been lost, only those human genes located on chromosomes 7 and 10 should be expressed in this hybrid. Employing gel electrophoresis, human enzymes are often separated and identified from rodent enzymes. These enzymes represent excellent gene markers and have been assigned to each of the human chromosomes except the Y. The enzymes β-glucuronidase (βGUS) and glutamic oxaloacetic transaminase (GOT$_S$) whose genes are encoded on chromosomes 7 and 10, respectively, are expressed in this hybrid, while the other enzyme markers representing the remaining human chromosomes were not expressed. The subunit structure of enzymes (Hopkinson et al., 1976) is also studied by examining the electrophoretic phenotype of enzymes in hybrids. The βGUS electrophoretic pattern has been separated into 2 parental

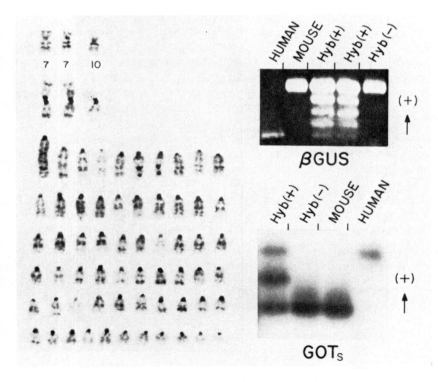

Fig. 2. Chromosomes and enzymes of a man-mouse cell hybrid. Chromosomes and enzymes were studied as reported: Shows and Brown (1975a); Lalley et al. (1977); Shows (1974).

bands and 3 man–mouse interspecific bands, indicating a tetrameric structure for this enzyme. The 3-banded pattern of GOT_S similarly demonstrates a dimeric structure for this enzyme. Enzyme expression, genes coding for individual enzymes on each human chromosome, and a discussion of the subunit nature of human enzymes as determined in cell hybrids have been reviewed (Shows, 1975, 1978).

Since human chromosomes 'segregate' in cell hybrids and human gene markers and chromosomes are recognized, gene linkages and gene assignments can be determined. As an example, Table 1 illustrates the linkage relationships, chromosome assignment, and regional mapping of genes coding for the enzymes α-fucosidase (αFUC), enolase-1 (ENO_1), and peptidase-C (PEPC). Part A of Table 1 shows that αFUC, ENO_1, and PEPC segregate together in hybrid clones when compared to 4 additional enzymes which segregate independently and show no linkage. Part B demonstrates that αFUC, ENO_1, and PEPC segregate concordantly with chromosome 1 but not with other chromosomes, indicating assignment of the *αFUC*,

TABLE 1

Mapping strategy for somatic cell hybrids

A. *Gene linkage relationships*

Cell hybrid clones	Human enzyme markers						
	αFUC	ENO_1	PEPC	MDH_S	βGAL	PEPS	HEX_B
A	+	+	+	−	−	−	+
B	−	−	−	−	+	−	+
C	+	+	+	−	+	+	−
D	+	+	+	+	−	−	−
E	−	−	−	+	+	+	+

B. *Chromosome assignment strategy*

	Gene markers	Human chromosomes				
	αFUC, ENO_1, PEPC	1	2	3	4	5
A	+	+	−	−	−	+
B	−	−	−	+	−	+
C	+	+	−	+	+	−
D	+	+	+	−	−	−
E	−	−	+	+	+	+

C. *Regional localization methodology*

	Gene markers			Human chromosomes					
	αFUC	ENO_1	PEPC	1p	1q	2	3	4	5
A	+	+	−	+	−	−	−	−	+
B	−	−	+	−	+	−	+	−	+
C	+	+	−	+	−	−	+	+	−
D	+	+	−	+	−	+	−	−	−
E	−	−	+	−	+	+	+	+	+

Examples are based on results we have obtained in the mapping of chromosome 1 (Shows and Brown, 1975b; Koch et al., 1978). It is important that enzymes and chromosomes be tested on the same cell passage.

ENO_1, and *PEPC* genes to this chromosome. Part C demonstrates the methodology for mapping the chromosome 1 genes to specific chromosomal regions. Utilizing translocations or deletions of the short arm (p) and long arm (q) of chromosome 1, the segregation data in Table 1 illustrate the assignment of *αFUC* and ENO_1 to the short arm 1p, and *PEPC* to the long arm 1q.

The X-chromosome gene map

Utilizing the somatic cell hybridization strategy, and to a lesser extent, pedigree analysis, deletion mapping, and molecular techniques, the human gene map is developing into a comprehensive genetic signature of man. The current map of the human X chromosome illustrates this point in Figure 3 and compares data derived from cell hybridization and family studies. Over 100 X-linked traits have been described in man (McKusick, 1975). With such numbers and if the traits were common, it would be expected that a detailed gene map could be generated. However, this is not the case since only the traits listed in Figure 3 are common enough in man to determine linkage relationships in family studies. By classical pedigree analyses, 2 clusters of X-linked loci have been described. One cluster centers around the closely linked color blindness, hemophilia, and glucose-6-phosphate dehydrogenase

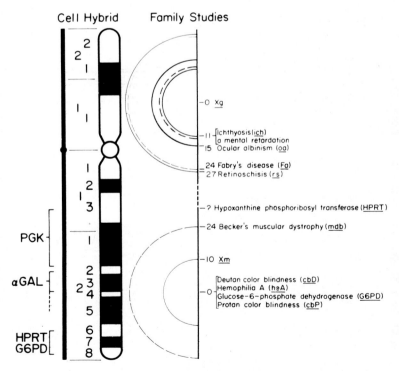

Fig. 3. The X chromosome gene map. Chromosome banding patterns based on the Paris Conference (1972); gene localization based on Brown et al. (1976) and Shows et al. (1977); the family map is based on Race and Sanger (1974).

(G6PD) loci; the second cluster of X-linked genes centers around the Xg blood group locus. These 2 groups of loci are far enough apart to be unlinked by classical recombination studies. Hypoxanthine phosphoribosyl transferase (HPRT) is also sex-linked but is not closely linked to either *Xg* or *G6PD*. With the knowledge that these loci are X-linked, they have been localized to specific regions utilizing the somatic cell hybrid strategy and a series of X-autosome translocations. Localization of X-linked genes has been reviewed (Shows and Brown, 1975a; Shows, 1977) and involves selection and analyses of cell hybrids with different regions of the X translocated to autosomes. Hybrids with different regions of the X chromosome express only those genes that are coded on the X region that is retained. Chromosome locations for *HPRT*, *G6PD*, α-galactosidase *(αGAL)*, and phosphoglycerate kinase *(PGK)* have been determined in this way. Figure 3 demonstrates the regions of the X chromosome that encode these 4 enzymes. The banding patterns of human chromosomes have been standardized at the Paris Conference (1972). When comparing the results obtained from cell hybrid and family studies, it is striking that *HPRT* and *G6PD* are closely located at the q terminus of the X on the physical map from hybrid studies but are not closely linked by recombination studies in families. This could be explained by considerable recombination at the end of the long arm of the X. α-Galactosidase, another X-linked enzyme marker, is deficient in Fabry's disease. Location of the *αGAL* gene to the Xp22–Xp24 region by cell hybrid studies

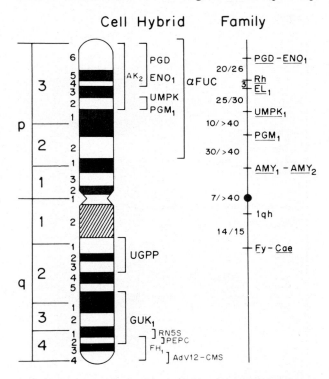

Fig. 4. Chromosome 1 gene map. Based on Hamerton (1976); Burgerhout et al. (1977); Jongsma and Burgerhout (1977).

suggests that the X_q cluster is located on the long arm of the X or very near to the centromere. These studies demonstrate how family and cell hybrid data can be combined to map the human genome.

Gene map of chromosome 1

With the cell hybrid strategy, chromosome translocations and breaks, and family studies, a detailed map of chromosome 1 is also rapidly developing. Figure 4 demonstrates the physical map determined by cell hybrid studies and the map derived by family studies. The map of chromosome 1 compares favorably for cell hybrid and family studies with regard to distances and linear order. Using cell hybridization methodology, several gene loci have been assigned to the short arm of 1. From family studies, it had been shown that some of these loci and others not expressed in cultured cells were closely linked. Assignment of one marker by cell hybrid strategy from this Mendelian linkage group indicates assignment of all loci within it. In this way both cell hybrid and family studies have complemented and stimulated each other in the mapping of this chromosome. This is best illustrated by the assignment of the important gene for the Rh blood group to the p32–pter region. Although the Rh antigens are not expressed in cell hybrids, family studies demonstrated the linkage of *PGD-Rh-PGM₁*. Assignment of *PGD* and *PGM₁* to the p32–pter region by cell hybrid studies implies assignment of *Rh* to the same region.

THE HUMAN GENE MAP

The gene map of each human chromosome is presented in Table 2. The majority of genes and their regional localizations have been assigned by cell hybridization techniques. Family studies have contributed significantly to gene assignments and particularly so when a marker or a closely linked locus is first assigned using cell hybrids. A growing number of genes are being assigned by gene dosage methods. Quantitative measurement of gene products might reflect an increased or decreased gene dosage, as in 3 copies of a gene (trisomy) or 1 copy of a gene (deletion). A small number of genes have also been assigned by in situ hybridization using procedures for annealing complementary nucleic acid to specific chromosome sites. In the future it can be expected that comparative mapping will play a significant role. The co-segregation of linkage groups in one species will suggest similar assignments in another species.

A wide range of traits have been mapped including genes coding for enzymes and proteins, surface antigens and blood groups, viral markers, RNA markers, susceptibility to drugs and toxins, gene regulatory markers, blood clotting factors, and diseases and syndromes. Important cell surface antigens are the Rh blood group assigned to 1p32–1pter, the ABO blood group assigned to 9q34, and the major histocompatibility complex which has been assigned to 6p12–6p22 (Table 2). Several additional important cell surface antigens have been assigned to different chromosomes with no suggestion that a specific chromosome or region generally codes for cell surface antigens. The major histocompatibility complex on chromosome 6 does, however, code for a cluster of HLA, complement components, and blood

TABLE 2

The gene map of each human chromosome

Chromosome	Most consistent smallest region	Gene marker	Gene symbol	E.C. No.	Status	System
1	pter–p32	Enolase-1	ENO_1	4.2.1.11	C	S, F
	pter–p34	Phosphogluconate dehydrogenase	PGD	1.1.1.44	C	S, F
	pter–p36	Adenovirus-12 chromosome modification site-1p	Adv-12-CMS-1p		P	S
	p32–p34	α-L-Fucosidase	αFUC	3.2.1.51	C	S, F
	pter–p32	Rhesus blood group	Rh		C	F
	pter–p32	Adenylate kinase-2	AK_2	2.7.4.3	C	S
	pter–p32	Uridine monophosphate kinase	UMPK	2.7.4.4.	C	S, F
	p21–p33	Phosphoglucomutase-1	PGM_1	2.7.5.1	C	S, F
	1p	Amylase₁ (salivary)	AMY_1	3.2.1.1	C	F
	1p	Amylase₂ (pancreatic)	AMY_2	3.2.1.1	C	F
	q21–q23	UDP glucose pyrophosphorylase-1	$UGPP_1$	2.7.7.9	C	S
	q32–qter	Guanylate kinase-1	GUK_1	2.7.4.8	C	S
	q41–qter	Peptidase-C	PEPC	3.4.11.–	C	S
	q42	Adenovirus-12 chromosome modification site-1q	AdV-12-CMS-1q		P	S
	q32–qter	Fumarate hydratase (soluble)	FH_S	4.2.1.2	C	S
	q42	5S RNA	RN5S		C	A
	1p	Elliptocytosis	El_1		C	F
	1q	Duffy blood group	Fy		C	F
		Zonular pulverulent cataract	Cae		C	F
		Scianna blood group	Sc		P	F
		Retinitis pigmentosa-1	RP_1		P	F
	pter–p21	Glucose dehydrogenase	GDH	1.1.1.47	P	S
		Dombrock blood group	Do		T	F
		Antithrombin III	AT-3		T	F
		Aniridia type II	AN-2		T	F
2	p23	Acid phosphatase-1 (red cell)	ACP_1	3.1.3.2	C	S, F
	pter–p23	Malate dehydrogenase (soluble)	MDH_S	1.1.1.37	C	S
	p11–p22	Galactose enzyme activator	Gal^+-Act		P	S
	2q	Isocitrate dehydrogenase (soluble)	IDH_S	1.1.1.42	C	S
		Arylhydrocarbon hydroxylase	AHH	1.14.14.1	P	S
		UDP glucose pyrophosphorylase-2	$UGPP_2$	2.7.7.9	P	S
		Interferon	If-1		P	S
		MNSs blood group	MNSs		P	F
3		β-Galactosidase	βGAL	3.2.1.23	I	S
		Glutathione peroxidase-1	GPX_1	1.11.1.9	P	S
		Herpes virus sensitivity	HVS		P	S
		Temperature sensitive complement	tsAF8		P	S

This table is based on the Third International Workshop on Human Gene Mapping (1975) and the Fourth International Workshop on Human Gene Mapping (1977).

Enzyme gene symbols are based on the report by Giblett et al. (1976).

Symbols: C = result confirmed by 2 or more independent reports. P = results reported for the first time. I = inconsistent results of 2 or more laboratories. T = tentative results. S = results determined by somatic cell hybridization. F = results determined by family studies. D = results determined by gene dosage. A = results from DNA/RNA annealing.

TABLE 2 (continued)

Chromo-some	Most consistent smallest region	Gene marker	Gene symbol	E.C. No.	Status	System
4	p14–p21	Phosphoglucomutase-2	PGM_2	2.7.5.1	C	S
	pter–q21	Peptidase-S	PEPS	3.4.11.–	C	S
	q11–q13	Group specific protein	Gc		P	F
		Phosphoribosylpyrophosphate amidotransferase	PRPP-ATF		P	S
		Albumin	Alb		P	F
5	cen–q13	Hexosaminidase-B	HEX_B	3.2.1.30	C	S
		Arylsulfatase-B	ARS_B	3.1.6.1	P	S
		Diphtheria toxin sensitivity	DTS		C	S
		Interferon-2	If-2		C	S
		Leucyl-tRNA synthetase	LEURS		P	S
6	pter–p12	Glyoxalase-1	GLO_1	4.4.1.5	C	S
	p12–p22	Major histocompatibility complex				
		HLA-A,B,C,D	HLA		C	S, F
		C2, C4, C8	C		C	S, F
		Rogers blood group	Rg		C	F
		Chido blood group	Ch		C	F
		Properdin factor B	Bf		C	F
	p12–qter	Phosphoglucomutase-3	PGM_3	2.7.5.1	C	S
	q12–q15	Malic enzyme (soluble)	ME_S	1.1.1.40	C	S
	q21	Superoxide dismutase (mitochondrial)	SOD_M	1.15.1.1	C	S
		Glutamic oxaloacetic trans-aminase (mitochondrial)	GOT_M	2.6.1.1	P	S
		Pepsinogen	Pg	3.4.23.–	P	F
7	p13–cen	β-Glucuronidase	βGUS	3.2.1.31	C	S
	p22–q22	Malate dehydrogenase (mitochondrial)	MDH_M	1.1.1.37	C	S
	q35	Hageman factor	HaF		P	F
	7q	SV40 site 1	SV40-1		P	S
	7q	Kidd locus	Jk		P	D
		Colton blood group	Co		P	F, D
		Hydroxyacyl-CoA dehydrogenase	HADH	1.1.1.35	P	S
		Surface antigens	SA7		P	S
		Uridine phosphorylase	UP	2.4.2.3	P	S
8	p11	Glutathione reductase	GSR	1.6.4.2	C	S, D
9	7p	Adenylate kinase-3	AK_3	2.7.4.10	C	S
	7p	Aconitase (soluble)	$ACON_S$	4.2.1.3	C	S
	q34	ABO blood group	ABO		C	D
	q34	Adenylate kinase-1	AK_1	2.7.4.3	C	S, F, D
	q34	Nail-patella syndrome	NPa		C	D
		Argininosuccinate synthetase	ASS	6.3.4.5	C	S
		Galactose-1-phosphate uridyl transferase	GALT	2.7.7.12	I	S

TABLE 2 (continued)

Chromosome	Most consistent smallest region	Gene marker	Gene symbol	E.C. No.	Status	System
10	pter–q24	Hexokinase-1	HK_1	2.7.1.1	C	S
	pter–q24	Pyrophosphatase (inorganic)	PP	3.6.1.1	C	S
	q24–q26	Glutamic oxaloacetic trans-aminase (soluble)	GOT_S	2.6.1.1	C	S
		Adenosine kinase	ADK	2.7.1.20	C	S
		Glutamate-α-semialdehyde synthetase	$GSAS$	6.3.4.4	P	S
		Polykaryocytosis promoter	$FUSE$		P	S
		External membrane protein-130	$EMP\text{-}130$		P	S
11	pter–p13	Lactate dehydrogenase-A	LDH_A	1.1.1.27	C	S
	pter–p13	Lethal antigen	AL		P	S
	p12–cen	Acid phosphatase-2 (tissue)	ACP_2	3.1.3.2	C	S
	cen–q22	Esterase-A_4	ESA_4	3.1.1.1	C	S
	11p	Species antigen	$SA\text{-}1$		P	S
12	pter–p12	Triosephosphate isomerase	TPI	5.3.1.1	C	S
	pter–p12	Glyceraldehyde-3-phosphate dehydrogenase	$GAPDH$	1.2.1.21	C	S
	p12	Lactate dehydrogenase-B	LDH_B	1.1.1.27	C	S
	p21	Peptidase-B	$PEPB$	3.4.11.–	C	S
	pter–q14	Serine hydroxymethyltransferase	$SHMT$	2.1.2.1	P	S
		Enolase-2	ENO_2	4.2.1.11	C	S
		Citrate synthase	CS	4.1.3.7	C	S
13	q3	Esterase-D	ESD	3.1.1.1	C	S
	q	Retinoblastoma	RB		C	D
	13p	Ribosomal RNA	$rRNA$		P	A
14	q12–q20	Nucleoside phosphorylase	NP	2.4.2.1.	C	S
	q21–qter	Tryptophenyl-tRNA synthetase	$TRPRS$	6.1.1.2	C	S
		External membrane protein-195	$EMP\text{-}195$		P	S
	14p	Ribosomal RNA	$rRNA$		P	A
15	q14–q21	β_2-microglobulin	$\beta_2 M$		C	S
	q22–qter	Hexosaminidase-A	HEX_A	3.2.1.30	C	S
	q22–qter	Mannosephosphate isomerase	MPI	5.3.1.8	C	S
	q22–qter	Pyruvate kinase-M2	PK_{M2}	2.7.1.40	C	S
	q21–qter	Isocitrate dehydrogenase (mitochondrial)	IDH_M	1.1.1.42	C	S
	q11–qter	α-Mannosidase-A	MAN_A	3.2.1.24	P	S
	15p	Ribosomal RNA	$rRNA$		P	A
16	16q	Adenine phosphoribosyl transferase	$APRT$	2.4.2.7	C	S
	16q	Thymidine kinase (mitochondrial)	TK_M	2.7.1.75	P	S
	cen–q22	Cholinesterase (serum)-1	$E1$	3.1.1.8	P	F
	cen–q22	α-Haptoglobin	αHp		P	D
		α-Hemoglobin	$Hb\alpha$		P	S
		Lecithin-cholesterol acyltransferase	$LCAT$	2.3.1.43	C	F

TABLE 2 (continued)

Chromo-some	Most consistent smallest region	Gene marker	Gene symbol	E.C. No.	Status	System
17	q21	Thymidine kinase (soluble)	TK_S	2.7.1.75	C	S
	q21–q22	Galactokinase	$GALK$	2.7.1.6	C	S
	q21–q22	Adenovirus-12 chromosome modification site-17	*Adv. 12-CMS-17*		P	S
		Collagen-1	COL_1		I	S
		SV40 site 2	*SV40-2*		P	S
18	q23–qter	Peptidase-A	*PEPA*	3.4.11.–	C	S
19	pter–q13	Glucosephosphate isomerase	*GPI*	5.3.1.9	C	S
		Poliovirus sensitivity	*PVS*		C	S
		Peptidase-D	*PEPD*	3.4.13.9	C	S
	pter–q13	α-Mannosidase-B	MAN_B	3.2.1.24	C	S
20	p11–qter	Adenosine deaminase	*ADA*	3.5.4.4	C	D
		Desmosterol-to-cholesterol enzyme	*DCE*		P	S
		Inosine triphosphatase	*ITP*	3.6.1.19	C	S
21	q22	Superoxide dismutase (soluble)	SOD_S	1.15.1.1	C	S
		Antiviral protein (Antiviral response)	*AVP*		C	S
		Phosphoribosyl glycinamide synthetase	*GAPS*	6.3.4.13	P	S
	21p	Ribosomal RNA	*rRNA*		P	A
		Ag Lipoprotein	*Ag*		P	F
22	22p	Ribosomal RNA	*rRNA*		P	A
		Arylsulfatase-A	ARS_A	3.1.6.1	C	S
		Aconitase (mitochondrial)	$ACON_M$	4.2.1.3	C	S
		NADH Diaphorase	DIA_1	1.6.2.2	P	S
X	q13–q22	Phosphoglycerate kinase	*PGK*	2.7.2.3	C	S
	q22–q24	α-Galactosidase	*αGAL*	3.2.1.22	C	S
	q26–qter	Hypoxanthine phosphoribosyl transferase	*HPRT*	2.4.2.8	C	S
	q26–qter	Glucose-6-phosphate dehydrogenase	*G6PD*	1.1.1.49	C	S
		Xg antigen	*Xg*		P	F
		Tyrosine aminotransferase regulator	*TATr*		P	S
		Phosphorylase kinase	*PHK*	2.7.1.38	P	F
		Ornithine transcarbamylase	*OTC*	2.1.3.3	P	F
		Surface antigen	*SAX*		C	S
		Color blindness	*cb*		C	F
		Hemophilia	*heA*		C	F
Y		Y histocompatibility antigen	*H-Y*		C	F

group genes (Bodmer, 1976). Non-clustering was also extended to proteins which make up the external membrane, as for example, 2 external membrane proteins, *EMP-130* and *EMP-195*, which we have assigned to chromosomes 10 and 14, respectively (Owerbach et al., 1977).

The majority of genes assigned to the map code for enzymes. Each chromosome except the Y encodes enzyme genes which provide simple biochemical markers to identify each human chromosome. These markers make it feasible to map a large variety of markers including various syndromes and, in particular, metabolic disorders. The location of enzyme structural genes on human chromosomes does not suggest any pattern of organization. Genes coding for lysosomal and mitochondrial enzymes, for example, are dispersed randomly on different human chromosomes, and those that are on the same chromosome are not closely linked. This observation also holds for genes encoding enzymes that function in several metabolic pathways. These findings suggest that enzyme structural genes of related function or cell location are generally not located on a single chromosomal region. Isolated gene clusters suggesting a biological significance do, however, exist; for example, the close linkage of thymidine kinase and galactokinase located on chromosome 17 in man and linked in chimpanzee, mouse, and Chinese hamster (see Ruddle and Meera Kahn, 1976, and Warburton and Pearson, 1976). Tight linkage of genes derived from gene duplication has played a significant role in evolution and accounts for the clustering of the amylase loci, the hemoglobin β, δ, and γ peptide chains, and the immunoglobulin genes.

Several interesting viral markers have been mapped; for example, the polio virus sensitivity gene on 19, herpes virus sensitivity on 3, and SV40 and adenovirus 12 markers located on several different chromosomes (Table 2). Other mapped viral markers include interferon on 5, antiviral protein on 12, and integration and transformation sites on 17. A human gene coding for a polykaryocytosis promoter has recently been assigned to chromosome 10 (Wright and Shows, 1978).

Several important proteins that have been mapped are the genes coding for α-hemoglobin on 16, α-haptoglobin on 16, albumin on 4, collagen on 17, and histones on 7.

In situ hybridization has been instrumental in mapping the 5S RNA to 1q42, and ribosomal RNA genes to the short arms of chromosomes 13, 14, 15, 21, and 22. tRNA synthetase genes have been assigned to chromosomes 5 and 14.

MAPPING INBORN ERRORS

Assignment of genes associated with metabolic diseases and genetic dissection of components necessary for the final expression of inborn errors are applications of the gene mapping strategy. If mutant genes coding for enzyme deficiencies that are associated with a metabolic defect can be mapped, then this information can be used in genetic counseling, prenatal diagnosis, and possible genetic therapy through gene transfer. The gene assignments of several metabolic disorders are listed in Table 3. Many of these enzyme deficiencies in Table 3 are the result of a structural gene mutation since a structurally altered enzyme can be identified. If this is known for an enzyme associated with a disease, then mapping of the normal structural gene

TABLE 3

Gene mapping of inborn errors

Disorder	Enzyme deficiency	Locus	Chromosome assignment	Evidence[a] for processing gene
Lipid metabolism:				
GM$_1$ gangliosidosis	β-Galactosidase	βGAL	3	+
GM$_2$ gangliosidosis (Tay Sachs)	β-Hexosaminidase-A	HEX_A	15	+
GM$_2$ gangliosidosis (Sandhoff's)	β-Hexosaminidase-A & -B	HEX_B	5	+
Fabry's disease	α-Galactosidase	αGAL	X	+
Metachromatic leukodystrophy	Arylsulfatase-A	ARS_A	22	+
Maroteaux-Lamy syndrome	Arylsulfatase-B	ARS_B	5	+
Carbohydrate metabolism:				
Galactosemia	Galactose-1-phosphate uridyl transferase	$GALT$	9	
Galactokinase deficiency	Galactokinase	$GALK$	17	
Mannosidosis	α-Mannosidase-B	MAN_B	19	+
Fucosidosis	α-Fucosidase	αFUC	1	+
β-Glucuronidase	β-Glucuronidase	βGUS	7	+
Nucleic acid metabolism:				
Lesch-Nyhan syndrome	Hypoxanthine phosphoribosyl transferase	$HPRT$	X	
Hyperuricemia	Adenine phosphoribosyl transferase	$APRT$	16	
Erythrocyte abnormalities:				
Hexokinase deficiency	Hexokinase	HK	10	
Glucosephosphate isomerase deficiency	Glucosephosphate isomerase	GPI	19	
G6PD deficiency	Glucose-6-phosphate dehydrogenase	$G6PD$	X	
Triosephosphate isomerase deficiency	Triosephosphate isomerase	TPI	12	
Phosphoglycerate kinase deficiency	Phosphoglycerate kinase	PGK	X	
Phosphogluconate dehydrogenase deficiency	6-Phosphogluconate dehydrogenase	PGD	1	
Glutathione reductase deficiency	Glutathione reductase	GSR	8	
Hemoglobinopathies	α chain	$Hb\alpha$	16	
Hemolytic disease	Adenylate kinase	AK_1	9	
Other abnormalities:				
Combined immunodeficiency	Adenosine deaminase	ADA[b]	20[b]	
Acid phosphatase deficiency	Lysosomal acid phosphatase	ACP_2	11	+
Lecithin:cholesterol acyl transferase deficiency	Lecithin:cholesterol acyl-transferase	$LCAT$	16	

Based on Fourth International Workshop on Human Gene Mapping (1978); Harris (1975); Shows et al. (1978); Shows et al. (1977); Hamers et al. (1977); Chern (1977); Champion and Shows (1977b); Turner et al. (1974).

[a]Champion and Shows (1978).

[b]Assignment of combined immunodeficiency is only tentative since there are instances where combined immunodeficiency (CID) occurs without a deficiency of ADA; however, CID occurs when ADA is deficient.

through conventional methods will identify the chromosome and region on which the mutant gene is encoded in an affected individual. This strategy applies for the mapping of several disorders listed in Table 3; as for example, mannosidosis (Champion and Shows, 1977a; Ingram et al., 1977) and GM_1 gangliosidosis (Shows et al., 1978; Bruns et al., 1978). Knowing the structural gene assignment of an enzyme, somatic cell hybrids can be employed to map a mutant gene responsible for an enzyme deficiency by fusing deficient cells with rodent cells. If in these hybrids the known structural gene chromosome is present but the affected enzyme continues to be deficient while the other human chromosomes segregate independently, then the mutant gene is most likely located on this chromosome. This procedure does not demonstrate that the mutation occurred at the structural gene but indicates that the mutant gene is located on the same chromosome. Using this strategy we have assigned Tay Sachs disease to chromosome 15 and Sandhoff-Jatzkewitz disease to chromosome 5 (Shows et al., 1977), as well as mannosidosis to chromosome 19 (Champion and Shows, 1977b).

It is possible that an enzyme deficiency may result from a mutant gene on a chromosome different from the structural gene. By investigating this possibility in cell hybrids and using enzyme deficient cells, chromosome segregation will dissect out the genetic components associated with the disorder. If the mutant gene and the structural gene are both present in a hybrid clone, then the enzyme should not be expressed. When the mutant gene segregates and the structural gene is retained, the enzyme should be expressed. This strategy identifies and maps a second gene necessary for the final expression of the enzyme. It is also possible that the mouse genome can correct the deficiency. If this occurs, then a gene different from the structural gene is implicated. In the man–mouse hybrids (above) using Tay Sachs and Sandhoff cells, all other chromosomes segregated and the deficient enzymes never regained activity supporting the mutant gene assignment to chromosomes 15 and 5, respectively.

We have observed correction of abnormal enzymes in hybrids formed from the fusion of rodent cells and cells from an individual with mucolipidosis II (Champion and Shows, 1978). Mucolipidosis II (ML II) is a fatal, early childhood, inherited disorder with several deficiencies or electrophoretic abnormalities of several lysosomal enzymes. In these hybrids the abnormal enzyme phenotypes observed in ML II cells for β-galactosidase, β-hexosaminidase-A and -B, α-galactosidase, arylsulfatase-A and -B, α-mannosidase, α-fucosidase, β-glucuronidase, and acid phosphatase were corrected in cell hybrids. The primary defect of ML II is not known, but the multiple enzyme defects would suggest the mutation of a gene product important in the expression of a large number of lysosomal enzymes rather than structural gene mutations of all the individual lysosomal enzymes. Post-translational modification of the lysosomal enzymes is suggested from the hybrid data and from the restoration of normal electrophoretic phenotypes of several of the enzymes after neuraminidase treatment (Champion and Shows, 1977c). These results demonstrate that the mouse genome corrected the affected human enzyme expression and suggest that the ML II mutation is a processing defect common to the final expression of multiple lysosomal enzymes.

The chromosome assignment of enzyme deficiencies listed in Table 3 refers to the assignment of the mutant gene. In many cases the mutation is at the structural locus and the locus designation is that of the structural gene coding for the enzyme.

Evidence for a processing gene separate from the structural gene is indicated in the last column (Table 3) and is indicated from the correction of abnormal enzymes observed in ML II-mouse cell hybrids (Champion and Shows, 1978). Evidence for additional genes being associated with the final expression of the other enzymes listed in Table 3 has not been obtained. By employing the gene map, the somatic cell hybrid strategy, and cells expressing mutant genes, it is now possible to genetically dissect metabolic diseases and identify chromosome assignments of structural genes, enzyme deficiencies, and other genes which are important for the final realization of an enzyme.

It is clear from the chromosome assignments listed in Table 3 that current genetic data do not support a single isolated chromosome or region for disorders associated with lipid metabolism, carbohydrate metabolism, nucleic acid metabolism, or for glucose metabolism in erythrocyte disorders. Several of the enzymes in Table 3 are localized in the lysosome (those that have evidence for a processing gene). As observed for other related gene products, these lysosomal enzyme genes are not located in a region on the same chromosome.

THE MAP AND ITS USES

A knowledge of the human gene map is important for understanding the organization of the human genome. Such information will be useful in understanding human biology, disease, and evolution. Understanding the intricacies of the map should reveal insights into the important question of genetic control mechanisms which influence gene expression and cellular development. The identification of a processing gene common to several lysosomal enzymes is such an example of a gene which influences expression and biogenesis of an organelle, the lysosome. As developmental markers become available for mapping, relationships between control and structural genes will become evident and a genetic organization relating to developmental processes may be revealed. Presently there are few human developmental markers that can be effectively used in an experimental way. The map is useful in identifying different complementation groups that may be responsible for an enzyme deficiency. If several genes are identified from complementation studies using cells deficient for the same enzyme, then gene assignment for the several genes would indicate genetic relationships and genes that are involved in the final expression of an enzyme. Developmental markers for somatic cell genetic studies will most likely be found in clinical abnormalities. Now that several enzyme loci have been mapped, individuals with clinical diseases that involve quantitative abnormalities of an enzyme can be examined for abnormal chromosomes and enzymes. Cultured cells from these individuals and with these characteristics can be investigated and cell hybrids isolated for the independent segregation of structural genes and the quantitative marker. In those individuals with cytogenetic abnormalities, the map is useful in relating which loci have been rearranged. Relocation of a gene to another chromosome may influence its expression, as observed in position effects in Drosophila. Such examples may be useful for identifying control mechanisms in man.

The human gene map has its most obvious application perhaps in genetic counseling and the diagnosis of inherited disorders that are not recognizable in utero by biochemical characteristics. Knowing which loci are closely linked to the genetic defect and which are detectable in utero can be very valuable for diagnosis. If the linked loci have allelic variants and if the linkage arrangement of the allelic variants and the mutant locus are known in the parents, then it is highly possible to make a diagnosis in utero. Observing in utero an allelic variant known to be on the same chromosome as the mutant not expressed in utero predicts the fetus has inherited the disease. Along these same lines and of interest for the future is gene therapy. Knowing where specific genes are located will be necessary for possible gene repair. If functional gene loci can be inserted into the human genome, then the gene transfer techniques now being investigated (Burch and McBride, 1975; Willecke et al., 1976) may be useful in supplying a normal gene for incorporation into the genome.

Construction of gene maps for mammalian species provides an opportunity to study the evolution of chromosomes and organization of genomes. This is achieved by comparing chromosome morphology, gene assignments, close linkage of genes, and relationships between non-linked genes. The retention of closely linked genes between diverse species would indicate evolutionary stability of a chromosomal region. The conserved linkage of specific genes throughout millions of years would suggest that segments of the mammalian genome may perhaps encode genes for essential functions. The retention of close linkage might also indicate structural, functional, regulatory, or temporal relationships between the genes in a stable region. Close linkage of genes in experimental organisms is also useful in predicting linkage in man and in identifying homologous genes and chromosome regions in laboratory organisms for experimental genetic studies.

CONCLUDING REMARKS

The current gene map has been achieved through a combination of biochemical and cellular methodologies in addition to classical Mendelian genetics. These methodologies include the cell hybridization approach which has greatly stimulated human gene mapping and made significant contributions along with in situ hybridization and gene dosage procedures. Each approach has stimulated and complemented the other. A combination of these has assigned over 150 autosomal loci and 100 X-linked genes. These methods have located genes on each human chromosome, determined linear gene order, and located genes on small chromosome regions. The accelerated rate in which human genes are being assigned points to achieving a detailed gene map of man. Once formulated, the gene map should be useful for understanding the biology and development of man, for mapping inborn errors, for prenatal diagnosis and genetic counseling, and possibly in therapy. Finally, knowledge of the gene map is basic for understanding the evolution of man, the organization of the human genome, and the control of human gene expression.

ACKNOWLEDGMENTS

The collaboration of my colleagues is greatly appreciated: Drs. J. A. Brown, M. J. Champion, C. DeLuca, P. A. Lalley, G. Koch, D. Owerbach and C. Wright. The expert assistance of M. Byers, E. Cooper, R. Eddy, A. Goggin, L. L. Haley, L. Scrafford-Wolff and C. Young is gratefully acknowledged.

REFERENCES

Bishop, J. O. (1974): *Cell, 2*, 81.

Bodmer, W. F. (1976): *Cytogenet. Cell Genet., 16*, 24.

Brown, J. A., Goss, S., Klinger, H. P., Miller, O. J., Ohno, S. and Siniscalco, M. (1976): *Cytogenet. Cell Genet., 16*, 54.

Bruns, G. A. P., Mintz, B. J., Leary, A. C., Regina, V. M. and Gerald, P. S. (1978): *Cytogenet. Cell Genet.* In press.

Burch, J. W. and McBride, W. (1975): *Proc. nat. Acad. Sci. (Wash.), 72*, 1797.

Burgerhout, W. G., Leupe-de Smit, S. and Jongsma, A. P. M. (1977): *Cytogenet. Cell Genet., 18*, 267.

Chern, C. J. (1977): *Proc. nat. Acad. Sci. (Wash.), 74*, 2948.

Champion, M. J. and Shows, T. B. (1977a): *Proc. nat. Acad. Sci. (Wash.), 74*, 2968.

Champion, M. J. and Shows, T. B. (1977b): In: *Abstracts, Vth International Conference on Birth Defects, Montreal*, Abstr. nr. 176. Excerpta Medica, Amsterdam.

Champion, M. J. and Shows, T. B. (1977c): *Amer. J. hum. Genet., 29*. 149.

Champion, M. J. and Shows, T. B. (1978): *Nature (Lond.), 270*, 64.

Evans, H. J., Buckland, R. A. and Pardue, M. L. (1974): *Chromosoma (Berl.), 48*, 405.

Ferguson-Smith, M. A., Aitken, D. A., Trulean, C. and De Grouchy, J. (1976): *Hum. Genet., 34*, 35.

Giblett, E. R., Harris, H., Meera Khan, P., Lovrien, E. W., Mellman, W. J., Partridge, C. W. H. and Shows, T. B. (1976): *Cytogenet. Cell Genet., 16*, 65.

Hamers, M. N., Westerveld, A., Meera Khan, P. and Tager, J. M. (1977): *Hum. Genet., 36*, 289.

Hamerton, J. L. (1976): *Cytogenet. Cell Genet., 16*, 7.

Harris, H. (1975): In: *The Principles of Human Biochemical Genetics, 2nd Ed.*, p. 368. North-Holland Publishing Company, Amsterdam.

Hopkinson, D. A., Edwards, Y. H. and Harris, H. (1976): *Ann. hum. Genet., 39*, 383.

Human Gene Mapping, IIIrd International Workshop on (1975): *Birth Defects: Orig. Art. Ser., XII*, 7. The National Foundation, New York. Also in *Cytogenet. Cell Genet.* (1976), *16*.

Human Gene Mapping, IVth International Workshop on (1977): *Birth Defects: Orig. Art. Ser.* The National Foundation, New York. In press. Also in *Cytogenet.* (1978), *18*, in press.

Ingram, P. H., Bruns, G. A. P., Regina, V. M., Eisenman, R. E. and Gerald, P. S. (1977): *Biochem. Genet., 15*, 455.

Jongsma, A. P. M. and Burgerhout, W. G. (1977): *Cytogenet. Cell Genet., 18*, 245.

Judd, J. H., Shen, M. W. and Kaufman, T. C. (1972): *Genetics, 71*, 139.

Klebe, R. J., Chen, T. R. and Ruddle, F. H. (1970): *J. Cell Biol., 45*, 74.

Koch, G., Brown, J. A. and Shows, T. B. (1978): *Somatic Cell Genet.*, in press.

Lalley, P. A., Brown, J. A., Eddy, R. L., Haley, L. L., Byers, M. G., Goggin, A. P. and Shows, T. B. (1977): *Biochem. Genet., 15*, 367.

Littlefield, J. W. (1964): *Science, 145*, 709.

McKusick, V. A. (1975): *Mendelian Inheritance in Man, 4th Ed.* The Johns Hopkins Press, Baltimore.

Minna, J. D., Lalley, P. A. and Francke, U. (1976): *In Vitro, 12*, 276.

Ohta, T. and Kimura, M. (1971): *Nature (Lond.), 233*, 118.

Owerbach, D., Doyle, D. and Shows, T. B. (1977): *Amer. J. hum. Genet., 29*, 84A.

Paris Conference (1972): *Birth Defects: Orig. Art. Ser., 8*, 7. The National Foundation, New York.

Pontecorvo, G. (1975): *Somatic Cell Genet., 1*, 397.

Race, R. R. and Sanger, R. (1974): *Blood Groups in Man, 6th Ed.*, p. 594. Blackwell Scientific Publications, Oxford.

Ruddle, F. H. (1972): *Advanc. hum. Genet., 3*, 173.

Ruddle, F. H. and Creagan, R. P. (1975): *Ann. Rev. Genet., 9*, 407.

Ruddle, F. H. and Meera Kahn, P. (1976): *Cytogenet. Cell Genet., 16*, 31.

Searle, A. G., Berry, R. J., Beechey, C. V. (1970): *Mutat. Res., 9*, 137.

Shows, T. B. (1974): *Cytogenet. Cell Genet., 13*, 143.

Shows, T. B. (1975): In: *Isozymes, Vol. III: Developmental Biology*, p. 619. Editor: C. L. Markert. Academic Press, New York.

Shows, T. B. (1977): In: *Birth Defects Symposium VII*. Editors: H. L. Vallet and I. H. Porter. Academic Press. In press.

Shows, T. B. (1978): In: *Isozymes: Current Topics in Biological and Medical Research, Vol. 2*, p. 108. Editors: M. C. Rattazzi, J. G. Scandalios and G. S. Whitt. Alan R. Liss Inc., New York.

Shows, T. B. and Brown, J. A. (1975a): *Proc. nat. Acad. Sci. (Wash.)*, 72, 2125.

Shows, T. B. and Brown, J. A. (1975b): *Cytogenet. Cell Genet.*, 14, 421.

Shows, T. B., Brown, J. A., Scrafford-Wolff, L. and Meisler, M. (1978): *Cytogenet. Cell Genet.*, in press.

Shows, T. B., Champion, M. J. and Lalley, P. A. (1977): *Amer. J. hum. Genet.*, 29, 99A.

Szybalski, W., Szybalska, E. H. and Ragni, G. (1962): *Nat. Cancer Inst. Monogr.*, 1, 75.

Turner, B. M., Beratis, N. G., Turner, V. S. and Hirschhorn, K. (1974): *Clin. chim. Acta*, 57, 29.

Warburton, D. and Pearson, P. L. (1976): *Cytogenet. Cell Genet.*, 16, 75.

Willecke, K., Lange, R., Kruger, A. and Reber, T. (1976): *Proc. nat. Acad. Sci. (Wash.)*, 73, 1274.

Wright, C. and Shows, T. B. (1978): *Cytogenet. Cell Genet.*, in press.

Human inherited diseases with altered mechanisms for DNA repair and mutagenesis *

JAMES E. CLEAVER

Laboratory of Radiobiology, University of California, San Francisco, Calif., U.S.A.

A group of human hereditary diseases has become recognized over the past decade which have in common defects in some of the multiple branches of biochemical pathways by which DNA is repaired and mutations generated. The symptoms of these diseases frequently involve a higher incidence of cancer than the general population, but the associated disorders in the central nervous system, in hematopoietic, immunological, ocular, and cutaneous tissues, and in embryological development, indicate how widespread are the influences of defects in DNA repair. The certainty with which DNA repair defects can be correlated with these diseases is not uniform, and the degree of defectiveness is not as great in some diseases as others. In some diseases the repair defects may actually be secondary to other defects that have indirect influence on the efficiency of repair. At the cellular level repair defects can be detected by their effects of increasing the sensitivity of cells to killing by DNA damaging agents (Table 1) and an alteration in the frequency of induced mutations.

The best established example of a human DNA repair deficiency is xeroderma pigmentosum (XP) (Cleaver, 1968, 1969) which shows an approximately 10-fold increase in sensitivity to ultraviolet (UV) light (Table 1). Other diseases show smaller responses to DNA damaging agents with the exception of Fanconi's anemia which shows a 5- to 15-fold increase in sensitivity to DNA cross-linking agents (Fujiwara et al., 1977). Just as prokaryotic mutations in DNA repair and radiation sensitivity genes have enabled multiple biochemical pathways of repair to be elucidated, corresponding human mutations have enabled a similar elucidation to be begun in human and other mammalian cells, albeit often with a heavy use of analogies with prokaryotic systems that may occasionally hinder as much as help. Our current knowledge of the various human repair deficiency diseases warrants consideration to illumine the relevance of DNA repair and replication to general theories of mutagenesis and carcinogenesis.

DNA REPAIR PROCESSES IN HUMAN CELLS

The main DNA repair process in human cells is excision repair, which has multiple

* Work supported by the U.S. Energy Research and Development Administration.

TABLE 1

Sensitivity of cells from various human diseases[a] (fibroblast survival curves except where noted otherwise)

Disease		Ratio of 10% survival doses		Agent
XP	A	7	$(15-30)^b$	UV
	C	6	$(3-9)^b$	UV
	D	7–12	$(28-20)^b$	UV
	V	1– 1.4	$(1.4-1.7)^b$	UV
AT		1.0		UV
		3.2		X-rays
FA		1.4	$(4.2)^b$	UV
		1.0	$(1.0)^b$	X-rays
		5–15		Mitomycin C
Cockayne's		4.2		UV
		1.0		X-rays
Retinoblastoma (D-deletion)		1.6		X-rays
Progeria		$1.6-2.3^c$		X-rays
Bloom's		2.0		UV
Down's		2^d (approx.)		X-rays

[a]Ratios derived from published curves, for references see sections on each disease. [b]Adenovirus survival. [c]Adenovirus V antigen. [d]Chromosome aberrations (Sasaki et al., 1970).

branches according to the chemical nature of the damage (Fig. 1). Some of the changes in DNA replication that occur in damaged cells are also described as a repair process, post-replication repair, but strictly speaking this is a transient perturbation of DNA replication that scarcely warrants being called repair. Additionally, genetic exchange between homologous double-stranded DNA molecules has been identified at the chromosomal level, sister chromatid exchange (SCE) (Perry and Evans, 1975; Latt, 1977). Two other processes may occur in human cells, but their existence is not generally agreed upon: photoreactivation, and inducible 'SOS' repair. A brief summary of these processes is required before consideration of repair defects in human diseases.

Excision repair is extremely versatile and can mend an almost infinite variety of UV light, X-ray, and chemically-induced forms of damage in DNA (Cleaver, 1973; Regan and Setlow, 1974b). This system excises damaged single-strand regions of DNA and usually replaces them accurately with a new sequence of bases. Excision repair has multiple branches according to whether the damage consists of single bases, larger lesions or cross-links, and whether damage is excised as nucleotides, bases or a complex combination in the case of cross-links (Figs. 1, 2, and 6). The early events in excision which involve recognition of damaged sites and nuclease action are the ones that show most variation. The first steps of *nucleotide excision repair* (Friedberg et al., 1976) involve endonucleolytic cleavage of a single poly-nucleotide strand on the 5′ side of the damaged site by one of a number of possible

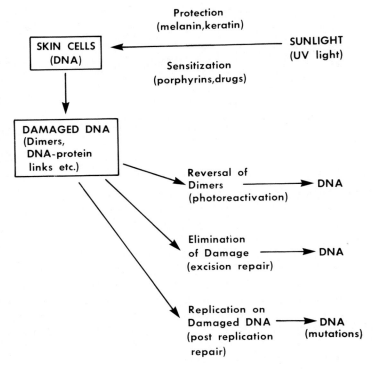

Fig. 1. Various branches for excision repair, post-replication repair and photoreactivation of ultraviolet-light-induced damage in DNA.

endonucleases. The first step of *base excision repair* (Friedberg et al., 1976; Lindahl, 1976) involves cleavage of the glycosidic linkage between a damaged base and the deoxyribose residue followed by cleavage of the polynucleotide strand by apurinic/apyrimidinic endonuclease(s). The first step of cross-link excision repair involves unlinking of one arm of the cross-link by either endonuclease or glycosidase action to produce a region of DNA with damage in closely spaced positions on opposite strands (Fujiwara et al., 1977, Fig. 6). These initial steps are followed by replacement of the damaged sites by repair replication and ligation to produce a patch. It is possible that large and small excision repair patches (Regan and Setlow, 1974b) are correlated with nucleotide and base excision repair, respectively. Repair of single strand and double strand breaks in DNA may proceed by a repair process involving enzymatic modification of the termini adjacent to the break and sealing by repair replication and ligation.

DNA is now known to be organized around histone particles, nucleosomes, 'nu bodies' (Olins et al., 1976) and the DNA closely wrapped around the histones is nuclease resistant. A number of cofactors may therefore be needed to dissociate DNA from histones and render the DNA susceptible to nuclease action before the first steps of repair can occur (Cleaver, 1977a,d; Bodell, 1977; Wilkins and Hart,

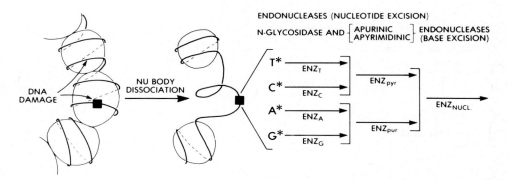

Fig. 2. Excision repair indicating an initial process of nucleosome dissociation followed by the first steps of multiple branches of excision repair involving endonucleases and glycosidases which may have different specificity for different damaged bases (A, T, G, C) or kinds of base (purines and pyrimidines).

1974; Mortelmans et al., 1976). This dissociation may be common to the repair of many kinds of damage, and be defective in XP (Fig. 2) (Mortelmans et al., 1976).

Excision repair, nucleotide or base, is generally regarded as being error-free in normal cells, but it may be altered under some conditions (e.g. through a defective repair polymerase) to become error-prone. Cross-link excision repair, however, because of the need to perform repair replication on one strand of DNA with damage still on the opposite strand, may be error-prone and generate mutations (Ishii and Kondo, 1975; Finkelberg and Siminovitch, 1977, personal communication).

Replication on damaged DNA (including post-replication repair)

Errors, some of which result in mutations, are likely to be introduced into DNA during replication on damaged templates. The biochemical changes in DNA replication observed in damaged cells include delays or blocks in chain growth (Lehmann, 1972a,b; Edenberg, 1976), gaps in newly synthesized DNA (Lehmann, 1972a,b; Lehmann et al., 1975), slow gap filling by caffeine sensitive processes (Lehmann et al., 1975), changes in replicon numbers (Buhl et al., 1973; Rudé and Friedberg, 1977), single strand exchanges (Waters and Regan, 1976; Menighini and Hanawalt, 1976), and double strand exchanges (SCEs, Perry and Evans, 1975; Wolff et al., 1974). The molecular mechanisms involved in these processes are poorly understood, and most interpretations are dominated, perhaps too much, by the model of post-replication repair in bacteria introduced by Rupp and Howard-Flanders. This model (Fig. 3) suggested that gaps are left opposite dimers in newly synthesized strands, and these are filled in slowly by de novo replication and single strand recombination. In animal cells, gap filling by de novo replication appears predominant (Lehmann, 1972a), but these features of post-replication repair are transient responses and only occur during the first few hours following damage. DNA that is synthesized several hours after being damaged, possibly on DNA that had begun replication at origins that were inactive when damaged, does not appear to suffer any delays or strand interruptions (Buhl et al., 1973; Lehmann, 1972b) even though the rates of DNA synthesis per cell are still reduced (Rudé and Friedberg, 1977).

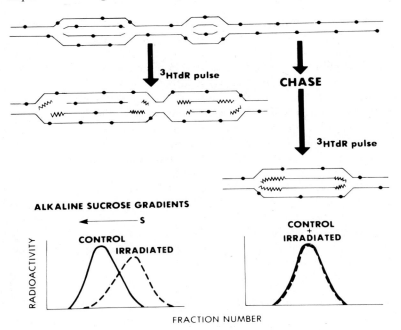

Fig. 3. Post-replication repair mechanism showing gaps formed opposite dimers in DNA synthesized soon after damage occurred, but the absence of gaps in DNA synthesized later.

These two kinds of observations imply that a severe perturbation in DNA replication involving the complete cessation of replication in many replicons occurs in damaged cells. These changed patterns of replicon synthesis occupy more time than the transient changes in DNA sizes associated with post-replication repair that are seen at early times. These phenomena are more severe in excision defective cells implying that excision of damage in unreplicated DNA may affect the perturbations in DNA replication. The points in DNA replication at which errors or mutations are introduced into newly synthesized DNA are at present impossible to identify.

Photoreactivation. This repair system is specific for UV-induced damage in DNA (pyrimidine dimers) and consists of a single enzyme (DNA photolyase) that binds to dimers and, in the presence of visible light, monomerizes them without removing any material from DNA (Cook and McGrath, 1967; Cook, 1972). This repair system functions in embryonic birds and placental mammals but in human cells in culture its function can only be demonstrated to a limited extent, with difficulty, under one restricted experimental condition (Sutherland and Oliver, 1976; Mortelmans et al., 1977). When special conditions are established that enable photoreactivation to be detected, its capacity appears to be correlated with the capacity for excision repair (Sutherland et al., 1975a,b). Photoreactivation observed, rarely, in mammalian cells may therefore be some secondary property of proteins whose primary function is in excision repair. Under most experimental conditions photoreactivation does not occur, and is not a factor to take into account, but whether it may occur under some situation in vivo is an open question.

Inducible 'SOS' repair.   Excision repair and photoreactivation are constitutive in most organisms, but prokaryotes also have a system which is synthesized de novo in response to DNA damage from a variety of agents. This inducible 'SOS' repair process is involved in prokaryotic mutagenesis and appears to be induced to rescue cells that cannot repair their DNA by the constitutive systems, especially those involving recombination (Witkin, 1976; Sedgwick, 1976). An important feature of bacterial SOS repair is the induction of new proteins in response to DNA degradation in damaged cells (Gudas, 1976), and this degradation is a unique feature of bacterial responses to DNA damage. Cell survival resulting from the induction of SOS repair is therefore achieved at the expense of high mutation frequencies among survivors.

Inducible SOS repair has provided the main explanation for non-linear dose response curves seen in bacterial mutagenesis (Fig. 4) (Ishii and Kondo, 1975). But the corresponding dose response curves in mammalian cells are usually linear (Fig. 5) (Hsie et al., 1975a,b; Cox and Masson, 1976; Maher et al., 1976a,b; Van Zeeland and Simons, 1976; Cleaver, 1977b). Inducible SOS repair may therefore be confined to prokaryotes and absent or of minor importance in eukaryotic mutagenesis which probably involves constitutive mechanisms.

REPAIR AND REPLICATION DEFECTS IN HUMAN DISEASES

The discovery that XP was a disease exhibiting defects in DNA repair (Cleaver, 1968, 1969) stimulated a search for other diseases which might also exhibit repair deficiencies. The searches concentrated on photosensitive diseases (Cleaver, 1970a; Lehmann et al., 1977), chromosome breakage syndromes (German 1972), high cancer diseases (Lehmann et al., 1977), but extended at times to less specific phenotypes such as hypertension (Pero and Norden, 1976), and poor reproductive ability (Hoar and Rudd, 1976). At the present time I think we can consider that DNA repair or DNA replication defects are associated with most cases of XP, ataxia telangiectasia (AT) and Fanconi's anemia (FA). To a lesser extent repair or replication defects may be seen in cases of Cockayne's syndrome, Bloom's syndrome, D-deletion retinoblastoma, Down's syndrome, and progeria.

In addition to possible defects seen in the homozygous condition of these inherited diseases there may be many other genes which modify cellular responses to mutagen- or carcinogen-induced damage in the homozygous or heterozygous state. These genes may complicate the phenotypes seen in cases of XP, AT, etc., and may give rise to carcinogen-sensitive responses that are not closely linked with an individual's phenotype and clinical condition.

REPAIR DEFICIENT DISEASES

Xeroderma pigmentosum and the de Sanctis Cacchione syndrome

The clinical features of this disease are an extreme sensitivity to sunlight exhibited as erythema, abnormal pigmentation, and a high incidence of sunlight-induced skin cancers of all cell types. Two main clinical forms are recognized: the common or

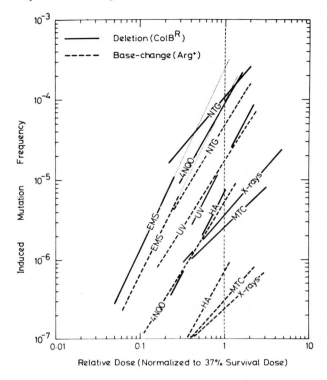

Fig. 4. Mutation frequency versus dose (as ratio of D_{37} for each chemical or radiation) in *E. coli* indicating that the slope for most agents is greater than one indicating cumulative effect of inducible SOS repair system. (Reproduced from Ishii and Kondo (1975).)

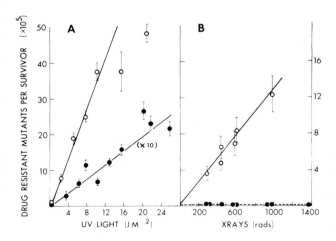

Fig. 5. Mutation frequency versus dose for UV light and ionizing radiation in Chinese hamster cells. O, cells resistant to 6-thioguanine, ●, cells resistant to ouabain. The curve shape for each radiation is linear in contrast to *E. coli* (Fig. 4). (Reproduced from Cleaver (1977b), by courtesy of the Editor of *Genetics*.)

classical form of XP in which there are only skin symptoms, and a form in which there can be a wide range of additional neurological abnormalities. The extreme of the neurological form, the de Sanctis Cacchione syndrome (Robbins et al., 1974), shows choreoathetosis, senso-neural deafness, sexual dysfunction, and mental retardation. The common and neurological forms are genetically distinct, both are autosomal recessive (Robbins et al., 1974; Cleaver and Bootsma, 1975), and a tentative allocation of linkage with the ABO blood group genes on chromosome 9 has been made (El-Hefnawi et al., 1965).

Most XP cells are more sensitive than normal cells to killing (Cleaver, 1970b; Arlett et al., 1975) (Table 1), chromosome aberration production (Sasaki, 1973) and mutagenesis from UV light (Maher et al., 1976a,b) and many other mutagens (Cleaver, 1971, 1973; Regan and Setlow, 1974b). The frequencies of SCEs in undamaged XP cells is the same as in normal cells (Wolff et al., 1975), but is higher than in normal cells following exposure to alkylating agents and other chemical mutagens (Wolff et al., 1977). This latter observation is probably due to the extreme sensitivity of SCE production to small amounts of unexcised damage in DNA (Cleaver, 1977c; Goth-Goldstein, 1977).

The 2 classifications made on the basis of clinical symptoms (i.e., patients with and without central nervous system disorders) have been further subdivided on the basis of biochemical observations in heterokaryons made by cell hybridization.

Most forms of XP are defective to various degrees in excision repair of UV damage. At least 5 mutually complementing groups have been identified by in vitro cell hybridization (Table 2) (Cleaver and Bootsma, 1975; Kraemer et al., 1976), but there is no certainty that this list is complete, or that the properties which thus far characterize each group will be found to apply universally (De Weerd-Kastelein et al., 1976). Two more complementation groups may have been identified recently (Bootsma, 1977, personal communication).

TABLE 2

Some characteristic properties of excision repair and post-replication repair defective XP cells

Disease	Skin	CNS	Complementation group	Exsision repair (% of normal)
XP (de Sanctis Cacchione)	+	+	A	2–5
XP + Cockayne's syndrome[a]	+	+	B	3–7
XP	+	—	C	5–20
XP	+	+	D	25–50
XP	+	—	E	40–50
XP variant	+	—	V	100

[a]Patient shows symptoms of both diseases.

The biochemical defect in excision repair defective XP cells was originally inferred as being a UV endonuclease which initiates excision of UV-induced pyrimidine dimers from DNA (Cleaver, 1969) which was consistent with subsequent observation of a reduced ability of XP cells to excise pyrimidine dimers (Setlow et al., 1969; Cleaver and Trosko, 1970). It is most likely that the defect involves the nucleotide excision repair pathway, which results in failure to repair a large number of different kinds of

TABLE 3

Representative carcinogens producing damage which is predominantly reparable or irreparable by XP cells.

Reparable damage		Irreparable damage
Single base damage[a,b] (base excision repair)	Cross-link damage	'Large' carcinogen adducts[a,b] (nucleotide excision repair)
X-rays		
Bromouracil photoproducts	Mitomycin C[d]	UV light
Methylmethane sulfonate	Nitrogen mustard[c]	4-nitroquinoline-1-oxide
N-methyl-N'-nitro-N-nitrosoguanidine	Psoralen[e]	Bromobenz(a)anthracene
Methyl nitrosourea		Benz(a)anthracene epoxide
ICR 170		1-Nitropyridine-1-oxide
		Acetylaminofluorene

[a]Cleaver, 1973; [b]Regan and Setlow, 1974; [c]Cleaver, 1971; [d]Fujiwara et al., 1977; [e]Day, 1975.

chemically induced lesions (Table 3). Base excision repair and interstrand cross-link repair appear functionally normal at least in some early steps (Table 3).

The existence of several complementation groups defining the enzymatic steps defective in XP cells has not been satisfactorily interpreted, but may indicate (a) that there is a complex system of genetic control of repair or (b) that there are multiple subunits for the human UV endonuclease, or (c) that a number of cofactors are required for repairing damage in chromatin, or (d) that the process of cell hybridization alters gene expression such that complementation in vitro is not a simple indicator of the number of different alleles involved.

Experiments based on the ability of XP cell extracts to excise pyrimidine dimers from pure DNA in vitro indicate that XP groups A and C do contain functional UV endonuclease (Mortelmans et al., 1976), but lack some factor(s) that are required to excise dimers from chromatin (Fig. 2). A variety of chromatin proteins appear to be involved in controlling the accessibility of damage in chromatin to nucleases, resulting in different regions of DNA being repaired at different rates (Wilkins and Hart, 1974; Bodell, 1977; Cleaver, 1977d). The association of low levels of apurinic endonuclease with certain XP complementation groups (Kuhnlein et al., 1976) and the low, but uniquely medium dependent level of photoreactivation in XP cells (Sutherland et al., 1975; Sutherland and Oliver, 1976) also point to a complexity of enzymatic defects in XP cells. The initial steps of DNA repair in man may therefore be considerably more complicated than in microorganisms because of the structure of eukaryotic chromatin, and XP may represent a defect in cellular control of DNA repair rather than a defect in a specific enzyme.

XP variant (XP V)

This form of XP was defined as a classification for clinically diagnosed common XP patients whose excision repair and sensitivity to cell killing appeared normal (Cleaver, 1972). Subsequently, XP variant cells have been shown to be sensitized to UV-induced killing by growth in caffeine after irradiation, whereas normal and excision defective XP cells are not (Arlett et al., 1975; Maher et al., 1976b). The biochemical defect in XP variant cells increases the UV mutability more than UV-induced cell killing (Maher et al., 1976a,b). The defect appears to involve both a prolonged post-replication repair (Lehmann et al., 1975) and a slow rate of completion of a few excision repair patches, when repair replication on one strand of DNA occurs close to damage on the opposite strand (Dingman and Kakunaga, 1976; Fornace et al., 1976). These observations suggest that the defect in XP variant cells may involve a polymerase that has difficulty replicating past damaged sites, resulting in effects both on post-replication repair and excision repair. It is possible therefore that the increased mutagenesis in XP variant cells might arise from excision repair that has become error-prone rather than the observed delays in post-replication repair.

Ataxia telangiectasia

This disease exhibits progressive cerebellar ataxia, telangiectases of skin and conjunctiva, proneness to sinopulmonary infection, immunological deficiencies, a tendency to develop lymphatic malignancy and recessive inheritance. Some patients are hypersensitive to conventional doses of radiation therapy.

Cellular characteristics include multiple chromosome aberrations in lymphocytes and fibroblasts, and increased sensitivity to cell killing by X-rays (Table 1) (German, 1972; Taylor et al., 1975). SCE frequencies are induced to the same extent as in normal cells by a variety of chemical mutagens (Galloway, 1977). Fibroblasts can mend UV damage normally (Cleaver, 1968; Paterson et al., 1976), and rejoin single-strand breaks (Paterson et al., 1976) and double-strand breaks (Lehmann and Stevens, 1977). Excision of some unknown X-ray-induced lesions are slower than normal in some AT cell lines (Paterson et al., 1976). These lesions are ones which are induced with equal efficiency in oxygen or nitrogen (i.e., oxygen enhancement ratio (OER) of 1.0) but both normal and AT cells are more sensitive to irradiation in oxygen than nitrogen (OER = 2 to 3) (Ritter, 1977, personal communication). The lesions, and repair defects responsible for the increased X-ray sensitivity of AT cells may therefore not be those detected in earlier experiments. Also, even though AT cells appear to respond normally to UV damage, they do have a slightly reduced ability to support proliferation of UV-damaged adenovirus (Rainbow, 1977, personal communication). The biochemical defect associated with the clinical features and the X-ray sensitivity may therefore involve some defects in DNA repair, but both the heterogeneity of the disease and complexity of cellular responses preclude simple characterization of the repair defects.

Bloom's syndrome

This disease exhibits low birth weight, sensitivity to sunlight, a prominent nose, hypoplastic malar areas and retruded mandible, a high risk of acute leukemia, and recessive inheritance, and a high incidence of chromosome aberrations (German, 1972) and SCEs (Chaganti et al., 1974). Fibroblasts perform excision repair of UV damage normally (Cleaver, 1970a), and appear to have a slightly reduced DNA chain growth rate (Hand and German, 1975). One report has however demonstrated an increased sensitivity of Bloom's cells to UV-induced cell killing but because

Bloom's cells have substantially different cell cycle parameters from normal cells, the observed sensitivity might be the consequence of different distributions of cells in the cell cycle (Gianelli et al., 1977). The biochemical defects in this disease have yet to be identified.

Cockayne's syndrome

This disease exhibits dwarfism, premature senility, retinal pigment degeneration, optic atrophy, deafness, mental retardation, sensitivity to sunlight and autosomal recessive inheritance.

Cellular characteristics include normal sensitivity to X-rays but increased sensitivity to ultraviolet light (Table 1) (Schmickel et al., 1977). Despite the increased sensitivity, Cockayne's cells in vitro excise pyrimidine dimers normally, and no other biochemical defect has been identified. Symptoms of Cockayne's syndrome are found in the one XP patient that constitutes complementation group B (Robbins et al., 1974) (Table 2), and the contributions of the unique features of each disease to the biochemical properties of cells from this patient remain to be elucidated.

Fanconi's pancytopenia (anemia)

This disease exhibits hypoplasia of all blood elements, pigmentary changes in the skin, malformation of the heart, kidneys and extremities, a tendency to develop acute leukemia and certain kinds of solid tumors and autosomal recessive inheritance. Heterozygotes may also show a higher than normal incidence of malignancy.

Cellular characteristics include a high frequency of spontaneous chromosome aberrations, a high frequency of chromosome aberrations after exposure to DNA cross-linking agents (Sasaki, 1975) but a normal frequency of sister chromatid exchanges (Latt, 1977). Cells are 5- to 15-fold more sensitive to killing by cross-linking agents (Fujiwara et al., 1977). There may also be a slight defect in excision repair of UV damage resulting in a failure of cells to rejoin excision-related breaks (Poon et al., 1974). Cells appear to perform normal levels of unscheduled synthesis after UV irradiation and treatment with cross-linking agents (Sasaki, 1975), even though cells have a reduced ability to support the survival of gamma- and UV-irradiated adenovirus at high radiation doses (Rainbow and Howes, 1977).

The biochemical defect of FA cells appears to be an inability to perform an early step in the removal of interstrand DNA-DNA cross-links (Fujiwara et al., 1977) (Fig. 6). The first step in removal of interstrand cross-links may proceed by base excision (i.e. glycosidase action) rather than endonucleolytic cleavage because XP cells can remove these cross-links (Figs. 6 and 7, Table 3) (Cleaver, 1971; Day, 1975; Fujiwara et al., 1977). Observation of slightly increased sensitivity to high UV or X-ray doses may be due to the production of interstrand cross-links or closely spaced lesions on opposite strands at these doses (Poon et al., 1974; Rainbow and Howes, 1977). Subsequent steps of repair involve repair replication of damaged sites on each strand produced by the cleavage of the cross-link (Fig. 7). Because these steps necessitate repair replication on one strand complementary to a region of DNA that is also damaged it is likely that this kind of excision repair has a high possibility of errors or mutations. This view of excision repair of cross-links is supported by

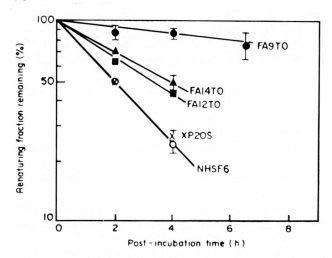

Fig. 6. Removal of interstrand DNA cross-links produced by mitomycin C in normal human, XP and FA cells. O, normal fibroblasts; X, XP20S Xeroderma pigmentosum group A cells; ●, ▲, ■, Fanconi's anemia cells. (Reproduced from Fujiwara et al. (1977), by courtesy of the Editor of the *Journal of Molecular Biology.*)

observations in *E. coli* (Ishii and Kondo, 1975) and FA cells (Finkelberg and Siminovitch, 1977, personal communication) that mutation frequencies are lower than normal in cells unable to remove cross-links.

Progeria (Hutchinson-Gilford's syndrome)

This disease exhibits a striking degree of premature senility and patients often die of coronary artery disease before the age of 10. Patients show facial features of extremely rapid senility, are of small stature, have almost complete absence of subcutaneous fat, and blood vessels show arteriosclerosis.

Cellular characteristics include a normal ability to perform excision repair of UV damage (Cleaver, 1970a) and reduced ability to support survival of X-ray irradiated adenovirus (Rainbow, 1977). Progeric cells that show premature aging in vitro have reduced ability to rejoin X-ray-induced DNA breaks (Epstein et al., 1973, 1974; Regan and Setlow, 1974a), but a clear demonstration of repair defects has not been made.

SOME IMPLICATIONS OF REPAIR DEFICIENCIES

Probably only for XP is there a ready interpretation of the relationships between biochemical and clinical observations. In most other diseases the involvement of repair defects is not clearly established as a consistent feature of the majority of the cases and XP is probably the only disease for which the involvement of repair defects is certain. AT, FA, and Cockayne's syndrome do, however, appear to be

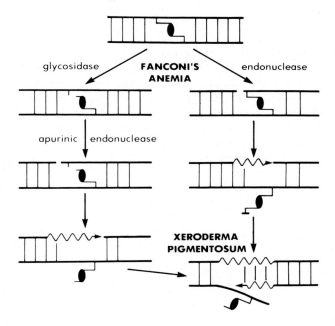

Fig. 7. Mechanisms for removal of cross-links in DNA by a 2-step excision repair, indicating 2 branches for removal of 1 arm of the cross-link by endonuclease or glycosidase action.

the most promising diseases of current interest. The immunological disorders in AT may imply a role for DNA repair in the immune response, and the developmental and neurological disorders in XP, AT, FA and Cockayne's may imply a role for DNA repair in maintaining normal embryological development.

XP is a striking illustration for the mutational theory of carcinogenesis in which a high frequency of malignancy is induced by defective repair of UV-induced damage in cells of the skin. As such it can be used as a model of other kinds of cancers induced by environmental DNA-damaging agents. But it is interesting to note that XP, AT and FA do not lend any support to theories of aging involving DNA damage and repair because the clinical symptoms and cellular characteristics of these diseases represent normal rates of aging. In progeria, however, in which premature aging is characteristic, the involvement of repair defects is very uncertain. Also, the reduced frequency of mutagenesis in FA cells (Finkelberg and Simonovitch, 1977, personal communication) points to a greater complexity in the relationship between mutagenesis and carcinogenesis than the simple correlation that XP provides.

If XP and other recessive genes associated with DNA repair also have small effects in the heterozygous state, it is conceivable that many more examples of carcinogenesis in man than those described here may be influenced by repair genes. The evaluation of these possible contributions in the induction of human cancer, and in particular the role played by DNA repair defects in many human high cancer diseases would seem to be especially important.

SUMMARY

A variety of human diseases involving clinical symptoms of increased cancer risk, and disorders of the central nervous system, and of hematopoietic, immunological, ocular, and cutaneous tissues and embryological development have defects in biochemical pathways for excision repair of damaged DNA. Excision repair has multiple branches by which·damaged nucleotides, bases, and cross-links are excised and requires cofactors that control the access of repair enzymes to damage in DNA in chromatin. Diseases in which repair defects are a consistent feature of their biochemistry include xeroderma pigmentosum, ataxia telangiectasia and Fanconi's anemia.

REFERENCES

Arlett, C. F., Harcourt, S. A. and Broughton, B. C. (1975): *Mutat. Res., 33*, 341.
Bodell, W. J. (1977): *Nucl. Acids Res., 4*, 2619.
Buhl, S. N., Setlow, R. B. and Regan, J. D. (1973): *Biophys. J., 13*, 1265.
Chaganti, R. S. K., Schonberg, S. and German, J. (1974): *Proc. nat. Acad. Sci. (Wash.), 71*, 4508.
Cleaver, J. E. (1968): *Nature (Lond.), 218*, 652.
Cleaver, J. E. (1969): *Proc. nat. Acad. Sci. (Wash.), 63*, 428.
Cleaver, J. E. (1970a): *J. invest. Derm., 54*, 181.
Cleaver, J. E. (1970b): *Int. J. radiat. Biol., 18*, 557.
Cleaver, J. E. (1971): *Mutat. Res., 12*, 453.
Cleaver, J. E. (1972): *J. invest. Derm., 58*, 124.
Cleaver, J. E. (1973): *Cancer Res., 33*, 362.
Cleaver, J. E. (1977a): In: *Human Molecular Cytogenetics, ICN-UCLA Symposia on Molecular and Cellular Biology, Vol.* 7. Editors: R. S. Sparks, D. Cummings and C. F. Fox. Academic Press, New York.
Cleaver, J. E. (1977b): *Genetics, 87*, 129.
Cleaver, J. E. (1977c): *J. Toxicol. environ. Hlth, 2*, 1387.
Cleaver, J. E. (1977d): *Nature (Lond.), 270*, 451.
Cleaver, J. E. and Bootsma, D. (1975): *Ann. Rev. Genet., 9*, 19.
Cleaver, J. E. and Trosko, J. E. (1970): *Photochem. Photobiol., 11*, 547.
Cook, J. S. (1972): In: *Molecular and Cellular Repair Processes*, pp. 79–94. Editors: R. F. Beers Jr, R. M. Herriott and R. C. Tilghman. Johns Hopkins University Press, Baltimore.
Cook, J. S. and McGrath, J. R. (1967): *Proc. nat. Acad. Sci. (Wash.), 58*, 1359.
Cox, R. and Masson, W. K. (1976): *Mutat. Res., 37*, 125.
Day, R. F., III (1975): *Mutat. Res., 33*, 311.
De Weerd-Kastelein, E. A., Keijzer, W., Sabour, M., Parrington, J. M. and Bootsma, D. (1976): *Mutat. Res., 37*, 307.
Dingman, C. W. and Kakunaga, T. (1976): *Int. J. radiat. Biol., 30*, 55.
Edenberg, H. (1976): *Biophys. J., 16*, 849.
El-Hefnawi, E., Maynard-Smith, S. and Penrose, L. S. (1965): *Ann. hum. Genet., 28*, 273.
Epstein, J., Williams, J. R. and Little, J. B. (1973): *Proc. nat. Acad. Sci. (Wash.), 70*, 977.
Epstein, J., Williams, J. R. and Little, J. B. (1974): *Biochem. biophys. Res. Commun., 59*, 850.
Fornace Jr, A. J., Kohn, K. W. and Kann Jr, H. E. (1976): *Proc. nat. Acad. Sci. (Wash.), 73*, 39.
Friedberg, E. C., Cook, K. H., Mortelmans, K. and Rude, J. (1976): In: *Research in Photobiology*. Editor: A. Castallani. Plenum Press, New York. In press.
Fujiwara, Y., Tatsumi, M. and Sasaki, M. S. (1977): *J. molec. Biol., 113*, 635.
Galloway, S. (1977): *Mutat. Res., 45*, 343.
German, J. (1972): *Progr. med. Genet., 8*, 61.
Gianelli, F., Benson, P. F., Pawsey, S. A. and Polani, P. E. (1977): *Nature (Lond.), 265*, 466.
Goth-Goldstein, R. (1977): *Nature (Lond.), 267*, 81.
Gudas, L. J. (1976): *J. molec. Biol., 104*, 567.

Hand, R. and German, J. (1975): *Proc. nat. Acad. Sci. (Wash.)*, *72*, 758.

Hoar, D. I. and Rudd, N. L. (1976): In: *Abstracts, Vth International Congress of Human Genetics, Mexico City, 1976*, Abstr.nr. 196. Excerpta Medica, Amsterdam.

Hsie, A. W., Brimer, P. A., Mitchell, T. J. and Gosslee, D. G. (1975a): *Somatic Cell Genet.*, *1*, 247–261.

Hsie, A. W., Brimer, P. A., Mitchell, T. J. and Gosslee, D. G. (1975b): *Somatic Cell Genet.*, *1*, 383.

Ishii, Y. and Kondo, S. (1975): *Mutat. Res.*, *27*, 27.

Kraemer, K. H., Andrews, A. D., Barrett, S. F. and Robbins, J. H. (1976): *Biochim. biophys. Acta (Amst.)*, *442*, 147.

Kuhnlein, U., Penhoet, E. E. and Linn, S. (1976): *Proc. nat. Acad. Sci. (Wash.)*, *73*, 1169.

Latt, S. (1977): In: *Human Molecular Cytogenetics, ICN-UCLA Symposia on Molecular and Cellular Biology, Vol. 7*. Editors: R. S. Sparks, D. Cummings and C. F. Fox. Academic Press, New York.

Lehmann, A. R. (1972a): *J. molec. Biol.*, *66*, 319.

Lehmann, A. R. (1972b): *Europ. J. Biochem.*, *31*, 438.

Lehmann, A. R., Kirk-Bell, S., Arlett, C. F., Harcourt, S. A., de Weerd-Kastelein, E. A., Keijzer, W. and Hall-Smith, P. (1977): *Cancer Res.*, *37*, 904.

Lehmann, A. R., Kirk-Bell, S., Arlett, C. F., Paterson, M. C., Lohmann, P. H. M., de Weerd-Kastelein, E. A. and Bootsma, D. (1975): *Proc. nat. Acad. Sci. (Wash.)*, *72*, 219.

Lehmann, A. R. and Stevens, S. (1977): *Biochim. biophys. Acta (Amst.)*, *474*, 49.

Lindahl, T. (1976): *Nature (Lond.)*, *259*, 64.

Maher, V. M., Ouellette, L. M., Curren, R. D. and McCormick, J. J. (1976a): *Nature (Lond.)*, *261*, 326.

Maher, V. M., Ouelette, L. M., Curren, R. D. and McCormick, J. J. (1976b): *Biochem. biophys. Res. Commun.*, *71*, 228.

Menighini, R. and Hanawalt, P. C. (1976): *Biochim. biophys. Acta (Amst.)*, *425*, 428.

Mortelmans, K., Cleaver, J. E., Friedberg, E. C., Paterson, M. C., Smith, B. P. and Thomas, G. H. (1977): *Mutat. Res.*, *44*, 443.

Mortelmans, K., Friedberg, E. C., Slor, H., Thomas, G. and Cleaver, J. E. (1976): *Proc. nat. Acad. Sci. (Wash.)*, *73*, 2757.

Olins, A. L., Carlson, R. D., Wright, E. B. and Olins, D. E. (1976): *Nucl. Acids Res.*, *3*, 3271.

Paterson, M. D., Smith, B. P., Lohmann, P. H. M., Anderson, A. K. and Fishman, A. L. (1976): *Nature (Lond.)*, *260*, 444.

Pero, R. W. and Norden, A. (1976): *Proc. nat. Acad. Sci. (Wash.)*, *73*, 2496.

Perry, P. and Evans, H. J. (1975): *Nature (Lond.)*, *258*, 121.

Poon, P. K., O'Brien, R. L. and Parker, J. W. (1974): *Nature (Lond.)*, *250*, 223.

Rainbow, A. J. (1977): *Biochem. biophys. Res. Commun.*, *74*, 714.

Rainbow, A. J. and Howes, M. (1977): *Int. J. radiat. Biol.*, *31*, 191.

Regan, J. D. and Setlow, R. B. (1974a): *Biochem. biophys. Res. Commun.*, *59*, 858.

Regan, J. D. and Setlow, R. B. (1974b): *Cancer Res.*, *34*, 3318.

Robbins, J. H., Kraemer, K. H., Lutzner, M. A., Festoff, B. W. and Coon, H. G. (1974): *Ann. intern. Med.*, *80*, 221.

Rudé, J. M. and Friedberg, E. C. (1977): *Mutat. Res.*, *42*, 433.

Ruddle, F. H. and Meera-Khan, P. (1976): *Cytogenet. Cell Genet.*, *16*, 31.

Rupp, W. D. and Howard-Flanders, P. (1968): *J. molec. Biol.*, *31*, 291.

Sasaki, M. S. (1973): *Mutat. Res.*, *20*, 291.

Sasaki, M. W. (1975): *Nature (Lond.)*, *257*, 501.

Sasaki, M. W., Toda, K. and Ozawa, A. (1976): In: *Proceedings, Japan-U.S. Seminar on Biochemistry of Cutaneous Epidermal Differentiation, Sendai, Japan*.

Sasaki, M. S., Tonomura, A. and Matsubara, S. (1970): *Mutat. Res.*, *10*, 617.

Schmickel, R. D., Chu, E. H. Y., Trosko, J. E. and Chang, C. C. (1977): *Pediatrics*, *60*, 135.

Sedgwick, S. G. (1976): *Mutat. Res.*, *41*, 185.

Setlow, R. B., Regan, J. D., German, J. and Carrier, W. L. (1969): *Proc. nat. Acad. Sci. (Wash.)*, *64*, 1035.

Sutherland, B. M. and Oliver, R. (1976): *Biochem. biophys. Acta (Amst.)*, *442*, 348.

Sutherland, B. M., Rice, M. and Wagner, E. K. (1975): *Proc. nat. Acad. Sci. (Wash.)*, *72*, 103.

Sutherland, B. M., Runge, P. and Sutherland, J. C. (1974): *Biochemistry*, *13*, 4710.

Taylor, A. M. R., Harnden, D. G., Arlett, C. F., Harcourt, S. A., Lehmann, A. R., Stevens, S. and Bridges, B. A. (1975): *Nature (Lond.)*, *258*, 427.

Van Zeeland, A. A. and Simons, J. W. I. M. (1976): *Mutat. Res.*, *35*, 129.

Waters, R. and Regan, J. D. (1976): *Biochem. biophys. Res. Commun.*, *72*, 803.

Weichselbaum, R. R., Nove, J. and Little, J. B. (1977): *Nature (Lond.)*, *266*, 726.

Wilkins, R. J. and Hart, R. W. (1974): *Nature (Lond.)*, *247*, 35.

Witkin, E. (1976): *Bact. Rev.*, *40*, 869.

Wolff, S., Bodycote, J. and Painter, R. B. (1974): *Mutat. Res.*, *25*, 73.

Wolff, S., Bodycote, J., Thomas, G. H. and Cleaver, J. E. (1975): *Genetics*, *81*, 349.

Wolff, S., Rodin, B. and Cleaver, J. E. (1977): *Nature (Lond.)*, *265*, 347.

Wolff, S. and Perry, P. (1975): *Exp. Cell Res.*, *93*,23.

Relationships between aneuploidy and development

MARIE-ODILE RETHORÉ

INSERM, Institute of Progenesis, Paris, France

Each species is characterized by the number and morphology of the chromosomes contained in the cell nuclei, i.e. by its karyotype. However, in each generation accidents modify either the number or the morphology of one or several chromosomes. Among these accidents, only those which modify the quantity of genetic information become responsible for a pathological state. Within the general population somewhat less than one newborn child out of a hundred suffers from an autosomal or sexual chromosome imbalance.

Chromosome alterations which respect the total amount of genetic material are termed balanced. They do not alter the carriers' phenotype, but they do severely compromise their progeny. In the general population one person out of 700 is carrier of a balanced chromosome rearrangement.

GENETIC INFORMATION IN CHROMOSOMAL DISEASES

The originality of diseases due to chromosome aberrations lies in the fact that the genetic change is purely *quantitative:* omission of part of the information in monosomy or, conversely, repetition in trisomy.

The following observations prove the integrity of the *quality* of the information contained in an aneuploid genome:

In heterokaryotic monozygotic twins (Lejeune et al., 1962), the aneuploid child is malformed while the normal twin shows no sign of the defect. The genetic information is the same in these 2 children derived from the same ovum. Thus, it is clear that only the imbalance resulting from the aneuploidy is responsible for the disease.

In subjects carying a balanced translocation, t(14q21q) for example, the normal phenotype shows that the translocation has not led to any disorder and that the carrier has a genome of normal quality. The disease observed in the child who receives this t(14q21q) translocation *together with* a free chromosome 21 as a result of defective segregation proves that only the excess of genetic material is at fault since the same material is tolerated perfectly well if evenly distributed.

Among children born to women trisomic for chromosome 21, the third example, almost half are trisomic 21 like their mother, the others having a normal karyotype (Rethoré et al., 1970a). The normal phenotype of the latter shows clearly that the maternal chromosome 21 is qualitatively normal and that only the presence of an extra copy of this same chromosome is responsible for the disease in the other children.

Differences in gene balance have been demonstrated directly in patients with various states of trisomy or monosomy (Table 1). The first demonstration was provided by Ferguson-Smith et al. in 1973 who observed a reduction of 45% in the activity of erythrocytic acid phosphatase (ACP-1) in a child monosomic for the segment 2p23 → 2pter. In the following year, Povey et al. confirmed the localization of the ACP-1 gene on chromosome 2 by means of cell hybridization; in 1975 Magenis et al. observed a 50% increase in the activity of this enzyme in a patient trisomic for the same chromosome segment. This is the only instance in which mapping for a gene controlling an enzyme activity was first demonstrated by an enzymatic assay in a patient with an unbalanced karyotype. In all other instances gene assignment was first obtained by cellular hybridization. Then the demonstration of the enzymatic disturbance allowed a more precise localization of the gene, the degree of precision being inversely proportional to the length of the altered segment.

TABLE 1

Demonstrations of changes in enzyme activities in chromosomal imbalance

Authors	Tissues examined	Changes in enzyme activity	Chromosomal imbalance of the patients
Ferguson-Smith et al., 1973	RBC	↓ ACP-1	Monosomy: 2p23 → 2pter
Magenis et al., 1975	RBC	↑ ACP-1	Trisomy: 2p23 → 2pter
Mayeda et al., 1974	RBC	↓ LDH-B	Monosomy: 12p
Malpuech et al., 1975	RBC	↓ LDH-B	Monosomy: 12p11 → 12p12.2
Rethoré et al., 1975, 1976, 1977a, b	RBC	↑ LDH-B	
	Fibroblasts	↑ G-3-PD	Trisomy: 12pter → 12q12
		↑ TPI	
Tenconi et al., 1975	RBC	↓ LDH-B	Monosomy: 12p11 → 12p13
Marimo and Giannelli, 1975	Embryos	↑ APRT	Trisomy: 16
Allerdice and Tedesco, 1975	RBC	↑ GALT	Trisomy: 3q21 → 3qter
Junien et al., 1976	Embryos	↑ G-6-PD	Triploids 69,XXY;
		↑ PGK	69,XXX and 69,XYY
Sinet et al., 1976	RBC	↑ SOD-1	{Trisomy: 21
			{Trisomy: 21q21 → 21q21.1
Ferguson-Smith et al., 1976	RBC	↑ AK-1	Trisomy: 9q33 → 9qter
De la Chapelle et al., 1976	RBC	↑ E-GSR	Trisomy: 8
		↓ E-GSR	Monosomy: 8pter → 8p21
Sinet et al., 1977	RBC	↑ E-GSR	Trisomy: 8pter → 8q22.1
		↑ E-GSR	Trisomy: 8p11 → 8p22
Hellkuhl and Grzeschik, 1976	RBC	↑ GOT-1	Trisomy: 10q24 → 10q25

RBC = red blood cells. ACP-1 = erythrocytic acid phosphatase. LDH-1 = Lactate dehydrogenase B. G-3-PD = glyceraldehyde-3-phosphate dehydrogenase. TPI = triose-phosphate isomerase. APRT = adenine phosphoribosyl transferase. GALT = galactose-1-phosphate uridyltransferase. G-6-PD = glucose-6-phosphate dehydrogenase. PGK = phosphoglycerate kinase. SOD-1 = superoxide dismutase-1. AK-1 = adenylate kinase. E-GSR = glutathione reductase. GOT-1 = cytoplasmic glutamate oxaloacetic transaminase.

CONSEQUENCES OF QUANTITATIVE CHANGES

By modifying the rhythm of the normal processes of organogenesis, genetic imbalance hinders the development of the egg to a greater or lesser degree. Some of these disorders are incompatible with intra-uterine life while others allow pregnancy to continue but lead to a syndrome combining a dysmorphic state with mental deficiency.

Chromosomal imbalance and intra-uterine life

From various systematic studies of the products of spontaneous miscarriages it seems that a chromosomal imbalance is responsible for more than 50% of early abortions (Grouchy, 1976; Boué et al., 1975). Monosomy for the X chromosome by itself accounts for almost one fourth of all abnormalities. This frequency is all the more surprising if it is compared with the frequency of 0.4% observed in newborn girls and if the low mortality of the Turner syndrome is taken into consideration. In contrast, the other abnormalities of the sex chromosomes are much less frequent in the products of spontaneous miscarriage than in children born at term.

TABLE 2

Lethal autosomal trisomies

Supernumerary autosome	Number of cases observed
Group A, No. 1	0
2	12
3	2
Group B, No. 4	4
5	0
Group C, No. 6	1
7	14
8	15
9	12
10	10
11	1
12	3
Group D, No. 13	10
14	32
15	32
Group E, No. 16	104
17	0
18	20
Group F, No. 19	1
20	5
Group G, No. 21	34
22	37

Results from 5 studies: Boué (France), Carr (Canada), Creasy (Great Britain), Kajii (Switzerland) and Therkelsen (Denmark). (From Boué et al. (1976), by courtesy of the Editor of *Annales de Génétique*.)

Trisomy for an entire autosome accounts for a little more than half of the abnormalities observed in abortuses. In most cases (Table 2) it concerns trisomy of chromosome 16, a condition not found in children born alive. Among the G trisomies, trisomy of chromosome 22 is observed as often as that of chromosome 21 even though trisomy 22 seems to be very rare at term. Among the D trisomies, those of chromosomes 14 and 15, which are those most rare in children born alive, are much more frequent than those of chromosome 13. In group C aneuploidies, trisomy of chromosome 8 seems the most frequent. This condition, which is rarely observed in the homogeneous state in live subjects, is relatively frequent, especially in boys, and is well tolerated when it is in a mosaic form.

Triploidies (69,XXX; 69,XXY; 69,XYY) account for almost 20% of the abnormalities, and tetraploidies for 5%. Among the latter, the constitution 92,XXX is by far the most frequent. Unbalanced changes of structure leading to partial trisomy or monosomy are practically never observed, but perhaps this is because they are not detectable by the techniques at hand.

The almost total absence of complete autosomal monosomic states suggests that the true frequency of aneuploidy must be much greater, even if it cannot be estimated with accuracy, most of the ova being eliminated even before pregnancy is recognized According to Boué et al. (1975), less than 1 zygote out of 2 will be unaffected.

Chromosomal diseases

The frequency of chromosomal imbalance at birth is in the order of 0.5%, the sexual aneuploidies accounting for one third of the anomalies. Survival depends on the extent of the visceral malformations which are, usually, associated in various non-specific combinations.

The common denominator in all autosomal chromosomal diseases is mental deficiency, which varies from one patient to another depending on the intrinsic quality of the genetic material. In other words, these differences, which can be great, reflect the interaction between the quality of the patient's genome and the effect of gene dosage.

The characteristic sign in these diseases is a group of *minor morphological alterations* such as, for example, hyper- or hypotelorism, slanting of the palpebral fissures, deformations of the ear lobes, the dermatoglyphics, etc. For a given chromosomal accident the same embryonic systems are always affected, and the deviation from the norm is always in the same direction, i.e. exaggerated development of specific embryonic buds or, in case of the opposite imbalance, hypoplasia of the same embryonic buds. The semeiological value of a given symptom becomes greater if its frequency in the general population is low and if its countertype is found in patients with the opposite chromosome imbalance. Thus the discriminatory value of the single palmar crease which is generally considered to be important is in fact rather low since its frequency in the general population is 1% (Rethoré and Lafourcade, 1974). Conversely, brachymesophalangia of all fingers observed in patients trisomic for the short arm of chromosome 9a has real diagnostic value because the second phalanges are abnormally long in subjects monosomic for the same chromosome segment.

Detailed comparisons of phenotype and karyotype show that complex groups of malformations result from trisomy or monosomy of very small chromosome segments. This is the case, for example, for the 4p- syndrome and 21 trisomy.

The 4p–syndrome   This morbid entity, described by Wolf et al. in 1965, is accompanied by debility and severe growth retardation. The malformation syndrome is clearly defined, the dysmorphisms affecting the whole body. Although the clinical aspect is stereotyped from one patient to another, this is not so for the chromosomal lesion, which may vary from a complete deletion of 4p to a limited deletion of the 4p16 sub-band.

Two observations of r(4) by Chavin-Colin et al. (1977) and Fraisse et al. (1977) are particularly informative in this respect. In the first, the ring chromosome 4 was almost complete and the 4p16 sub-band seemed to be present at least in part. The patient's phenotype had none of the features observed in the 4p–syndrome. In the second observation the diagnosis of 4p–was possible even before karyotype analysis. Only the 4p16 sub-band was deleted in the r(4). To account for these 2 observations it has to be admitted that the 4p16 sub-band is not terminal and/or that the 4p–syndrome is due to monosomy limited to just one part of the 4p16 sub-band.

21-trisomy   Banding of the chromatids reveals 2 regions on the long arm of chromosome 21: *the proximal region* from 21q11 to 21q22, divided into 2 sub-bands and *the distal region*, divided into 3 sub-bands 21q22.1, 21q22.2 and 21q22.3.

An analysis of various conditions (Aula et al., 1973; Niebuhr, 1974; Wahrman et al., 1974; Williams et al., 1975; Poissonnier et al., 1976; Raoul et al., 1976) shows that the presence in triplicate of the 21q22 region or even only that of the 21q22.1 sub-band is enough to induce the complete clinical picture of 21-trisomy and a 1.5 increase of SOD-1 activity (Sinet et al., 1976). Monosomy for this same region is responsible for the countertype phenotype individualized by Lejeune et al. in 1964 and observed in patients with a r(21). In contrast, trisomy or monosomy for the proximal region of chromosome 21 induce syndromes which are entirely different from 21-trisomy or of its countertype (Lafourcade and Rethoré, 1976).

A completely different situation is observed in other chromosomal diseases.

Chromosome 8 trisomies   Observations on patients with various chromosome 8 rearrangements show that the phenotype of complete trisomy is fragmented in the segmentary trisomies, i.e. trisomy of the short arm (8p22→8p11), trisomy of the short arm and of the proximal region of the long arm (8pter→8q22.1), and trisomy of the distal region of the long arm (8p23→8qter). Although all these trisomic states are accompanied by mental deficiency, only 8p trisomy leads to severe mental retardation. It is accompanied by specific symptoms – a large nose, a large mouth, and microcephaly – which are not found in complete trisomy.

Three symptoms are common to the different chromosome changes: vertebral abnormalities, depression of the mesosternum and bulging brow. This indicates that several zones of chromosome 8 carry genes which play a role in bone growth. The other symptoms can be divided into 3 groups which correspond to the short arm, the proximal part of the long arm and the distal part of the long arm (Rethoré et al., 1977b).

Alterations of chromosome 9 While the phenotype induced by trisomy of the short arm is taken as a model, the symptoms observed in the case of monosomy of the same segment are the opposite:

9p trisomy (Rethoré et al., 1970b): a rounded skull with open anterior fontanelles, enophthalmos, palpebral fissures slanted downward and outward, a large nose, a short upper lip exposing the upper incisors, brachymesophalangia, excess of arches on the finger tips.

9p monosomy (Alfi et al., 1973): craniostenosis and trigonocephaly, exophthalmos, palpebral fissures slanted upward and outward, a short nose, a long upper lip overlapping the lower lip, adherent ears, elongated intermediate phalanges, excess of whorls on the fingertips.

Symptoms of 9p trisomy are found in complete 9 trisomy (Feingold and Atkins, 1973) – enophthalmos, large nose – but they are associated with other signs observed in 9q trisomy (Turleau et al., 1975), i.e. narrow eyes, and retromicrognathism. The visceral malformations are more numerous and more severe.

The facial dysmorphism of babies with a r(9) (Fraisse et al., 1974) is similar to that observed in children monosomic for 9p. In contrast, the symptoms of trisomy were found in an adolescent (Jacobsen et al., 1973). The phenotypic variations reflect the coexistence of monosomic cells and of partial trisomic cells in subjects with a ring chromosome.

The patient accumulation of observations and the improvement of techniques will allow the effects of each segment of the genome to be determined with precision and a better knowledge of the human factorial map.

REFERENCES

Alfi, O., Donnel, G. N., Crandall, B. F., Derencsenyi, A. and Menon, R. (1973): *Ann. Génét., 16*, 17.
Allderdice, P. W. and Tedesco, T. A. (1975): *Lancet, 2*, 39.
Aula, P., Leisti, J. and Von Koskull, H. (1973): *Clin. Génét., 4*, 241.
Boué, J., Boué, A. and Lazar, P. (1975): In: *Aging Gametes: International Symposium, Seattle 1973*, p. 330. Karger, Basel.
Boué, J., Daketsé, M. J., Deluchat, C., Ravisé, N., Yvert, F. and Boué, A. (1976): *Ann. Génét., 19*, 233.
Chavin-Colin, F., Turleau, C., Limal, J. M. and De Grouchy, J. (1977): *Ann. Génét., 20*, 105.
De Grouchy, J. (1976): In: *Aspects of Genetics in Paediatries. Scientific Proceedings, 3rd Unigate Workshop*. Donald Barltrop Ed., London.
De La Chapelle, A., Icen, A., Aula, P., Leisti, J., Turleau, C. and De Grouchy, J. (1976): *Ann. Génét., 19*, 253.
Feingold, M. and Atkins, L. (1973): *J. med. Genet., 10*, 184.
Ferguson-Smith, M. A., Aitken, D. A., Turleau, C. and De Grouchy, J. (1976): *Hum. Genet., 34*, 35.
Ferguson-Smith, M. A., Newman, B. F., Ellis, P. M., Thomson, D. M. G. and Riley, I. D. (1973): *Nature New Biol., 243*, 271.
Fraisse, J., Lauras, B., Couturier, J. and Freyçon, F. (1977): *Ann. Génét., 20*, 101.
Fraisse, J., Lauras, B., Ooghe, M. J., Freyçon, F. and Rethoré, M. O. (1974): *Ann. Génét., 17*, 175.
Hellkuhl, B. and Grzeschik, K. H. (1976): *Hum. Genet., 33*, 109.
Jacobsen, P., Mikkelsen, M. and Rosleff, M. (1973): *Clin. Genet., 4*, 434.
Junien, C., Rubinson, H., Dreyfus, J. C., Meienhofer, M. C., Ravisé, N., Boué, J. and Boué, A. (1976): *Hum. Genet., 33*, 61.
Lafourcade, J. and Rethoré, M. O. (1976): In: *Abstract Volume, V International Congress of Human Genetics, Mexico, 1976, Abstr. Nr. 25.*
Lejeune, J. (1966): In: *Journées Parisiennes de Pédiatrie*, 75. Flammarion Ed., Paris.

Lejeune, J., Berger, R., Rethoré, M. O. Archambault, L., Jérome, H., Thieffry, S., Aicardi, J., Broyer, M., Lafourcade, J., Cruveillier, J. and Turpin, R. (1964): *C.R. Acad. Sci. (Paris)*, *259*, 4, 187.

Lejeune, J., Lafourcade, J., Scharer, K., De Wolff, E., Salmon, Ch., Haines, M. and Turpin, R. (1962): *C.R. Acad. Sci. (Paris)*, *254*, 4404.

Magenis, R. E., Koler, R. D., Lovrien, E., Bigley, R. H., Duval, M. C. and Overton, K. M. (1976): In: Human Gene Mapping, IIIrd International Workshop (1975): *Cytogenet. Cell Genet.*, *16*, 326.

Malpuech, G., Kaplan, J. C., Rethoré, M. O., Junien, C. and Geneix, A. (1975): *Lyon méd.*, *233*, 275.

Marimo, B. and Giannelli, F. (1975): *Nature (Lond.)*, *256*, 204.

Mayeda, K., Weiss, L., Lindahl, R. and Dully, M. (1974): *Amer. J. hum. Genet.*, *26*, 59.

Niebuhr, E. (1974): *Humangenetik*, *21*, 99.

Nielsen, J. (1975): *Humangenetik*, *26*, 215.

Poissonnier, M., Saint Paul, B., Dutrillaux, B., Chassaigne, M., Gruyer, P. and De Blignieres-Strouk, G. (1976): *Ann. Génét.*, *19*, 69.

Povey, S., Swallow, D. M., Bobrow, M., Craig, I. and Van Heyningen, V. (1974): *Ann. hum. Genet. 38*, 1.

Raoul, O., Carpentier, S., Dutrillaux, B., Mallet, R. and Lejeune, J. (1976): *Ann. Génét.*, *19*, 187.

Rethoré, M. O., Aurias, A., Couturier, J., Dutrillaux, B., Prieur, M. and Lejeune, J. (1977b): *Ann. Génét.*, *20*, 5.

Rethoré, M. O., Junien, C., Malpuech, G., Baccichetti, C., Tenconi, R., Kaplan, J. C., De Romeuf, J. and Lejeune, J. (1976): *Ann. Génét.*, *19*, 140.

Rethoré, M. O., Kaplan, J. Cl., Junien, C., Cruveillier, J., Dutrillaux, B., Aurias, A., Carpentier, S., Lafourcade, J. and Lejeune, J. (1975): *Ann. Génét.*, *18*, 81.

Rethoré, M. O., Kaplan, J. C., Junien, C. and Lejeune, J. (1977a): *Hum. Genet.*, *36*, 235.

Rethoré, M. O. and Lafourcade, J. (1974): In: *Journées Parisiennes de Pédiatrie*, pp. 379–390. Flammarion Ed., Paris.

Rethoré, M. O., Lafourcade, J., Prieur, M., Caille, B., Cruveiller, J., Tanzy, M. and Lejeune, J. (1970a): *Ann. Génét.*, *13*, 42.

Rethoré, M. O., Larget-Piet, J. L., Abonyi, D., Boeswilwald, M., Berger, R., Carpentier, S., Cruveiller, J., Dutrillaux, B., Lafourcade, J., Penneau, J. and Lejeune, J. (1970b): *Ann. Génét.*, *13*, 217.

Sinet, P. M., Bresson, J. L., Couturier, J., Laurent, C., Prieur, M., Rethoré, M. O., Taillemite, J. L., Toudic, D., Jérome, H. and Lejeune, J. (1977): *Ann. Génét.*, *20*, 13.

Sinet, P. M., Couturier, J., Dutrillaux, B., Poissonnier, M., Raoul, O. Rethoré, M. O., Allard, D., Lejeune, J. and Jérome, H. (1976): *Exp. Cell Res.*, *97*, 47.

Tenconi, R., Baccichetti, C., Anglani, F., Pellegrino, P. A., Kaplan, J. C. and Junien, C. (1975): *Ann. Génét.*, *18*, 95.

Turleau, C., De Grouchy, J., Chavin-Collin, F., Roubin, M., Brissaud, P. E., Represse, G., Safar, A. and Borniche, P. (1975): *Humangenetik*, *29*, 23.

Wahrman, J., Goitein, R. and Richler, C. (1974): In: *Leiden Chromosome Conference, 1974*, p. 87 (Abstr.).

Williams, J. D., Summitt, R. L., Martens, P. R. and Kimbrell, R. A. (1975): *Amer. J. hum. Genet.*, *27*, 478.

Wolf, U., Reinwein, H., Porsch, R., Schroter, R. and Baitsch, H. (1965): *Humangenetik*, *1*, 397.

DEVELOPMENTAL MECHANISMS

Chairman: James D. Ebert, Woods Hole, Mass.

The cell periphery in morphogenesis*

MERTON R. BERNFIELD

Department of Pediatrics, Stanford University School of Medicine, Stanford, Calif., U.S.A.

Morphogenesis, the developmental process by which form is generated, involves the precise and integrated organization of cells into unique multicellular configurations. Although the ultimate shape of each organ is unique, the cellular behavior involved in the formation of these specific structures is not. All morphogenesis in metazoan animal embryos involves a limited repertoire of cellular behavior: localized cell proliferation, localized cell death, change in cell shape (accounting for both the motility of single cells and the movements in cell populations), cell adhesion, and the localized deposition of extracellular materials. Every cell, regardless of type, possesses the potential for expressing these behavioral properties. However, the extent to which each of these properties is utilized in the formation of a specific structure varies with the type of structure and only a few of these types of behavior may be primarily involved in the formation of any single organ.

The properties are recognized as behavioral phenotypes and the molecules involved undoubtedly represent several gene products. But, because these are universal cellular properties, the gene products are unlikely to be characteristic of a specific cell type. Recent work has identified some of these gene products, which should ultimately allow identification of the structural genes involved. We are unaware, however, of any regulatory genes and although each of the properties is influenced by cell and tissue interactions (see paper by E. D. Hay, *This Volume*), we have little knowledge of the precise way in which the properties are influenced by these interactions.

Emphasizing these types of behavior as separate and discrete processes is a simplification which obscures their inter-relationships in morphogenetic events and which provides an imprecise distinction between morphogenesis and differentiation. However, this categorization allows the events to be defined in terms of their component parts, facilitating experimental approaches to elucidate their mechanisms and providing a way in which abnormalities in morphogenesis may be understood.

Much evidence indicates that the cell periphery, the plasma membrane and its extracellular and cytoplasmic components, are involved in morphogenesis and this

* The original research reported in this review was supported by Grant HD06763 and Contract N01-CB-53903 from the United States Public Health Service and a grant from the National Foundation–March of Dimes.

topic is the subject of several recent volumes (Moscona, 1974; Clarkson and Baserga, 1974; Goldman et al., 1976; Poste and Nicolson, 1976). In this brief review, I will discuss the organization and properties of the cell periphery, illustrate how components of the cell periphery are involved in morphogenetic cell behavior and provide an experimental example of the involvement of the cell periphery in branching epithelial morphogenesis.

THE CELL PERIPHERY

During the past decade, our knowledge of the components and dynamics at the periphery of the cell has increased substantially. Although a detailed understanding of several aspects is lacking, the plasma membrane is no longer viewed as a static envelope for the cell which serves only as a barrier to the environment. It is coupled to various cytoplasmic and extracellular structures, it mediates complicated and precisely coordinated events, and is under complex controls. Thus, it is appropriate to view the plasma membrane as a major element in a dynamic multi-component cellular organelle. Although the organization of the cell periphery has not been examined in detail in embryonic cells, the basic principles appear to be common to nearly all cells. Detailed discussions of the basis for these principles are found in several recent reviews (Singer, 1974; Steck, 1974; Robbins and Nicolson, 1975; Edelman, 1976; Nicolson, 1976; Rothman and Lenard, 1977) and they will be only briefly described.

The plasma membrane

The constituents of the cell periphery are asymmetrically distributed between the 2 surfaces of the plasma membrane, resulting in a vectorially oriented composite structure. The plasma membrane consists of a bilayer of phospholipids with proteins and other lipids, principally cholesterol, embedded in it. The phospholipid molecules, with their ionic head groups and hydrocarbon fatty acyl chains, form a bilayer because of association of the hydrophobic hydrocarbon chains, while the hydrophilic head groups tend to interact with the aqueous intra- and extracellular environment. The head groups are at the 2 surfaces and the acyl chains are in the center of the bilayer, providing an effective diffusion barrier for the cell. The distribution of phospholipids within the bilayer itself is asymmetric, and in certain membranes, there are different proportions of various phospholipids in the inner and outer monolayers.

The proteins of the cell periphery are also organized asymmetrically and are of 2 general types. Those which have substantial interactions with the hydrocarbon region of the bilayer, the integral membrane proteins, are necessary for the integrity of the membrane and most of them apparently span the bilayer, presumably functioning in membrane transport. The other class are the peripheral membrane proteins, which associate with the lipid or with the integral proteins, but can be removed without disrupting the bilayer and thus are not essential to the basic membrane structure.

The structure of the plasma membrane is not static, being in a constant state of flux. Under physiologic conditions, the plasma membrane lipids are relatively fluid and diffuse rather freely in the lateral plane of the membrane. As stressed by Singer and Nicolson (1972) in their fluid mosaic model, the proteins are dispersed in this fluid lipid matrix, allowing them to move within the plane of the membrane. While this lateral mobility can be rapid, transverse rotation is very slow even for lipids and may not occur in the case of membrane proteins. In fact, the asymmetry of the proteins of the cell periphery is probably maintained by the lack of transmembrane diffusion.

Studies of cells in tissue culture have shown that interactions at the cell surface mediate the rate of cellular proliferation. Like cells in culture, cells in developing organisms exhibit the phenomenon of density-dependent inhibition of growth, in which proliferation markedly decreases when cells are in intimate proximity at high density. This effect seems to result from direct contact because the addition of isolated plasma membranes to intact cells mimics the effect of increased cell density on DNA synthesis (Whittenberger and Glaser, 1977). Several growth-promoting factors have been implicated in morphogenesis (e.g., nerve growth factor, epithelial growth factor, pancreatic mesenchymal factor, insulin) and these also seem to exert their proliferative effects by acting at the plasma membrane. The membrane recognition sites or receptors for these factors are under investigation, as are the mechanisms by which these interactions at the membrane generate the intracellular signals which result in stimulation of DNA synthesis and mitosis, but the mechanisms involved are unclear. The enzyme adenylate cyclase is localized within the plasma membrane and a major element in this sequence is thought to be the regulation of cytoplasmic cAMP levels at the level of the plasma membrane (Pastan et al., 1975).

Cell surface carbohydrate

The extracellular surface of the plasma membrane is covered by complex carbohydrate (see reviews by Cook and Stoddart, 1973; Hughes, 1973): The relatively short carbohydrate chains of glycoproteins and glycolipids, in which the carbohydrate is covalently linked to proteins and lipids held to or within the bilayer, may extend out more than 10 nm from the plasma membrane and are thought to function, in part, as specific receptors for hormones, growth factors and other agents. In the relatively large carbohydrate chains of proteoglycans, found within the basal lamina at the basal surface of embryonic epithelia (Bernfield and Banerjee, 1972), the carbohydrate is in glycosaminoglycans covalently bound to protein. An additional glycosaminoglycan, hyaluronic acid, is also found at the cell surface, but it may not be linked to protein. The glycosaminoglycans are highly anionic, flexible polymers which are involved in interactions with other extracellular components, principally collagen. The carbohydrate of the cell periphery is also distributed asymmetrically, being exclusively extracellular, is thought to orient proteins within the membrane and has been proposed to be involved in the mechanisms by which proteins are integrated into the membrane (Rothman and Lenard, 1977).

The carbohydrate chains of glycoproteins and glycolipids have been implicated in the mechanism of intercellular adhesion, although the precise events and molecules involved are unclear (see papers by N. LeDouarin and by S. Roth, *This Volume*). The major ideas are that adhesion is either mediated by physicochemical interactions between the carbohydrate chains, viz. calcium ion bridging, ionic forces or hydrogen bonding, or by a complementary interaction between cell surface molecules (Curtis, 1973). The high degree of specificity shown by certain instances of cellular adhesion has been attributed to multivalent ligands which are thought to bond with cell surface carbohydrate receptors (Moscona, 1976), and to specific cell surface enzymes which transfer glycosyl groups to the cell surface carbohydrate on apposing cells (Roseman, 1970; Schur and Roth, 1975).

The presence of proteoglycans at the basal cell surface of epithelia may be unique to organs undergoing branching morphogenesis. By special staining for anionic polysaccharides, the basal cell surface of branched embryonic epithelia shows highly ordered, geometrically arranged fibers and particles (Cohn et al., 1977). The fibers are apparently attached to the plasma membrane on one side and to the particles which extend 70–80 nm from the bilayer on the other side. This structure, the epithelial basal lamina, contains proteoglycan as well as other components, and the amount of glycosaminoglycan (GAG) decreases with advancing development (Banerjee and Bernfield, 1976). On the other hand, where examined, the basal laminae of mature epithelial organs contain no or trace amounts of GAG (Kefalides, 1973). Thus, the laminae of embryonic epithelia which undergo branching morphogenesis change during development from being GAG-rich to GAG-poor, a sequence which appears to result in a GAG-free lamina after the completion of morphogenesis.

Cytoplasmic fibers

The intracellular surface of the plasma membrane is associated with 2 major types of cytoplasmic fibers. The microtubules, 20–25 nm diameter fibers of polymerized units of the globular protein tubulin (see review Snyder and McIntosh, 1976; and the volume by Soifer, 1975), and the microfilaments, 5–7 nm diameter fibers of non-muscle actin in the F-actin form which are frequently associated into bundles underlying and parallel to the plasma membrane (see reviews by Pollard and Weihing, 1974; Clarke and Spudich, 1977; and the volume by Goldman et al., 1976). These fibers are thought to restrict the mobility of membrane components and to mediate their non-random movements, providing a way in which the organization of the components can be controlled through the membrane.

Evidence concerning the morphogenetic function of these cytoplasmic fibers is largely correlative, based on their localization within cells, their in vitro behavior and the selective action of drugs. These data indicate that the fibers are involved in mediating the 2 basic changes in cell shape: localized contraction and elongation.

The microtubules seem to play a cytoskeletal role, involved in moving cytoplasmic organelles, and by virtue of the elegant studies of Byers and Porter (1964), and more recently of Burnside (1971), are almost certainly involved in cell elongation. The effect of the alkaloid colchicine has been used as a diagnostic tool for the participation of microtubules in cellular processes because of its ability to bind specifically to tubulin and prevent its polymerization into tubules. For example, although there is meager morphological evidence for an association of microtubules with the plasma membrane, colchicine inhibits the mobility of cell surface receptors, suggesting that microtubules are linked in some way to the plasma membrane (Edelman, 1976).

The microfilaments serve as a major component of an actomyosin-like contractile system, and there is some evidence that they may also play a cytoskeletal role. The initial proposal that microfilaments are responsible for contractile events in non-muscle cells came from morphogenetic studies of tail retraction in ascidians (Cloney, 1966), and it is now generally accepted that actin fibers are involved in nearly all types of cell movement. A significant distinction, however, between muscle and non-muscle contractile systems is that the supramolecular assemblies formed by non-muscle actin systems can be transient and rapidly responsive to changes in the environment of the cell. Although not proven, there is substantial evidence supporting the direct attachment of microfilaments to the plasma membrane.

The multilobular shape of epithelia which form during branching morphogenesis appears to be dependent on the function of bundles of actin microfilaments (Spooner and Wessells, 1972). In mouse embryonic submandibular epithelia, the presence of the bundles correlates with the formation of interlobular clefts and recently formed clefts are reversibly lost within a few minutes after treatment with cytochalasin B, an agent which alters the ultrastructural organization of the bundles and which affects the gelation of F actin in vitro. The new clefts are lost over several hours by treatment with agents presumed to inhibit the contractility of the actin micro-filaments: i.e., papaverine, a smooth muscle relaxant that acts by reducing membrane permeability to calcium, and calcium-free medium (Ash and Spooner, 1973). Older, more established clefts resist these treatments, possibly because these clefts are stabilized by the presence of fibrous collagen. The epithelia maintain their lobular morphology and recover from cytochalasin treatment in the presence of levels of colchicine which disrupt microtubules, suggesting that microtubules are not involved in maintaining the clefts.

Cell junctions

The structure of the cell periphery at certain regions where the plasma membranes of adjacent cells come into close apposition is distinct from that of the cell periphery at other sites. These regions of local membrane specialization are the cell junctions and their structure and physiology have been recently reviewed (McNutt and Weinstein, 1973; Staehlin, 1974; Revel and Brown, 1975; Griepp and Revel, 1977). There are several types of cell junctions, and classifications of these junctions depend on the extent of involvement of the cell surface in the junction, the degree of separation of the membranes and the nature of the structure between the membranes. Junctions of a similar type can be found in many different cell types and the classification schemes have given rise to a terminology that can be confusing.

This brief comment on junctions will be limited to the general aspects of junctions in epithelial cell sheets, in which the junctions are predominantly at the lateral surfaces of the cells in the sheet. Toward the apical end of these cells are tight or occluding junctions, areas where the adjacent membranes are fused, which prevent passage of extracellular molecules to the space between the lateral surfaces of the cells. Firm adhesions between the cells are ascribed to the intermediate junctions and the desmosomes, areas of close proximity of adjacent membranes in which the extracellular interspace is filled with fine filamentous material. Actin microfilaments are associated with the cytoplasmic surface of the intermediate junctions, while 10–12 nm diameter fibers (tonofilaments), whose function is unclear, are at the cyto-plasmic surface of the desmosomes. Gap junctions have a narrow 2–4 nm gap between the apposed plasma membranes which contains elements spanning the gap. These junctions occur in nearly all developing cells and are thought to be the morphologic correlate of ionic coupling and metabolic cooperation in which occurs the flow of intracellular ions and of small molecules from cell to cell.

The invagination and folding of an epithelial cell sheet, as discussed above in the context of cleft formation, represents a morphogenetic event involving changes in the shape of the individual cells within the sheet. Because of the junctions between the cells, these shape changes are translated directly into the coordinated deformation of the entire cell population. Thus, the junctions provide the means for the activities of individual cells to be highly coordinated and for groups of cells to undergo precisely integrated morphologic changes.

BRANCHING EPITHELIAL MORPHOGENESIS

The generation of structural form of branched epithelial organs has been used as an experimental paradigm for understanding the basis for morphogenesis (Grobstein, 1967; Saxen, 1972; Spooner, 1975; Cunha, 1976). These organs achieve their distinctive morphologies by a common sequence and their morphogenesis is completely dependent on the presence of a closely associated, highly cellular loose connective tissue, or mesenchyme. The organs (e.g., lung, kidney, pancreas, mammary and salivary glands) arise from a sheet of tightly adherent epithelial cells as a rounded bud which protrudes into the surrounding mesenchyme. The epithelial protrusion undergoes a distinctive pattern of branching, resulting from the repetitive formation of clefts and of intervening lobules. This morphogenesis, primarily due to changes in cell shape and localized differences in mitotic rate, ultimately gives rise to a highly branched morphology that is characteristic of the organ type. This morphogenesis is completely dependent on the mesenchyme because in the absence of mesenchyme, the epithelia fail to continue branching and will slowly lose their shape.

When 13-day mouse embryo submandibular salivary glands are explanted in organ culture, the epithelium changes by repetitive cleft formation and growth during a period of a few days from a few lobes to a highly distinctive, tree-like epithelium, duplicating normal in vivo morphogenesis (Fig. 1). At the interface between the 13-day epithelium and its mesenchyme are amorphous extracellular materials and fibrous collagen, both superficial to the epithelial basal lamina. The collagen is in greater amounts in the clefts between lobules and on the stalk than at the distal aspects of the lobules (Grobstein and Cohen, 1965). The basal lamina encompasses the epithelium, but is thinner and interrupted at the distal aspects of the lobules where contacts between epithelial and mesenchymal cells may be seen (Coughlin, 1975).

Evidence for the involvement of these surface materials in morphogenesis is derived from organ culture studies of epithelia from which the materials were sequentially removed with enzymes (Bernfield et al., 1972, 1973; Banerjee et al., 1977). Treatment of whole glands with highly purified collagenase and microdissection removes the mesenchyme, as well as the amorphous materials and fibrous collagen, yielding an isolated epithelium retaining a basal lamina. These epithelia maintain their lobular shape when cultured recombined with mesenchyme (Fig. 2, A),

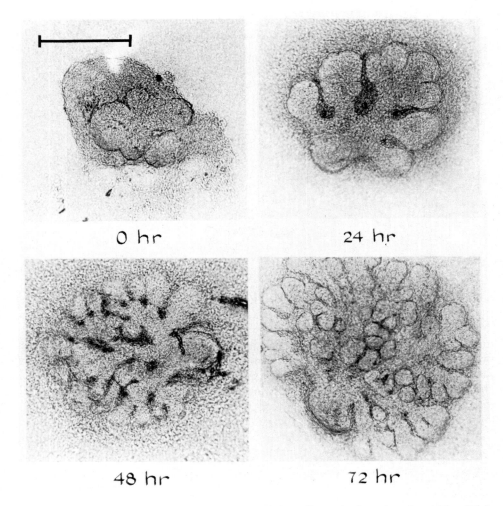

Fig. 1. Living whole 13-day mouse embryo submandibular salivary gland, explanted and immediately cultured (0 hr). The epithelium undergoes progressive branching morphogenesis within the surrounding mesenchyme (24, 48 and 72 hr). Bar is 0.5 mm.

and are normal ultrastructurally, showing a well-defined lamina, relatively smooth plasma membrane, normal epithelial junctions and bundles of microfilaments (Fig. 3). Thus, the amorphous materials and fibrous collagen are not required for the maintenance of a normal cell periphery and normal lobular morphology.

Brief treatment of the isolated epithelia with nanogram amounts of hyaluronidase, which degrades the GAG of proteoglycans, completely removes the lamina. When such epithelia are promptly placed in culture with mesenchyme, lobular morphology is rapidly lost and the epithelium becomes spherical, the shape with the least surface area for volume, as if the actin filaments were uniformly and randomly contracting (Fig. 2, B). The lamina, therefore, appears to be involved in maintaining normal

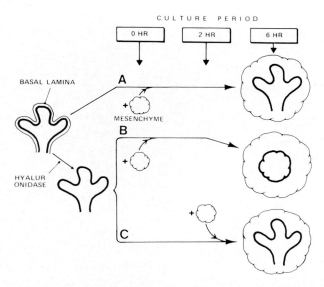

Fig. 2. Morphogenetic effects of removal and replacement of the basal lamina from 13-day mouse embryo submandibular epithelia. See text for description. (Reproduced from Bernfield and Banerjee (1977), by courtesy of Academic Press.)

morphology. Removal of the lamina is associated with major changes in the cell periphery: within 10 minutes, the plasma membrane is thrown into folds, cell junctions are lost, actin filament bundles become disorganized, and microtubules change their orientation (Fig. 4). Thus, removal of hyaluronidase-susceptible materials from the cell surface causes immediate alterations in the plasma membrane and the cytoplasmic fibers, a possible example of transmembrane control.

These changes are completely reversible by allowing the epithelium to regenerate a lamina during 2-hour culture in the absence of mesenchyme. Redeposition of the

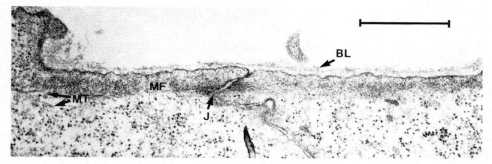

Fig. 3. Electron micrograph of the basal surface of a submandibular epithelium isolated free of mesenchyme with collagenase. The basal lamina (BL) covers the epithelial surface, the cells are closely adherent at the junctions (J) and linear arrays of microfilaments (MF) subjacent to the plasma membrane are frequently observed extending from one junctional complex to the other. A portion of some microtubules (MT) are seen. Tissue fixed with glutaraldehyde, post-fixed with OsO₄ and stained with uranyl acetate followed by lead citrate. Bar is 1 μm. (Reproduced from Banerjee et al. (1977), by courtesy of the Editors of the *Journal of Cell Biology*.)

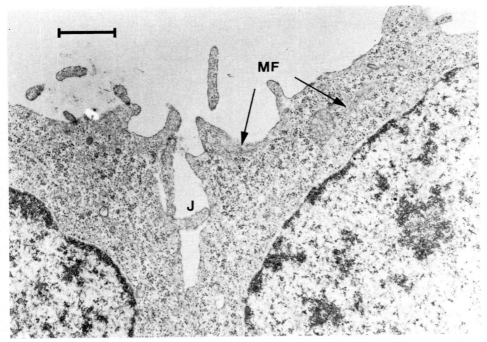

Fig. 4. Electron micrograph of the basal surface of a submandibular epithelium isolated free of mesenchyme with collagenase and then incubated for 10 minutes with 50 ng per ml testicular hyaluronidase. Small projections of the plasma membrane are seen which often contain microfilaments (MF) running parallel to the long axis of the projection. Short patches of microfilaments are also seen which show less organization than the arrays of filaments seen in Figure 3. The projections are most prominent at spaces between the cells where cell junctions (J) are usually seen. Fixed and stained as in Figure 3. Bar is 1 μm. (Reproduced from Banerjee et al. (1977), by courtesy of the Editors of the *Journal of Cell Biology*.)

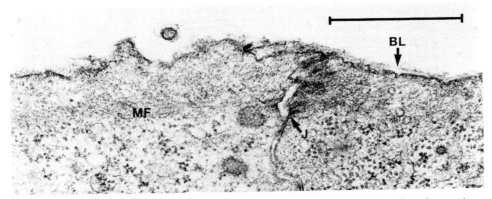

Fig. 5. Electron micrograph of the basal surface of a submandibular epithelium isolated free of mesenchyme with collagenase, incubated with hyaluronidase for 10 minutes and then cultured for 2 hours in the absence of mesenchyme. A basal lamina (BL) is seen covering most of the surface. Linear band-like arrays of microfilaments (MF) are seen subjacent to the plasma membrane extending from one junctional area (J) to the other. Fixed and stained as in Figure 3. Bar is 1 μm. (Reproduced from Banerjee et al. (1977), by courtesy of the Editors of the *Journal of Cell Biology*.)

lamina is accompanied by complete restoration of a normal cell periphery: the plasma membrane becomes smooth, the junctions return and the actin filament bundles reorganize (Fig. 5). Allowing restoration of the lamina prevents the loss of lobular morphology when the epithelia are cultured combined with mesenchyme (Fig. 2, C).

These observations suggest that the basal lamina is involved in maintaining a normal cell periphery and normal lobular morphology, pointing to the epithelial basal lamina as probable major factor in controlling morphogenesis. Although the mesenchyme is required for morphogenesis, it appears to be deleterious to epithelial recovery from removal of the lamina. The implication is that the mesenchyme may exert its morphogenetic effects, in part, by influencing the lamina.

The basal lamina may contain hyaluronic acid and proteoglycan organized into an extracellular scaffolding. Labeling studies reveal that the lamina in intact glands and the lamina which is rapidly replaced by the epithelium after enzymatic removal contain identical proportions of newly synthesized GAG (Fig. 6), and by staining for anionic polysaccharides, show an identical pattern of components in ordered periodic arrays associated with the plasma membrane (Cohn et al., 1977). These data suggest that the lamina contains discrete supramolecular complexes of GAG which accumulate as units of constant composition. The changes observed upon removal and redeposition of the lamina are comparable in type and in speed of reversibility to those found by Goldman and Knipe (1973) in cultured cells following their detachment and reattachment to a glass or plastic surface. Therefore, as suggested by Vracko (1974), the lamina may be a substratum-like framework to which the epithelial cells attach. This role would enable the lamina to be involved in the organization of the cell periphery while imposing a stable morphology on the

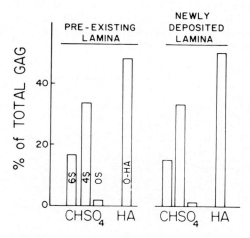

Fig. 6. ^{3}H-glycosaminoglycan in the basal lamina synthesized by isolated epithelia. Epithelia with or without a pre-existing lamina, prepared by treatment with collagenase or with collagenase followed by hyaluronidase, were labeled for 2.5 hours with ^{3}H-glucosamine. After removing basal surface materials with trypsin, the materials were digested with chondroitinase ABC, yielding disaccharides characteristic of the various glycosaminoglycans which were separated by paper chromatography. $CHSO_4$ is chondroitin sulfate, 6S, 4S and 0S representing chondroitin-6-sulfate, chondroitin-4-sulfate and chondroitin, respectively. HA is hyaluronic acid and 0-HA is its characteristic disaccharide.

epithelium. Because proteoglycans are in the laminae of branching embryonic epithelia, and since the GAG are highly flexible molecules, the scaffolding in organs undergoing this morphogenesis would be expected to be malleable and pliant.

However, the idea that structural form is imposed by a scaffolding at the cell surface, no matter how flexible or malleable, appears inconsistent with the fact that changes in form occur rapidly and continually during branching morphogenesis. This difficulty is resolved by the finding that the GAG in the basal lamina is itself undergoing rapid dynamic changes (Bernfield and Banerjee, 1977). In intact glands, the most rapid accumulation of label in GAG is at the distal ends of the lobules, the sites of greatest change in cell shape, and as shown by thymidine incorporation, the sites of most rapid cell proliferation (Fig. 7). Removing the label and chasing shows that the GAG label is rapidly lost from the distal aspects of lobules while it slowly accumulates within the clefts. This pattern of GAG metabolism is not altered by inhibition of cell proliferation or by inhibitors of collagen secretion or cross-linking. Detailed studies have shown that this change in GAG distribution results from a more rapid rate of deposition and loss of laminar GAG at the distal aspects of the lobules than in the clefts. Thus, in intact glands, laminar GAG is turning over most rapidly at sites where a rigid scaffolding would be inappropriate and least rapidly where morphologic stability would be required.

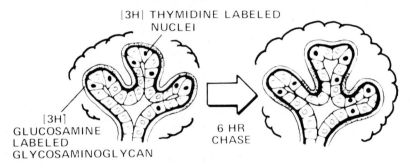

Fig. 7. Autoradiographic distribution of [3H]-glucosamine and [3H]-thymidine after 2 hours label and 6 hours chase of intact submandibular glands. See text for description.

This differential turnover rate could account for the site-specific differences in accumulation of labeled GAG and in amount of total GAG found at the basal surfaces of salivary, lung, mammary and kidney epithelia undergoing branching morphogenesis (Banerjee and Bernfield, 1976). This distribution consistently reflects the morphology of these organs: at the stage of the unbranched single buds, total and newly synthesized GAG are distributed uniformly over the basal surface. With tissue-specific changes in morphology, more total GAG is at the surfaces of the clefts and lateral aspects of lobules and branches, the morphogenetically quiescent sites, than at the distal aspects of lobules and branches, the sites where further branching will take place. In contrast, labeled GAG accumulates most rapidly at the distal ends of lobules and branches and least rapidly at the quiescent sites.

The epithelium alone is responsible for the synthesis, deposition and organization of the lamina, but the epithelium alone cannot undergo morphogenesis; mesenchyme is required. While these organs are growing and changing shape, the GAG in the lamina is turning over, and it appears that the mesenchyme is responsible for the degradation of the GAG. Biochemical studies show that intact mesenchymal cells have an activity which removes labeled GAG from the epithelial surface, producing a mixture of small GAG fragments. This activity appears to be involved in laminar GAG turnover because when epithelia are briefly labeled and then chased in the presence and absence of mesenchyme, rapid loss of GAG label from the distal aspects of the lobules, as seen in intact glands, is observed only in the presence of mesenchyme (Fig. 8). Thus, mesenchymal-induced GAG degradation correlates with morphogenesis: in the presence of mesenchyme, branching proceeds and site-specific loss of GAG is seen; in the absence of mesenchyme, no GAG loss is seen and branching ceases.

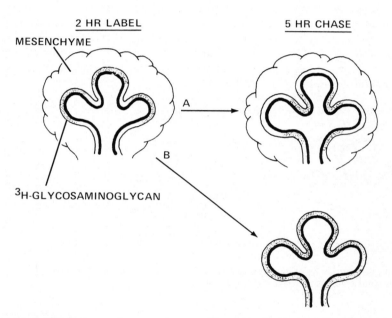

Fig. 8. Effect of mesenchyme on the autoradiographic distribution of ^{3}H-glucosamine at the basal surface of submandibular epithelia. Labeling of intact glands was for 2 hours (left column). Following isolation by collagenase treatment, the epithelia were chased in the presence (A) and absence (B) of mesenchyme for 5 hours (right column). See text for description.

A model for branching epithelial morphogenesis

We are now able to visualize a possible sequence of events at the cell periphery that leads to branching morphogenesis (Fig. 9). The organ primordium arises as a bulbous protrusion and expands in size due to growth, placing the bud in close proximity to the mesenchyme. The mesenchyme degrades the laminar GAG, and both the lobular expansion and GAG degradation cause thinning and interruptions of the lamina. Possibly due to reduced anchorage of the cells to the disappearing

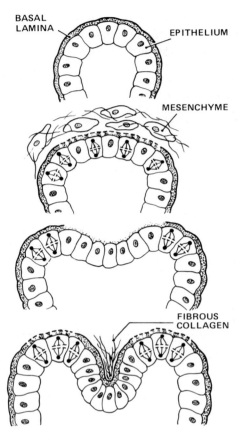

Fig. 9. Schematic model depicting a possible sequence of events in branching morphogenesis. See text for description.

lamina, the actin filaments at the basal end of the cell contract, the cells change shape, and by virtue of the junctions, the cell population invaginates. The beginning cleft becomes deeper due to the enlargement by cell division of the intervening lobules, and as it matures, becomes stabilized at its base by extracellular bundles of fibrous collagen. Within the cleft, laminar GAG degradation decreases due to reduced proximity of the lamina to the mesenchyme, allowing the laminar GAG to re-accumulate into an ordered array. The lobular morphology of the epithelium is maintained by adhesive junctions between the cells and the anchorage of the cells to the basal lamina. With continued mitosis, GAG turnover and new cleft formation, a tree-like epithelium gradually emerges.

CONCLUSIONS

Morphogenesis involves a limited repertoire of cellular behavior and present evidence indicates that the plasma membrane and its extra- and intracellular components are intimately involved in this behavior. The organization of the cell periphery has important implications for morphogenesis. The asymmetrical vectorial assembly of membrane proteins and lipids seems appropriately designed for the reception of extracellular signals and their transduction intracellularly. The fluid nature of the membrane allows easy adaptation to rapid changes in cell shape mediated by the cytoplasmic fibers. Transmembrane control of the membrane provides a way in which the cytoplasm can influence cell surface components, and vice versa. And finally, the junctions which provide both a firm attachment of the cells to each other and channels for transcellular passage of small molecules allow morphologic changes to occur coordinately in a cell population.

Studies of branching epithelial morphogenesis have provided a model for how precisely integrated and coordinated morphogenetic events may occur. Although clearly speculative, the model emphasizes the point that it now may be possible to understand, because of increased knowledge of the cell periphery, the individual processes involved in morphogenesis. By establishing the basis for normal organ morphogenesis, the etiology of birth defects, whether inherited or environmentally induced, will undoubtedly become apparent.

ACKNOWLEDGEMENTS

Parts of the work described here were performed in collaboration with Shib D. Banerjee, Ronald H. Cohn and R. Lane Smith. I thank Margareta Swenson-Rosenberg and Suzanne Tharpe for expert technical assistance, and Marjorie Weesner and Paige Patch for their help.

REFERENCES

Ash, J. F. and Spooner, B. S. (1973): *Develop. Biol.*, *33*, 463.
Banerjee, S. D. and Bernfield, M. R. (1976): *J. Cell Biol.*, *70*, 111a.
Banerjee, S. D., Cohn, R. H. and Bernfield, M. R. (1977): *J. Cell Biol.*, *73*, 445.
Bernfield, M. R. and Banerjee, S. D. (1972): *J. Cell Biol.*, *52*, 664.
Bernfield, M. R. and Banerjee, S. D. (1977): In: *Proceedings, First International Symposium on the Biology and Chemistry of Basement Membranes, Philadelphia, Pa.* Editor: N. A. Kefalides. Academic Press, New York. In press.
Bernfield, M. R., Banerjee, S. D. and Cohn, R. H. (1972): *J. Cell Biol.*, *52*, 674.
Bernfield, M. R., Cohn, R. H. and Banerjee, S. D. (1973): *Amer. Zool.*, *13*, 1067.
Burnside, B. (1971): *Develop. Biol.*, *26*, 416.
Byers, B. and Porter, K. (1964): *Proc. nat. Acad. Sci. (Wash.)*, *52*, 1091.
Clarke, M. and Spudich, J. A. (1977): *Ann. Rev. Biochem.*, *46*, 797.
Clarkson, B. and Baserga, R. (Eds.) (1974): *Control of Proliferation in Animal Cells, Vol. 1.* Cold Spring Harbor Laboratory, New York.
Cloney, R. A. (1966): *J. ultrastruct. Res.*, *14*, 300.
Cohn, R. H., Banerjee, S. D. and Bernfield, M. R. (1977): *J. Cell Biol.*, *73*, 464.
Cook, G. M. W. and Stoddart, R. W. (Eds.) (1973): *Surface Carbohydrates of the Eukaryotic Cell.* Academic Press, New York.
Coughlin, M. D. (1975): *Develop. Biol.*, *43*, 123.
Cunha, G. R. (1976): *Int. Rev. Cytol.*, *47*, 137.
Curtis, A. S. G. (1973): *Progr. Biophys. molec. Biol.*, *27*, 317.
Edelman, G. M. (1976): *Science*, *192*, 218.
Goldman, R. D. and Knipe, D. M. (1973): *Cold Spr. Harb. Symp. quant. Biol.*, *37*, 523.
Goldman, R., Pollard, T. and Rosenbaum, J. (Eds.) (1976): *Cell Motility, Book A, Vol. 3.* Cold Spring Harbor Laboratory, New York.

Griepp, E. B. and Revel, J. P. (1977): In: *Intercellular Communications*, p. 1. Editor: W. C. DeMello. Plenum Press, New York.

Grobstein, C. (1967): *Nat. Cancer Inst. Monogr.*, 26, 279.

Grobstein, C. and Cohen, J. (1965): *Science*, 150, 626.

Hughes, R. C. (1973): *Progr. Biophys. molec. Biol.*, 26, 191.

Kefalides, N. A. (1973): *Int. Rev. connect. Tissue Res.*, 6, 63.

McNutt, N. S. and Weinstein, R. S. (1973): *Progr. Biophys. molec. Biol.*, 26, 45.

Moscona, A. A. (Ed.) (1974): *The Cell Surface in Development*. John Wiley and Sons, New York.

Moscona, A. A. (1976): In: *Neuronal Recognition*, p. 205. Editor: S. H. Barondes. Plenum Press, New York.

Nicolson, G. L. (1976): *Biochim. biophys. Acta (Amst.)*, 457, 57.

Pastan, I. H., Johnson, G. S. and Anderson, W. B. (1975): *Ann. Rev. Biochem.*, 44, 491.

Pollard, T. D. and Weihing, R. R. (1974): *CRC Crit. Rev. Biochem.*, 2, 1.

Poste, G. and Nicolson, G. L. (Eds.) (1976): *The Cell Surface in Animal Embryogenesis and Development*, *Vol. 1*. North-Holland, New York.

Revel, J. P. and Brown, S. S. (1975): *Cold Spr. Harb. Symp. quant. Biol.*, 40, 443.

Robbins, J. C. and Nicolson, G. L. (1975): In: *Cancer, A Comprehensive Treatise*, p. 3. Editor: F. F. Becker. Plenum Press, New York.

Roseman, S. (1970): *Chem. Phys. Lip.*, 5, 270.

Rothman, J. E. and Lenard, J. (1977): *Science*, 195, 743.

Saxen, L. (1972): In: *Tissue Interactions in Carcinogenesis*, p. 49. Editor: D. Tarin. Academic Press, New York.

Schur, B. D. and Roth, S. (1975): *Biochim. biophys. Acta (Amst.)*, 415, 473.

Singer, S. J. (1974): *Ann. Rev. Biochem.*, 43, 805.

Singer, S. J. and Nicolson, G. L. (1972): *Science*, 175, 720.

Snyder, J. A. and McIntosh, J. R. (1976): *Ann. Rev. Biochem.*, 45, 699.

Soifer, D. (Ed.) (1975): *The Biology of Cytoplasmic Tubules*, Ann. N.Y. Acad. Sci., 253, 848 pp.

Spooner, B. S. (1975): *BioScience*, 25, 440.

Spooner, B. S. and Wessells, N. K. (1972): *Develop. Biol.*, 27, 38.

Staehelin, L. A. (1974): *Int. Rev. Cytol.*, 39, 191.

Steck, T. L. (1974): *J. Cell Biol.*, 62, 1.

Vracko, R. (1974): *Amer. J. Path.*, 77, 314.

Whittenberger, B. and Glaser, L. (1977): *Proc. nat. Acad. Sci. (Wash.)*, 74, 2251.

Embryonic induction and tissue interaction during morphogenesis *

ELIZABETH D. HAY

Harvard Medical School, Department of Anatomy, Boston, Mass., U.S.A.

Embryonic induction is a term used by embryologists today to refer to developmentally significant interaction between 2 tissues. In the Spemann and Grobstein sense of the term, the interacting tissues are closely associated but of dissimilar origin; a developmentally significant interaction is a change in one or both tissues which is progressive, stable and maturational in direction (Spemann, 1938; Grobstein, 1955, 1967).

In the classic sense of the term, then, hormone-cell interactions are not embryonic inductions because they are long-range (Fig. 1). I have also put tissue remodeling in a separate classification in the scheme shown here, even though tissue interaction can be involved in the process of cell death and matrix turnover (Saunders and Fallon, 1966; Kratochwil and Schwartz, 1976; Banerjee et al., 1977; Wessells, 1977). I have also classified the kind of cell–cell interaction that probably occurs within tissues separately from the kind of tissue to tissue interaction that we will be discussing here because the contacts and junctions that occur within a tissue are different than those which occur between tissues (Hay, 1968).

MORPHOLOGICAL AND BIOCHEMICAL EFFECTS OF INDUCERS

Our discussion of embryonic induction, then, will concern developmentally significant changes in closely associated tissues that seem to be brought about at close range by the products of one or both of the tissues (Fig. 1, A). The kinds of effects that such short-range inducers might have on the morphological and biochemical characteristics of the responding tissues are shown in Figure 2.

One of the most common effects of short-range inducers is on cell shape and/or motility. The ability of cells to adhere to and migrate along the matrix produced by another tissue could be considered to be an example of short-range tissue interaction (see Le Douarin, *This Volume*). The morphogenetic movements which we will be discussing, however, involve mainly changes in the shape of cells that are anchored to basement membranes (for example, the thickening and constriction of neural epithelium during neural tube formation).

* The original research reported in this review was supported by a grant, HD-00143, from the United States Public Health Service.

126

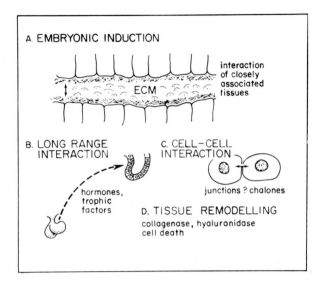

Fig. 1. Types of tissue interactions. A. Embryonic induction is a developmentally progressive interaction between closely associated, but dissimilarly derived tissues. B. Examples of long-range tissue interaction include hormones and trophic factors made by one tissue that circulate through the blood stream to reach the target tissue. C. Direct cell–cell interaction may occur within tissues by exchange of substances across 2 plasmalemmas that contact each other. D. Tissue remodeling includes digestion of products secreted by one tissue by enzymes produced by another tissue. Cells also may be killed in some cases by the influence of an adjacent tissue.

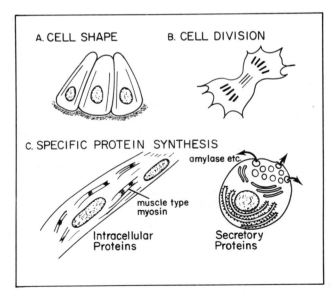

Fig. 2. Effects of inducers. A. Cell shape may be dependent on the presence or products of an adjacent tissue. B. Cell division in one tissue may be promoted by the presence of another tissue. C. Specific protein synthesis in one tissue may be enhanced by the products of an adjacent tissue.

Another common effect of short-range inducers is on cell division (Fig. 2, B). Since happy embryonic cells by nature are bound to be growing and properly induced embryonic tissues are bound to be happy, it is difficult to separate inducer effects on cell proliferation from those on cell differentiation. They go hand in hand.

Cell differentiation is often defined as the turning on of specific protein synthesis, as opposed to, say, the manufacture of proteins involved in mitosis and maintenance of cell shape. For example, the production of specific contractile proteins by muscle cells, chondromucoproteins by cartilage cells, and amylase by pancreatic acinar cells might be classified as cell differentiation (Fig. 2, C), whereas cell and tissue shape change is sometimes viewed as morphogenesis (Spooner, 1974; Wessells, 1977).

It has proved extremely difficult to discover just when specific protein synthesis is actually turned on in cells and whether or not inducers are involved in the turning on process itself. Rutter et al. (1968) have shown that pancreatic acinar cells are making amylase before the event Grobstein called induction in this system. In muscle differentiation, collagen and other 'inductive' molecules have been shown to enhance (directly or indirectly) myosin synthesis, but the machinery for myosin synthesis was probably already programmed in the myoblasts (Konigsberg and Hauschka, 1965; Ordahl and Caplan, 1976). In most of the inductive interactions that we will be discussing today, specific protein synthesis is probably not initiated by the inducers. The inducers seem to promote and stabilize differentiation. The actual genetic programs may be prepackaged in given parts of the egg, remaining dormant until their expression is encouraged by appriopriate tissue interaction (for further discussion of the question of determination see Hay and Meier, 1977; Wessells, 1977).

THE FIRST TISSUE INTERACTION:
PRIMARY EMBRYONIC INDUCTION

Let us turn now to the beginning of development to see how these principles apply. Most of the experiments that have been done on early development use the readily accessible amphibian egg (Fig. 3). The important point about cleavage in the amphibian egg, and probably also in the eggs of higher vertebrates, is that the cell cortex and cytoplasm create, in response to activation, preprogrammed reactions which are different in different parts of the egg (Needham, 1942). As cleavage proceeds, for example, nuclei in the lower pole of the egg will be combined with cytoplasm containing germ cell determinants, so that the resulting cells learn long before gastrulation that they are going to be oogonia and spermatogonia (Smith and Williams, 1975). Other examples of the cytoplasmic determination of parts of the egg undoubtedly exist, but are more difficult to recognize prior to gastrulation.

Gastrulation is a process whereby a hollow mass of cells resulting from cleavage subdivides itself into definitive germ layers or primitive tissues, of which there are 3 in most vertebrates (the familiar endoderm, mesoderm and ectoderm). In the amphibian (Fig. 3), gastrulation is accomplished by pushing in part of the outside lining cells through the so-called blastopore. The cells coming through the dorsal lip of the blastopore form a dorsal sheet of notochord and mesoderm, the so-called chordamesoderm, that induces the overlying ectoderm to fold up and fuse into a neuroectodermal tube which becomes the spinal cord.

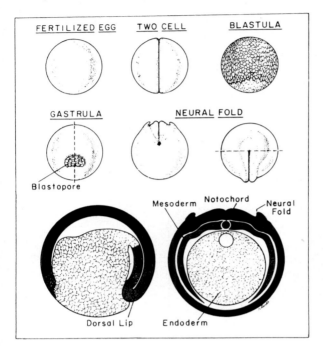

FERTILIZED EGG TWO CELL BLASTULA

GASTRULA NEURAL FOLD

Blastopore

Mesoderm Notochord Neural Fold

Dorsal Lip Endoderm

Fig. 3. Early stages in development of the amphibian egg. At the blastula stage, the center of the cleaving egg becomes hollowed out. At the gastrula stage the outer lining cells begin to invaginate along the dorsal lip of the blastopore. A sagittal section of a gastrula is shown in the lower left. At the neural fold or neurula stage the dorsal ectoderm is thrown into folds that fuse to form the neural tube. A cross section through a neurula is shown in the lower right. The notochord and adjacent mesoderm influence the formation of the neural folds, a tissue interaction known as primary induction because it is the first to occur.

How is this accomplished? The first principle, learned from the work of Spemann, Waddington and others in the first half of this century, is clearly this: the cells in the ectoderm overlying the chordamesoderm are already predisposed to become neural tube (Spemann, 1938; Needham, 1942). While certain other parts of the embryo at this stage are also competent to become neural tube (e.g., the ventral ectoderm), at later stages ectoderm loses the competence to neurulate. The second principle also stems from Spemann's era and relates to the first: the specificity of neural tube induction resides in the responding tissue and not in the inducing tissue. The effect of the chordamesoderm on neural tube formation by competent ectoderm can be mimicked by unrelated dead tissues, by albumin containing a variety of chemical compounds and even by non-specific culture conditions (Barth, 1941; Needham, 1942; Holtfreter, 1948).

The lack of specificity of the primary inducer has proved such a block to human thinking about the process of primary induction that little work has been done recently in this area (see Toivonen et al., 1976, for review). The work of Barth and Barth (1972) implicates ion gradients in early amphibian morphogenesis. The time may be ripe for exploring the possibility that the chordamesoderm produces an ion-filtering matrix under the neuroepithelium that is mimicked by albumin and dead tissues. Microtubule-dependent cell elongation of the type involved in neurulation has, in fact, been shown to be highly sensitive to intracellular ion concentrations (see Hay, 1973, 1977, for further discussion).

CLASSIFICATION OF SECOND-ORDER INDUCTIONS

Second-order inductions are those close-range tissue interactions which occur after the neural tube has formed. The neural tube, for example, influences the adjacent mesoderm to subdivide into paired epithelial balls, the somites (Lipton and Jacobson,

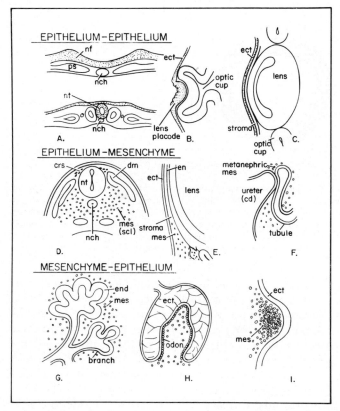

Fig. 4. Classification of short-range tissue interactions. A. Primary induction of neural tube by notochord and mesoderm. B. Induction of lens by optic cup. C. Enhancement of corneal stroma production by lens. D. Interaction of sclerotome with neural tube and notochord. E. Migration of mesenchyme into the corneal stroma. F. Interaction of ureteric bud with metanephric mesenchyme (this interaction is mimicked in vitro by spinal cord influence on metanephric mesenchyme). G. Salivary gland and pancreatic ducts are induced to branch and form acini by mesenchyme. H. In the developing tooth, mesenchyme induces the enamel epithelial cells to become columnar in shape and probably also helps digest the epithelial basement membrane. I. During feather formation, the mesenchyme condenses under the ectoderm which then thickens and develops feather characteristics. cd, presumptive collecting duct; crs, neural crest; dm, dermatome; ect, ectodermal epithelium; en, endothelium; end, endodermal epithelium; mes, mesenchyme; nch, notochord; nf, neural fold; nt, neural tube; ps, presumptive somite; odon, odontoblast; scl, sclerotome.

1974). In the head region, the neural tube evaginates to give rise to the optic cup which induces lens to form from overlying ectoderm and then the lens induces the remaining ectoderm to form the primitive cornea (Coulombre, 1965).

It is convenient to classify second-order inductions according to the morphology of the tissues involved as epithelial-epithelial, epithelial-mesenchymal, or mesenchymal-epithelial (Fig. 4). An epithelium is a tissue composed of contiguous cells that rest on a basement membrane and that have a free surface facing outside or on a cavity. Shortly after they are formed, the notochord and mesoderm become organized as epithelia with inner cavities. The endoderm and ectoderm are also epithelia at this stage and indeed, the initial tissue interactions in vertebrate embryos are mainly between epithelial sheets. The important point about this organization is the fact that the dissimilar epithelial tissues face each other with their basement membranes and subjacent epithelium-derived stromas apposed.

Mesenchymal cells arise secondarily from the epithelial sheets and migrate within, rather than on top of, extracellular matrices. The somites, for example, break apart after the neural tube is completely formed (Fig. 4, D) and give rise to the freely wandering cells of the sclerotome, which form the axial skeleton. These mesoderm-derived mesenchymal cells differentiate into cartilage under the influence of adjacent epithelia, in this case, neural tube and notochord. In the region of the developing eye, ectoderm-derived mesenchymal cells (neural crest) migrate into the primitive stroma created by the corneal epithelium where they are probably influenced by extracellular matrix to differentiate into fibroblasts (Fig. 4, E).

Subsequently, mesenchymal cells exert influences on epithelial cell differentiation. Mesenchyme-epithelium interaction in the developing salivary gland and pancreas (Fig. 4, G) is complex (Bernfield and Wessells, 1970; Bernfield et al., 1972; Banerjee et al., 1977). Mesenchyme instructs other endodermal epithelia in their morphogenesis and differentiation (Croisille and Le Douarin, 1965; Wolff, 1970). Epithelial differentiation in feather germs (Fig. 4, I) and many other skin derivatives is also influenced by mesenchyme (McLoughlin, 1961; Kratochwil, 1972). In the developing tooth (Fig. 4, H), it has been suggested by Slavkin et al. (1969, 1972) that mesenchyme-derived materials lying within the extracellular matrix influence epithelial differentiation into ameloblasts.

EVIDENCE FOR CELL-MATRIX INTERACTION IN SECOND-ORDER INDUCTION

Let us turn now to the question of the nature of second-order inducers and consider first the idea already alluded to, that structural components of the extracellular matrix influence cytodifferentiation. In both epithelium-created and mesenchyme-created extracellular matrices, the structural components consist of collagens of 4 or 5 different varieties, glycosaminoglycans of a half dozen or more varieties and an unknown number of partially characterized glycoproteins (Fig. 5).

The idea that the extracellular matrix is a vital component of the early embryo can be traced to earlier workers, but it was Grobstein's work in the mid-1950's that called attention to the possible role of the matrix in what we are defining here as embryonic induction. Grobstein (1955) isolated the epithelial and mesenchymal

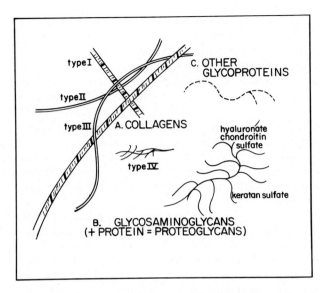

Fig. 5. Structural components of extracellular matrix (ECM). A. Collagens. Type I collagen occurs in skin and bone, type II in cartilage and type III in reticular connective tissue, either in the form of striated or non-striated fibrils. Type IV collagen is present in basement membranes and appears filamentous in the electron microscope. B. The principal glycosaminoglycans are hyaluronate, chondroitin, chondroitin sulfate, heparan sulfate, dermatan sulfate and keratan sulfate. Glycosaminoglycans are combined with protein to form proteoglycans in connective tissue. C. Other glycoproteins are also present in extracellular matrix, but these have not been completely characterized.

components of the salivary gland by trypsin digestion and recombined them in culture. Mesenchyme was able to affect epithelial branching even when located on the other side of a Millipore filter. In related experiments, Lash et al. (1957) found that transfilter induction was prevented if interacting tissues were not directly opposite each other on the filter. Thus, the inducer seemed unable to diffuse freely through the medium.

Grobstein decided to analyse the materials that might be trapped in the filter, using still another tissue interaction. He found that embryonic spinal cord transfilter to metanephric mesenchyme induces kidney tubules to form in vitro. Using methods that were readily available in the 1950's, he showed that spinal cord secretes a substance into the filter that reacts with histochemical stains for extracellular matrix (Grobstein, 1955, 1967). Subsequently, it has been shown that embryonic spinal cord secretes collagen and glycosaminoglycan (Cohen and Hay, 1971; Hay and Meier, 1974; Manasek and Cohen, 1977). But it was on the basis of the results of the histochemical stains that Grobstein suggested the matrix theory of embryonic induction.

It was Grobstein's contention that the matrix, and materials that might be trapped in it, mediated transfilter induction. Recently, Saxén and his collaborators have reexamined the interaction between (1) spinal cord and metanephric mesenchyme and (2) preameloblasts and mesenchyme using various types of filters (Wartiovaara et al., 1974; Lehtonen et al., 1975; Saxén et al., 1976; Thesleff et al., 1977). In some cases, cell processes extend all the way across Nucleopore filters and thin Millipore filters, but one would also expect newly secreted matrix to enter the filter pores. This group has opted against involvement of direct cell–cell contact in the in vivo interaction, at least in the case of the developing tooth. The reason is that the 2 interacting tissues involved in the interaction in vivo are separated by extracellular matrix at the time of the interaction (Thesleff et al., 1977).

Electron microscopy reveals no evidence of direct contact in vivo between mesenchymal and epithelial cells in the majority of the tissue interactions that we are discussing (Fig. 4). Mesenchymal cell processes have been reported to penetrate the epithelial basement membrane between odontoblasts and preameloblasts (Slavkin and Bringas, 1976), metanephric mesenchyme and kidney tubules (Lehtonen, 1975) and mesenchyme and salivary epithelium (Wessells, 1977). These may be special cases in that the basal lamina is probably in the process of being digested by the mesenchyme, at least in the case of tooth and salivary gland (Slavkin and Bringas, 1976; Banerjee et al., 1977).

Direct evidence that cell–cell contact is not involved in certain of the interactions that we are calling embryonic inductions can be obtained by substituting killed matrix for the living inducers. Collagen and other conditioned medium factors can replace the requirement of differentiating muscle cells for living mesenchyme in vitro (Konigsberg and Hauschka, 1965; Hauschka and White, 1972; White et al., 1975). Killed retinal products support scleral cartilage differentiation (Newsome, 1976). Frozen-killed dermis stimulates epidermal differentiation (Dodson, 1963) and frozen-killed lens substitutes for living lens in enhancing corneal epithelial differentiation in vitro (Dodson and Hay, 1971, 1974). Meier and Hay (1974a,b, 1975) found that isolated lens capsule, various collagens, purified type II collagen and certain glycosaminoglycans also enhance the ability of corneal epithelium to produce corneal stroma in vitro.

Perhaps the most important point to emerge from this study of corneal differentiation is that the basal epithelial cells in contact with extracellular matrix seem better able to maintain their columnar cell shape, differentiate and produce significant amounts of corneal stroma than cells grown on non-collagenous substrata (Fig. 6, Table 1). The interaction is believed to involve the cell surface because collagen does not enter the cells (Hay and Meier, 1976). In the living in vivo system, the epithelial cells are attached to a basal lamina, partly of their own making, to which the lens may contribute collagens and glycosaminoglycans. All 3 of the collagen types tested in vitro are stimulatory and all 3 are probably produced by both lens and corneal epithelium (see Hay et al., 1977). The particular glycosaminoglycans that are stimulatory are also produced by both the lens and corneal epithelium (Hay and Meier, 1974). The specificity of the epithelial response, that is, production of corneal stroma, seems to reside in the corneal epithelium and not in the so-called inducer.

Similarly, Nevo and Dorfman (1972) found that certain glycosaminoglycans, including cartilage proteoglycans such as chondromucoprotein, stimulate the production of chondroitin sulfate by isolated cartilage cells (see also Huang, 1974). The response of the chondrocytes is to make more chondrogenic products. Recently, Lash, Kosher and their colleagues have reported that collagen of both the type I and the type II varieties stimulate chondrogenesis in isolated sclerotome, a tissue which is already committed to becoming cartilage (Kosher and Church, 1975; Lash and Vasan, 1977). Here too, chondromucoprotein also has a stimulatory effect

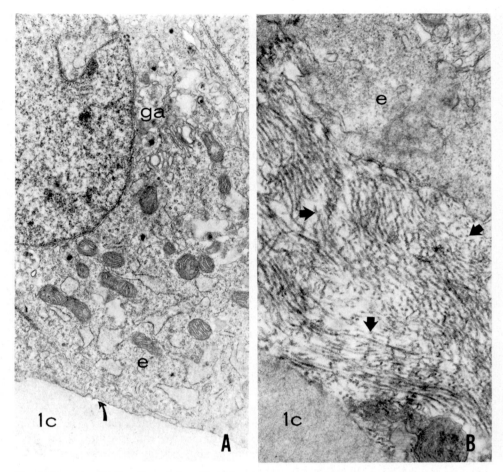

Fig. 6. Corneal epithelium from 5-day-old chick embryo grown on lens capsule for 24 hours. The outer layer of cells (not shown) is flattened in shape, similar to the periderm in vivo. The basal epithelial cells are columnar in shape and each has a prominent Golgi apparatus (ga) and endoplasmic reticulum, which are involved in the synthesis and secretion of corneal stroma. The new stroma produced in culture will appear in the space (curved arrow, figure A) between the base of the epithelium (e) and the lens capsule (lc). In figure B, a new stroma of collagen fibrils (arrows) can be seen. This stroma is rich in chondroitin sulfate and contains both types I and II collagen. The epithelium cultured on lens capsule (mainly type IV collagen), gels of type I collagen (Table 1) or gels of type II collagen synthesizes about twice as much collagen as epithelium grown on noncollagenous substrata. A. × 20,000. B. × 50,000. (Reproduced from Meier and Hay (1974a), by courtesy of the Editors of *Developmental Biology*.)

(Kosher et al., 1973). Treatment with enzymes that digest extracellular matrix interfere with the ability of neural tube and notochord to enhance somite chondrogenesis (O'Hare, 1972; Kosher and Lash, 1975; Strudel, 1976). Thus, in the epithelium–epithelium and epithelium–mesenchyme classes of tissue interaction, there is considerable evidence implicating extracellular matrix in what is being measured as induction in vitro; in general, the response to the presence of matrix is enhancement rather than initiation of differentiation.

TABLE 1

Synthesis of ECM by corneal epithelium

Substratum	24 hours in vitro		
	DNA[1]	c.p.m.[2]	c.p.m./DNA
Nucleopore filter	350	222	0.63
Millipore filter (triton-free)	370	515	1.39
Collagen gel	320	648	2.02

[1]DNA in ng (Prasad et al., 1973, *J. Lab. clin. Med.*, *80*, 598). Each value is the mean of 3 determinations of 4 epithelia each.
[2]c.p.m. in hydroxyproline (Juva and Prockop, 1966, *Analyt. Biochem.*, 15, 77). ^{3}H-proline added to cultures for last 6 hours. Each value is the mean of 3 determinations of 4 epithelia each. The epithelia were isolated from 5-day-old chick embryos as previously described by Meier and Hay (1974a,b, 1975).

Ironically, even though mesenchymal cells are renowned for their ability to produce collagen and glycosaminoglycan, there is no direct evidence for a role of matrix in the mesenchyme–epithelium class of induction. In feather development, the presence of a particular type of mesenchymal extracellular matrix is correlated with normal development; extracellular matrix may be guilty here, but only by association (Stuart and Moscona, 1967; Goetinck and Sekellick, 1972; Overton and Collins, 1976). In developing glands, collagenase treatment interrupts morphogenesis (Grobstein and Cohen, 1965; Wessells and Cohen, 1968), but it has now been shown that the enzymes used were impure (Bernfield et al., 1972). Even if they were pure, however, the case could not be proved by this approach alone because treatment with pure collagenase will obviously dislocate any potential inducers that might have been attached to the removed collagen. No direct analysis of possible roles of structural matrix components has been carried out for teeth, feathers or the other mesenchyme–epithelium interactions we mentioned.

OTHER FACTORS POSSIBLY OPERATING IN SECOND-ORDER INDUCTIONS

Some substances other than collagens and glycosaminoglycans have been implicated in mesenchyme–epithelium interactions. The proposal that RNA is transferred from tissue to tissue (Saxén and Toivonen, 1962; Slavkin and Croissant, 1973) has been challenged by the recent experiments of Grainger and Wessells (1974). There is some evidence that metabolites, such as mesenchymal cells might produce or concentrate, can affect epithelial differentiation (see Hay, 1963). There is a question, however, as to whether or not such substances (e.g., vitamin A) are actually found in the in vivo situation. In recent years, protein and polypeptide factors have received a considerable share of attention.

For example, Rutter and his collaborators have isolated a so-called mesenchymal factor from embryonic mesenchyme that stimulates pancreatic epithelial proliferation and differentiation (Rutter et al., 1964; Ronzio and Rutter, 1973; Levine et al., 1973; Pictet, 1975). This factor is a relatively insoluble, non-collagenous glycoprotein that interacts with the cell surface. Presumably, such pancreatic mesenchymal factors are not specific (Grobstein, 1967; see also Cunha, 1972). Interestingly, pancreatic epithelium will attach to Sepharose to which the mesenchymal factor has previously been covalently linked, but will not attach to albumin-coated Sepharose beads (Fig. 7).

Attachment of epithelial cells to a substratum (normally a basement membrane) may be of fundamental importance in the maintenance of cell shape and, directly or indirectly, cell proliferation and differentiation. Normal fibroblasts produce a so-called cell surface or LETS protein that seems to resemble a serum factor which promotes cell attachment to collagen (Yamada and Weston, 1975; Hynes, 1976; Pearlstein, 1976). Other differentiation-promoting factors which have not been fully characterized may be attached to extracellular matrix, for example, the so-called bone morphogenetic protein (Urist and Iwata, 1973). It is beyond the scope of this short review to consider all of the protein and polypeptide factors that have been implicated in the maintenance of epithelial and mesenchymal cell growth and differentiation (see Rutter, 1977). It should be pointed out, however, that one of the functions of collagen and other glycoproteins of the matrix could be to bind and concentrate trophic factors such as these (if they exist in vivo), just as glycosaminoglycans would be expected to bind and regulate juxtacellular ions. Finally, it should be mentioned that there may be as yet undiscovered mesenchyme-specific factors operating in skin and gut differentiation, for here an epithelium may actually modulate its differentiation in response to a particular mesenchyme (McLoughlin, 1961; Kollar and Baird, 1969, 1970a,b; Coulombre and Coulombre, 1971; Kratochwil, 1972).

RECEPTORS AND HORMONES

Since this chapter on induction was being followed by one on receptors and hormones by Dr. O'Malley, I think I should in closing comment on whether or not I think there is anything to be learned about embryonic induction from the study of hormone-receptor models.

Well, from the outset it is pretty clear we have at least one major problem in common to solve, and that is the fact that the specificity of the response usually, if not always lies, in the responding tissue. Estrogens circulate about, but they only cause oviduct cells to become oviduct cells. Insulin inactivates adenyl cyclase of fat cells, but probably spares oviduct cells. You might say, only the oviduct cells contain receptors in their nuclei for estrogen complexes; only the fat cells have cell surface receptors that, after binding insulin, inactivate adenyl cyclase. That's fine,

---

Fig. 7. Pancreatic epithelium from 12-day-old rat embryos grown with Sepharose beads covalently bound to mesenchymal factor (A, B) or to bovine serum albumin (C). In A and B, the cells have attached to the beads and electron microscopy reveals differentiating pancreatic acinar cells (A). Autoradiography shows ^{3}H-thymidine incorporation (arrow) by cells attached to factor-coated beads (B), whereas, there is little DNA synthesis (arrow) in control cells which do not attach to albumin-coated beads. Epithelia were cultured 18–24 hours in the presence of beads and then incubated for 6 hours with ^{3}H-thymidine (B, C) or in control medium for 6 days. On the factor-coated beads, the cells may be cuboidal in shape and they retain their polarity. A, × 3600. B and C, × 365. (Reproduced from Levine et al. (1973), by courtesy of the Editors of *Nature New Biology*.)

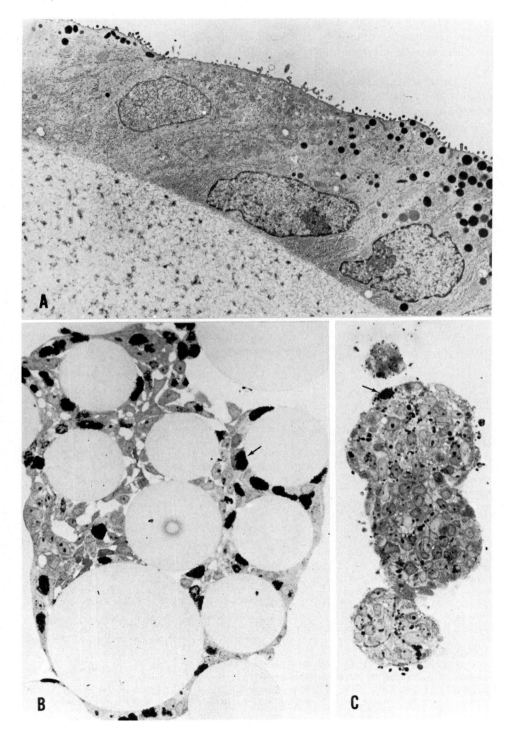

but you are still left with the fundamental question to answer and that is why do oviduct cells have receptors for estrogen and fat cells for insulin? Without solving that question, you have not totally solved the question of endocrine control mechanisms.

A generalization may emerge from comparison of the endocrine and induction systems. This is that nature seems to like to deal with the problem of progression in time by creating preprogrammed cells whose subsequent behavior can be modulated by adding relatively simple extraneous substances at just the right time.

Viewed in this context, the egg is never an undifferentiated cell, but is always preprogrammed. The task is to divide up the programs among the component cells that result from cleavage, so that when these cells are rearranged into tissues at gastrulation, they are ready to react to what may be trivial signals from each other. We know that the amphibian embryo first starts making collagen and glycosaminoglycan at about the time of gastrulation and these may be the only signals needed at first. Subsequent interactions may build on the same compounds or other secreted proteins and metabolites may be drawn into the act.

We are in an excellent position now to explore further the cellular mechanisms involved in the response of these preprogrammed embryonic cells to changes in their cell surface and immediate environment. The answer to the question of how the cells respond will enormously advance our understanding of congenital defects, even though for the time being we cannot solve the more fundamental question of how it came to be that some cells do one thing and others another when faced with the same inducer or, for that matter, the same hormone.

REFERENCES

Banerjee, S. D., Cohn, R. H. and Bernfield, M. R. (1977): *J. Cell Biol.*, *73*, 445.
Barth, L. G. (1941): *J. exp. Zool.*, *87*, 371.
Barth, L. G. and Barth, L. J. (1972): *Develop. Biol.*, *28*, 18.
Bernfield, M. R. and Wessells, N. K. (1970): *Develop. Biol.*, *Suppl.*, *4*, 195.
Bernfield, M. R., Banerjee, S. D. and Cohn, R. H. (1972): *J. Cell Biol.*, *52*, 674.
Cohen, A. M. and Hay, E. D. (1971): *Develop. Biol.*, *26*, 578.
Coulombre, A. J. (1965): In: *Organogenesis*, p. 219. Editors: R. L. DeHaan and H. Ursprung. Holt, Rinehart and Winston, New York.
Coulombre, J. L. and Coulombre, A. J. (1971): *Develop. Biol.*, *25*, 464.
Croisille, Y. and Le Douarin, N. M. (1965): In: *Organogenesis*, p. 421. Editors: R. L. DeHaan and H. Ursprung. Holt, Rinehart and Winston, New York.
Cunha, G. R. (1972): *Anat. Rec.*, *173*, 205.
Dodson, J. W. (1963): *Exp. Cell Res.*, *31*, 233.
Dodson, J. W. and Hay, E. D. (1971): *Exp. Cell Res.*, *65*, 215.
Dodson, J. W. and Hay, E. D. (1974): *J. exp. Zool.*, *189*, 51.
Goetinck, P. F. and Sekellick, M. J. (1972): *Develop. Biol.*, *28*, 636.
Grainger, R. and Wessells, N. K. (1974): *Proc. nat. Acad. Sci. (Wash.)*, *71*, 4747.
Grobstein, C. (1955): In: *Aspects of Synthesis and Order in Growth*, p. 233. Editor: D. Rudnick. Princeton University Press, Princeton.
Grobstein, C. (1967): *Nat. Cancer Inst. Monogr.*, *26*, 279.
Grobstein, C. and Cohen, J. (1965): *Science*, *150*, 626.
Hauschka, S. D. and White, N. K. (1972): In: *Research in Muscle Development and the Muscle Spindle*, p. 53. Editors: B. Q. Banker, R. J. Przybylski, J. P. van der Meulen and M. Victor. Excerpta Medica, Amsterdam.

Hay, E. D. (1963): *New Engl. J. Med., 268*, 114.
Hay, E. D. (1968): In: *Epithelial–Mesenchymal Interactions*, p. 31. Editors: R. Fleischmajer and R. E. Billingham. Williams and Wilkins Co., Baltimore, Maryland.
Hay, E. D. (1973): *Amer. Zool., 13*, 1085.
Hay, E. D. (1977): In: *First International Symposium on the Biology and Chemistry of Basement Membranes*. Editor: N. A. Kefalides. Academic Press, New York. In press.
Hay, E. D., Linsenmayer, T. F., Trelstad, R. L. and Von der Mark, K. (1977): In: *Current Topics in Eye Research*. Academic Press, New York. In press.
Hay, E. D. and Meier, S. (1974): *J. Cell Biol., 62*, 889.
Hay, E. D. and Meier, S. (1976): *Develop. Biol., 52*, 141.
Hay, E. D. and Meier, S. (1977): In: *Textbook of Oral Biology*. Editors: J. Shaw and S. Meller. W. B. Saunders, Co., Philadelphia. In press.
Holtfreter, J. (1948): *Symp. Soc. exp. Biol., 2*, 17.
Huang, D. (1974): *J. Cell Biol., 62* 881.
Hynes, R. O. (1976): *Biochim. biophys. Acta (Amst.), 458*, 73.
Kollar, E. and Baird, G. (1969): *J. Embryol. exp. Morph., 21*, 131.
Kollar, E. and Baird, G. (1970a): *J. Embryol. exp. Morph., 24*, 159.
Kollar, E. J. and Baird, G. R. (1970b): *J. Embryol. exp. Morph., 24*, 173.
Konigsberg, I. R. and Hauschka, S. D. (1965): In: *Reproduction: Molecular, Subcellular and Cellular*, p. 243. Editor: M. Locke. Academic Press, New York.
Kosher, R. A. and Church, R. L. (1975): *Nature (Lond.), 258*, 327.
Kosher, R. A. and Lash, J. (1975): *Develop. Biol., 42*, 362.
Kosher, R. A., Lash, J. W. and Minor, R. R. (1973): *Develop. Biol., 35*, 210.
Kratochwil, K. (1972): In: *Tissue Interactions in Carcinogenesis*, p. 1. Editor: D. Tarin, Academic Press, New York.
Kratochwil, K. and Schwartz, P. (1976): *Proc. nat. Acad. Sci. (Wash.), 73*, 4041.
Lash, J., Holtzer, S. and Holtzer, H. (1957): *Exp. Cell Res., 13*, 292.
Lash, J. and Vasan, N. S. (1977): In: *Cell and Tissue Interactions*. Editors: M. M. Burger and J. W. Lash. Raven Press, New York. In press.
Lehtonen, E. (1975): *J. Embryol. exp. Morph., 34*, 695.
Lehtonen, E., Wartiovaara, J., Nordling, S. and Saxén, L. (1975): *J. Embryol. exp. Morph., 33*, 187.
Levine, S., Pictet, R. and Rutter, W. J. (1973): *Nature New Biol., 246*, 49.
Lipton, B. H. and Jacobson, A. G. (1974): *Develop. Biol., 38*, 91.
Manasek, F. J. and Cohen, A. M. (1977): *Proc. nat. Acad. Sci. (Wash.),74*, 1057.
McLoughlin, C. B. (1961): *J. Embryol. exp. Morph., 9*, 385.
Meier, S. and Hay, E. D. (1974a): *Develop. Biol., 38*, 249.
Meier, S. and Hay, E. D. (1974b): *Proc. nat. Acad. Sci., 71*, 2310.
Meier, S. and Hay, E. D. (1975): *J. Cell Biol., 66*, 275.
Needham, J. (1942): *Biochemistry and Morphogenesis*. Cambridge, University Press.
Nevo, A. and Dorfman, A. (1972): *Proc. nat. Acad. Sci. (Wash.), 69*, 2069.
Newsome, D. A. (1976): *Develop. Biol., 49*, 496.
O'Hare, M. J. (1972): *J. Embryol. exp. Morph., 27*, 235.
Ordahl, C. P. and Caplan, A. I. (1976): *Develop. Biol., 54*, 61.
Overton, J. and Collins, J. (1976): *Develop. Biol., 48*, 80.
Pearlstein, E. (1976): *Nature (Lond.), 262*, 497.
Pictet, R. L. (1975): In: *Extracellular Matrix Influences on Gene Expression*, p. 531. Editors: H. C. Slavkin and R. C. Greulich. Academic Press, New York.
Ronzio, R. A. and Rutter, W. J. (1973): *Develop. Biol., 30*, 307.
Rutter, W. J. (1977): *Molecular Control of Proliferation and Differentiation*. Academic Press, New York
Rutter, W. J., Clark, W. R., Kemp, J. D., Bradshaw, W. S., Sanders, T. G. and Ball, W. D. (1968): In: *Epithelial-Mesenchymal Interactions*, p. 114. Editors: R. Fleischmajer and R. E. Billingham. Williams and Wilkins Co., Baltimore, Md.
Rutter, W. J., Wessells, N. K. and Grobstein, C. (1964): *Nat. Cancer Inst. Monogr., 13*, 51.
Saunders Jr, J. W. and Fallon, J. F. (1966): In: *Major Problems in Developmental Biology*, p. 289. Editor: M. Locke. Academic Press, New York.
Saxén, L., Lehtonen, E., Karkinen-Jaas Kelainen, M., Nordling, S. and Wartoivaara, J. (1976): *Nature (Lond.), 259*, 662.

Saxén, L. and Toivonen, S. (1962): *Primary Embryonic Induction*. Logos, London.

Slavkin, H. C. and Bringas, P. (1976): *Develop. Biol.*, *50*, 428.

Slavkin, H. C., Bringas Jr, P., Cameron, J., LeBaron, R. and Bavetta, L. A. (1969): *J. Embryol. exp. Morph.*, *22*, 395.

Slavkin, H. C., Bringas Jr, P., Croissant, R. and Bavetta, L. A. (1972): *Mechan. Aging and Develop.*, *1*, 139.

Slavkin, H. C. and Croissant, R. (1973): In: *The Role of RNA in Reproduction and Development*, p. 247. Editor: M. C. Niu and S. Segal. North-Holland Publishing Company, Amsterdam.

Smith, L. D. and Williams, M. A. (1975): In: *The Developmental Biology of Reproduction*, p. 3. Editors: C. L. Markert and J. Papaconstantinou. Academic Press, New York.

Spemann, H. (1938): *Embryonic Development and Induction*. Yale University Press, New Haven.

Spooner, B. S. (1974): In: *Concepts of Development*, p. 213. Editors: J. Lash and J. R. Whittaker. Sinauer Associates, Stamford.

Strudel, G. (1976): *Frontiers Matrix Biol.*, *3*, 77.

Stuart, E. S. and Moscona, A. A. (1967): *Science*, *157*, 947.

Thesleff, I., Lehtonen, E., Wartiovaara, J. and Saxén, L. (1977): *Develop. Biol.*, *58*, 197.

Toivonen, S., Tarin, D. and Saxen, L. (1976): *Differentiation*, *5*, 49.

Urist, M. R. and Iwata, H. (1973): *J. theoret. Biol.*, *38*, 155.

Wartiovaara, J., Nordling, S., Lehtonen, E. and Saxén, L. (1974): *J. Embryol. exp. Morph.*, *31*, 667.

Wessells, N. K. (1977): *Tissue Interactions in Development*. N. A. Benjamin, Inc., Menlo Park.

Wessells, N. K. and Cohen, J. H. (1968): *Develop. Biol.*, *18*, 294.

White, N. K., Bonner, P. H., Nelson, D. R. and Hauschka, S. D. (1975): *Develop. Biol.*, *44*, 346.

Wolff, E. (1970): *Tissue Interaction During Organogenesis*. Gordon and Breach, London.

Yamada, K. M. and Weston, J. A. (1975): *Cell*, *5*, 75.

Cell migrations during embryogenesis

An experimental analysis of the neural crest evolution by using the quail-chick marker system

NICOLE LE DOUARIN and CHRISTIANE LE LIEVRE

Institut d'Embryologie du C.N.R.S. et du Collège de France, Nogent-sur-Marne, France

Development has been divided into a *morphogenetic phase*, during which cells change shape and position to lay down the primitive plan of the body, and a *cytodifferentiation phase*, during which the individual cells acquire the special cellular and chemical features that characterize each particular tissue (Zwilling, 1968).

This division, although convenient, cannot be accepted as absolute because not only are there exceptions when the 2 processes occur simultaneously but also some kind of cytodifferentiation is a prerequisite for cells to engage in the shape changes that characterize the morphogenetic phase.

Regardless of the usefulness of this dichotomy, it has to be stated that most works on developmental problems have centered on the cytodifferentiation phase, neglecting the equally important problem of how the cells reach their definitive location. Thus, the mechanisms of cell migrations which occur during gastrulation and organogenesis, in spite of their fundamental nature, remain among the least understood of all developmental problems.

Although most cells seem to stay in place once histogenesis is complete, many kinds of cells can be stimulated to active mobility by removing a part of an organ or the complete organ. Stripping a piece of skin, for example, initiates locomotory activity in the cells of the marginal epidermis which will cover the wound. If differentiated tissues are explanted in vitro under suitable culture conditions, cells will migrate actively from the explant, demonstrating conclusively that virtually all tissue cells retain the capacity for locomotion.

The problem of mobility is interesting, both in relation to normal cells as also to the understanding of cancer. The extensive displacement of tumor cells when they become metastatic is apparently due in considerable part to the locomotory activity by individual tumor cells.

Our group has been interested in the analysis, during embryonic development in vivo, of cell migrations which play an important role in certain histogenetic

*This work was supported by the Centre National de la Recherche Scientifique, the Délégation Générale à la Recherche Scientifique, and by a Research Grant from the U.S. National Institute of Health (R01 DE0 4257 01CBY).

and organogenetic processes. We have especially investigated the migration of the *neural crest* cells and of the *blood stem* cells in the avian embryo (see reviews in Le Douarin, 1974, 1976, 1977a,b). This paper will be centered on the neural crest, a convenient model for investigating some of the general questions concerning the mechanisms of cell migration, such as: What factors start cells migrating? Which stop them? What are the pathways followed and are the cells motivated or passively guided in the course of their movements? How do the cells recognize the embryonic tissues in which they will become permanently located?

Although we are far from being able to answer all these questions satisfactorily, we will describe some experiments carried out on the autonomic nervous system which throw some light on them. At the same time, neural crest development provides one of the most spectacular systems in which an extensive migration of cells is a prerequisite for morphogenesis and histogenesis. This process will be described in the development of the head and neck in the avian embryo.

THE NEURAL CREST; METHODS FOR FOLLOWING ITS DEVELOPMENTAL FATE

The neural crest is a transitory structure which is characteristic of the vertebrate embryo. It arises from the neural fold, appears first in the head and progressively extends caudally during the closure of the neural tube. As soon as it is formed, the cells which participated in its constitution spread into the surrounding tissues and undergo extensive migrations in the developing embryo. They finally settle in various embryonic tissues and there differentiate into several cell types. Because of the diversity of its derivatives and the precise distribution of crest cells throughout the embryo, the neural crest has aroused the interest of many investigators. In common with most embryonic systems, the cells of the neural crest are un-differentiated when they begin to migrate and are, therefore, indistinguishable from the tissues through which they move. For this reason, experimental artefacts for studying their fate and the pathways they follow must be devised. The most suitable is to label the moving cells in one way or another. Labeling of the nuclei with tritiated thymidine was successfully used to follow the migration of the neural crest cells in the embryo of higher vertebrates by Weston (1963, 1970) and Johnston (1966). But although it is accurate and precise, it only provides information over a short period of time because the nuclear marker is unstable and becomes diluted through the rapid proliferation of the embryonic cells. Natural markers based on morpho-logical differences between 2 closely related species or between mutants of the same species are obviously more convenient. Some are available in amphibians but none had so far been used in higher vertebrates until one of us (Le Douarin, 1969–1973) devised a cell-marking technique and applied it to the migration of neural crest cells. It is based on a special feature of the interphase nucleus of the Japanese quail *(Coturnix coturnix japonica)*. In all embryonic and adult cell types of this species a large amount of heterochromatic DNA is associated with the nucleolus and can easily be visualized with the Feulgen-Rossenbeck stain or by the electron microscope after routine uranyl acetate-lead citrate staining. Such a disposition of the chromatin material does not usually occur in vertebrate cells in which the amount of nucleolus-

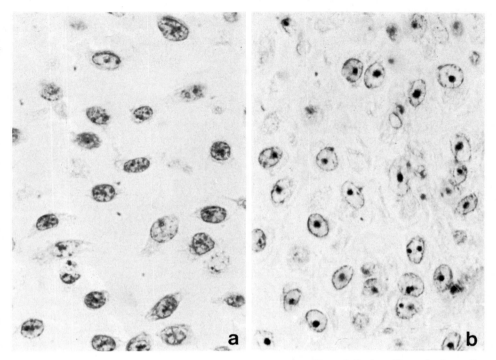

Fig. 1. Cartilage cells in the skull of 10-day-old embryos: (a) chick, (b) quail. Feulgen-Rossenbeck reaction. Note the presence of 1 or 2 large, heavily stained heterochromatic masses in the quail nuclei. G × 1280.

associated chromatin is small and usually undetectable by Feulgen-Rossenbeck staining. In chick or mouse cells, for example, the chromatin is evenly distributed in the nucleoplasm during the interphase and forms a fine network with only small dispersed chromocenters. The presence of heterochromatin condensations in the nucleus means that quail cells can be used as natural markers when combined in vitro or in vivo with chick or mouse tissues. The cells of the combined species retain their characteristics in the chimeras and can be identified whatever the duration of the association (Fig. 1).

The experimental procedure we used to follow the neural crest cell migration in vivo caused minimal disturbance to the normal course of development. Grafts of fragments of quail neural tube and associated neural folds were implanted isotopically into chick embryos of the same developmental stages. The chick neural primordium was excised by microsurgery, the endoderm, notochord and somites being left in situ. The quail neural tube and associated neural folds were isolated by incubating transverse sections of the quail embryo in Mg^{2+}-, Ca^{2+}-free Tyrode solution with 0.1 % trypsin added. Thus, the grafted neural anlage was completely uncontaminated by mesenchymal cells. In a second step, the quail neural primordium was grafted into the chick host in the groove resulting from the excision (Fig. 2).

To ensure that crest cells had not migrated at the time of the graft, we varied the level of the operation according to the developmental stage of the embryo. The more

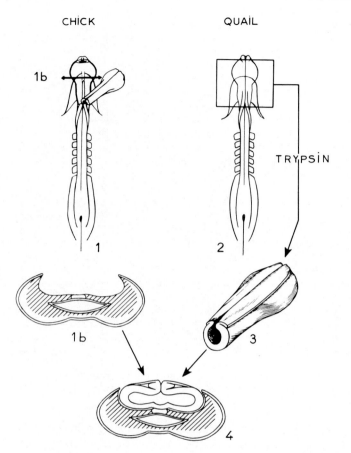

CHICK   QUAIL

Fig. 2. Operation technique for orthotopic grafts of quail neural tube and crest into a chick embryo: (1) removal of the prosencephalo-mesencephalic primordium from a 5-somite chick embryo; (2) preparation; and (3) isolation of the equivalent primordium from a 6-somite quail embryo; (4) cross section at the level of the graft.

cranial the level of the neural crest investigated, the younger the embryo. Operations involving the prosencephalon were done at the 2- to 5-somite stage, for the mesencephalon at the 4- to 6-somite stage, and for the rhombencephalon at the 6- to 12-somite stage. The experiments on the spinal cord were done at the level of the last somites formed.

Whatever the level of the graft, the grafted tissue was rapidly covered by healing host ectoderm and underwent normal histogenesis. In the head region where the operations were done at early developmental stages, malformations of the encephalon were sometimes seen, especially in the forebrain. The graft was often made unilaterally at this level, a procedure which in most cases ensured normal development of the head.

We were able to follow the migration of the implanted neural crest cells of the quail until they were fully differentiated. The stability of the labeling provided by the nuclear marker meant that quail cells could be recognized in sections of the host embryo either after Feulgen-Rossenbeck staining or in the electron microscope.

In the trunk region, the sensory and orthosympathetic ganglia and the aortic adrenergic plexus were entirely made up of quail cells at the level of the graft. In rachidian nerves and communicating ramus, the Schwann cells also showed the nuclear marker. On the other hand, when a quail neural tube was grafted into a White Leghorn chick, quail melanoblasts migrated into the host skin, the feathers of which exhibited the characteristic pigmentation of the donor. Observation of the well-known derivatives of the neural crest, such as sensory ganglia, orthosympathetic chains and melanocytes, indicated that in our experimental conditions the patterns of differentiation and migration of the grafted cells did not differ in the host from those of normal development. When this had been established, the normal fate of the crest was investigated at the cephalic and trunk levels of the neural axis. This enabled us to identify derivatives of the neural crest which had so far remained unknown.

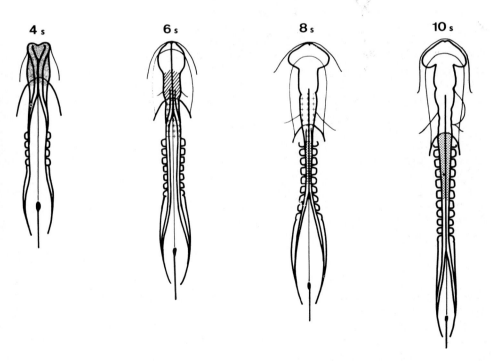

Fig. 3. Level and stage conditions of the graft. The graft was performed at various levels of the encephalic primordium, before neural crest cells start migrating, i.e. before:

the 6-somite stage at the prosencephalic level,
the 7-somite stage at the mesencephalic level,
the 10-somite stage at the anterior and medium rhombencephalic level,
the 12-somite stage at the posterior part of the rhombencephalon.

CONTRIBUTION OF THE NEURAL CREST TO HEAD
AND NECK MORPHOGENESIS

Various types of grafts were carried out as indicated in Figure 3. The cells originating from the grafted neural crest could subsequently be found in the following locations: the frontonasal area for prosencephalic grafts, the maxillary process and the first branchial arch for the mesencephalic grafts and the other branchial arches for the rhombencephalic grafts (Fig. 4). The differentiation of the neural crest cells was then followed and they appeared to give rise to the cartilage and membrane bones

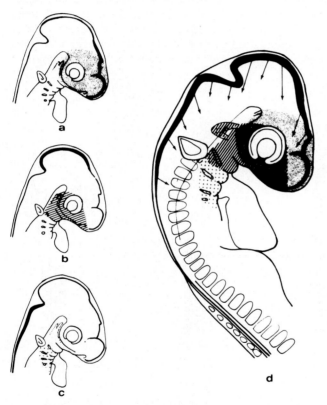

Fig. 4. Localization of neural crest-derived cells in the head and branchial regions of a stage 20 (Hamburger and Hamilton, 1951) chick embryo, according to their level of origin: (a) prosencephalon; (b) mesencephalon; (c) rhombencephalon; (d) derivatives of the whole cephalic neural crest.

Fig. 5. Mesectodermal derivatives of the grafted quail neural primordium in the chick host (Feulgen-Rossenbeck reaction). (a) Quail osteocytes in a mandibular bone of an 8-day chick embryo operated upon at the mesencephalic level (G × 600). (b) Feather germ of the facial skin of a 12-day chick embryo (G × 250). The graft was made at the mesencephalic level. The germ pulp and the dermis originate from the graft while the epithelium belongs to the host. (c) Cross section of the neck of a 9-day-old chick embryo. The graft was made at the rhombencephalic level (G × 150). ca = carotid artery, p = parathyroid. (d) Higher magnification of the same section. The wall of the carotid artery is formed by neural crest-derived (quail) cells except for the endothelium which is made up of chick cells (G × 600).

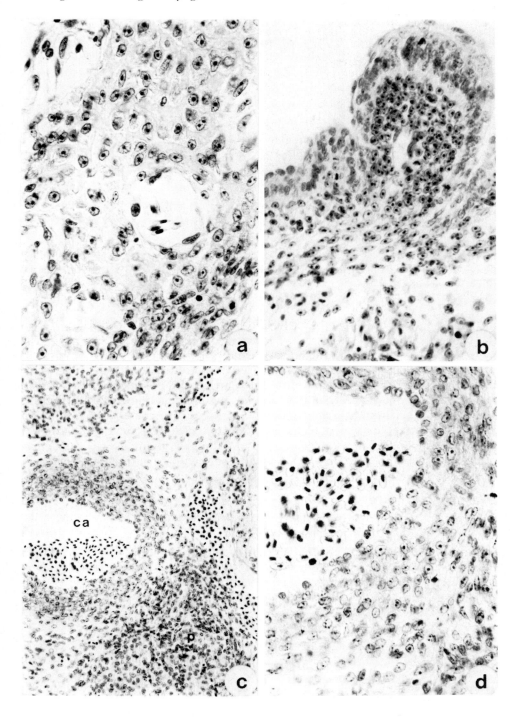

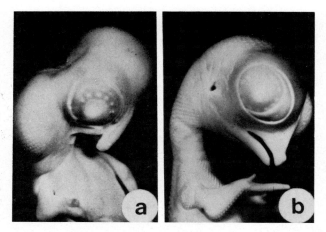

Fig. 6. Effect on the morphogenesis of the head and neck of removal of the cephalic neural primordium. (a) The mesencephalic and rhombencephalic primordia of this 8.5-day-old embryo were removed before the beginning of neural crest cell migration. Note the atrophy of the superior part of the beak, of the lids and interocular region, and of the ventral part of the neck. The inferior part of the beak, the mandible and tongue are missing (G × 3). (b) Control chick embryo at the same age.

of the face and of the visceral skeleton, to the dermis of the same regions and to the connective tissue of the face, the lower jaw and the tongue (Fig. 5a,b). The mesenchymal components of the salivary glands (thymus, parathyroid and thyroid) were also shown to be neurectodermal derivatives. In addition, the formation of the blood vessels which originate from the aortic arches and become the large arterial trunks arising from the heart entirely depends on an immigration of cells from the neural crest. Their wall is in fact composite in nature: the endothelial cells, which in our experiments are always of the host type, are of mesodermal origin. Shortly after its formation, the endothelial capillary of the developing arch becomes surrounded by neural crest cells which thereafter differentiate into the muscular and connective tissue wall of the arteries (Fig. 5c) (Le Lièvre and Le Douarin, 1975; Le Lièvre, 1978).

The rhombencephalic neural crest was found to give rise to glandular derivatives: the calcitonin-producing cells of the ultimobranchial body and the type I cells of the carotid body (see Le Douarin, 1974, 1976).

That the cephalic neural crest largely participates in head morphogenesis is confirmed by excision experiments in which the neural primordium is removed early from a chick embryo, for example, at the level of the mesencephalon and rhombencephalon, when the face, the lower jaw and the neck show important deficiencies (Fig. 6).

THE DEVELOPMENT OF THE AUTONOMIC NERVOUS SYSTEM

Transplantations of fragments of quail neural primordium were systematically carried out along the whole length of the neural axis. We have, in these experiments, especially focussed our interest on the formation of the autonomic nervous system.

Indeed, it provides an appropriate model to approach some of the questions we initially posed in relation to the developmental potentialities and the migration pathways of the neural crest cells.

The autonomic nervous system is divided into 2 trunks: *sympathetic* and *parasympathetic*. Both act on the same target cells antagonistically through 2 different neurotransmitters, a catecholamine for the sympathetic system and acetylcholine for the other. The ganglionic cells of both originate from the neural crest and, at an early developmental stage, migrate ventrally. Some cells stop in the dorsal structures of the trunk and give rise to the adrenergic sympathetic neurons and to the adrenomedullary paraganglia, while others migrate more ventrally and colonize the splanchnopleural mesenchyme to form the cholinergic parasympathetic enteric ganglia.

Two main questions arise concerning the development of the autonomic nervous system: (1) What are the factors controlling the precise and selective distribution

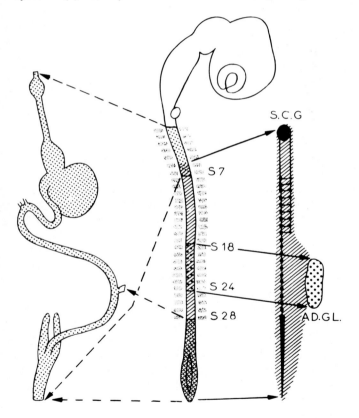

Fig. 7. Diagram showing the origin of adrenomedullary cells and autonomic ganglion cells. The spinal neural crest caudad to the level of the 5th somite gives rise to the ganglia of the orthosympathetic chain. The adrenomedullary cells originate from the spinal neural crest between the level of somites 18 and 24. The vagal neural crest (somites 1 to 7) gives rise to the parasympathetic enteric ganglia of the pre-umbilical region, the ganglia of the post-umbilical gut originating from both the vagal and lumbosacral neural crest. The ganglion of Remak is derived from the lumbosacral neural crest (posterior to the 28th somite level).

of the autonomic ganglioblasts in the trunk and in the viscera? (2) Are the neural crest cells pluripotential when they begin to migrate or are they already programmed to differentiate into adrenergic neurons, adrenomedullary cells or cholinergic neurons?

To investigate this problem we first determined the level of the neural axis from which the parasympathetic enteric ganglia, the orthosympathoblasts and the adrenomedullary cells originate in the normal development. This question is indeed controversial. It has generally been accepted that each level of the neural crest gives rise to both orthosympathetic and parasympathetic ganglia at the same transverse level of the embryo. In fact, using the quail–chick transplant technique to follow the migration of the neural crest cells we obtained a completely different picture of the phenomenon (Fig. 7).

The ganglion cells of the orthosympathetic system originate from the whole neural crest caudad to the level of the 5th somite. The particular region located at the level of somites 18–24 furnishes, in addition, the adrenomedullary cells of the suprarenal gland. The parasympathetic ganglia, which are responsible for the innervation of the gut, are derived from the vagal region of the neural primordium (level of somites 1–7) and the lumbosacral region behind the 28th somite. Therefore, the neural crest is divided into several sections: (a) one from which only enteric cholinergic ganglia originate (level 1–5 somites); (b) one from which only catecholaminergic cells arise; and (c) 2 others, which are able to give rise to both adrenergic and cholinergic cells (Le Douarin and Teillet, 1973; Le Douarin, 1977a; Le Douarin et al., 1976).

It was then of interest to investigate whether the neuroblasts originating from these various regions of the neural crest are already committed to differentiate into adrenergic and cholinergic neurons respectively. To answer this question, we have experimentally changed the pattern of crest cell migration.

We know that in normal development the autonomic neuroblasts of the cervicodorsal neural crest do not migrate into the intestine but give rise exclusively to catecholamine-producing cells. Thus, it seemed of interest to discover whether they could migrate into the intestine if transplanted at an early developmental stage at the vagal level of the neural crest. For this purpose, the 'adrenomedullary' level of the quail neural crest (from somites 18–24) was grafted into the 'vagal' region (from somites 1–7) of a chick embryo (Fig. 8). Conversely, the cephalic neural crest including mesencephalon or rhombencephalon of a quail was grafted at the adrenomedullary level of a chick in order to see whether the cephalic neuroblasts migrate into the suprarenal gland and differentiate into adrenomedullary cells. In the latter experiment, we found that the suprarenal glands of the host developed normally with strands of cells containing fluorogenic catecholamines. Post-staining of the same slide with Feulgen showed that the cells which fluoresce had the quail nucleus and were derived from the graft. At the electron microscope level, they also had both the electron-dense secretory granules characteristic of the adrenomedullary cells and the large DNA-rich nucleolus of the quail.

In the other experiment, in which a quail neural fragment from the level of the 18th–24th somite was grafted into a chick at the hindbrain level, we found that quail neural cells migrated into the gut and gave rise to enteric ganglia. In normal development, most of the cells originating from this part of the neural tube, form

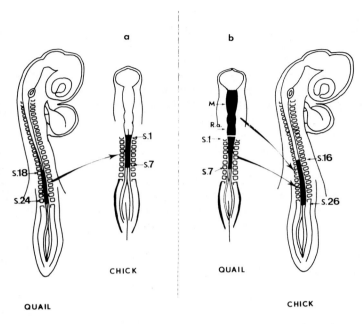

Fig. 8. Heterotopic grafts of quail neural primordium into the chick embryo. (a) The neural tissue is taken at the adrenomedullary level and grafted at the vagal level. (b) The quail primordium is removed from the mesencephalon and anterior rhombencephalon or at the vagal level and grafted into the adrenome-dullary region.

adrenergic ganglia or adrenomedullary cells. Thus, it was of interest to see whether they express their normal phenotype when they migrate into the gut. The application of the FIF technique according to Falck to these preparations showed that the neurons which differentiated in the intestine did not contain detectable catechol-amines (Le Douarin and Teillet, 1974). By applying a physiological test to these preparations we were able to demonstrate that, in fact, the neuroblasts originating from the adrenomedullary level of the neural crest differentiate into functional cholinergic neurons in the gut environment (Le Douarin et al., 1975).

It can be concluded from these experiments that the migration of neural crest cells is not random, but that preferential pathways exist in the developing body. In the dorsal region from somites 18–24 the crest cells are guided to the suprarenal glands, while at the hind brain level they are directed to the gut. In addition, it appears that the neuroblasts are not committed to differentiate into cholinergic or adrenergic neurons when they begin to migrate. Their evolution in terms of their capacity to synthesize neurotransmitters depends on the environment they meet either during their migration or after they have settled in their definitive location.

In order to investigate whether the crest cells undergo changes of developmental significance during their migration we have devised an experiment in which the neural crest is directly associated with the gut (Smith et al., 1977). We were able to show that the initial phase of migration that the neural crest cells undergo to reach the gut has no significant effect on their subsequent development. Ganglioblasts from the 'adrenomedullary' level of the neural axis differentiate into cholinergic cells not only after transplantation at the 'vagal' level of the neural primordium in vivo, as reported above, but also, after direct association with the gut. Therefore, the first extra-intestinal migration phase does not seem to have any developmental importance as regards the subsequent differentiation of the autonomic neuron precursor cells. The latter, on the contrary, depends entirely on the influence of the tissue environment in which the cells become localized at the end of their migration.

DISCUSSION AND CONCLUSIONS

This brief review of our studies on neural crest cells in vivo by using a natural cell marking technique shows that this transitory structure plays an important role in head and neck morphogenesis. It appears also that crest cells receive, after they have left their original site, informative signals which influence the expression of their final phenotype.

Our knowledge about the constitution of the environment in which the neural crest cells move is still uncertain. However, evidence concerning its chemical nature has now accumulated. Biochemical and radioautographic studies using ^{3}H-glucosamine (Pratt et al., 1975) have shown that, just prior to migration, a hyaluronate-rich, cell-free space appears along the cell migration pathway, between the peripheral ectoderm, the neural tube and the somite. Toole and coworkers have shown similar associations between cell migration and hyaluronate production and suggest that the hyaluronic acid may prevent interaction of the migrating cells with other components in their environment until they reach their final locations where hyaluronidase is produced (Toole, 1974).

The way by which the crest cells recognize the embryonic primordium into which they become localized and thus stop migrating remains an open question. Contact inhibition as described by Abercrombie (1961, 1970) in vitro is an obvious model for arresting cells, once they contact each other. However, the evidence is conflicting about whether cells in intact tissues move over each other's surfaces, or over a thin sheet of intervening intercellular material. Despite some information in the literature, careful investigation on this point is still needed, in particular to see whether there is a change in cell-to-cell contact relations when they cease migrating. Other ways by which cells might halt each other's movement through interactions are by transmission of a signal passing from an immobilized cell to a moving one with which it comes in contact, and by adhering specifically to other cells of the same kind (isotypic adhesion) or of another kind (heterotopic adhesion). Evidence has accumulated that specific cell adhesion (either by means of qualitatively specific sites or as a result of quantitative differences of adhesiveness) exists (Moscona, 1962; Roth, 1968, 1973; Steinberg, 1970; Boucaut, 1974a,b).

In respect of the neural crest, experiments are now in progress which indicate that specific sites of arrest for the cells are present in the embryo. These sites are recognized by the cells irrespective of the level of the neural axis from which they originate (Le Douarin, Teillet, Ziller, unpublished data). However, no information is available concerning the mechanism of cell-cell recognition which is responsible for the homing of crest cells to these particular places.

REFERENCES

Abercrombie, M. (1961): *Exp. Cell Res., Suppl. 8*, 188.
Abercrombie, M. (1970): *In Vitro, 6*, 128.
Boucaut, J. C. (1974a): *Ann. Embryol. Morphog., 7*, 7.
Boucaut, J. C. (1974b): *Ann. Embryol. Morphog., 7*, 119.
Hamburger, V. and Hamilton, H. L. (1951): *J. Morphol., 88*, 49.
Johnston, M. C. (1966): *Anat. Rec., 156*, 130.
Le Douarin, N. (1969): *Bull. biol. France Belg., 103*, 435.
Le Douarin, N. (1973): *Develop. Biol., 30*, 217.
Le Douarin, N. (1974): *Med. Biol., 52*, 281.
Le Douarin, N. (1976): In: *Embryogenesis in Mammals. Ciba Foundation Symposium 40, (New Series)*, p. 71. Editors: K. Elliott and M. O'Connor. Excerpta Medica–Elsevier–North-Holland, Amsterdam–Oxford–New York.
Le Douarin, N. (1977a): In: *Cell Interactions in Differentiation*, p. 171. Sigrid Juselius Symposium, Helsinki. Editors: M. Karkinen-Jääskeläinen, L. Saxén and L. Weiss. Academic Press, London.
Le Douarin, N. (1977b): In: *B and T Cells in Immune Recognition*, p. 1. Editors: F. Loor and G. E. Roelants. John Wiley and Sons, London.
Le Douarin, N., Renaud, D., Teillet, M. A. and Le Douarin, G. H. (1975): *Proc. nat. Acad. Sci. (Wash.), 72*, 728.
Le Douarin, N. and Teillet, M. A. (1973): *C. R. Acad. Sci., 277*, 1929.
Le Douarin, N. and Teillet, M. A. (1974): *Develop. Biol., 41*, 162.
Le Douarin, N., Teillet, M. A. and Le Lièvre, C. (1977): In: *Cell and Tissue Interactions*, p. 11. 30th Annual Meeting of the Society of General Physiologists, 1976, Marine Biol. Lab., Woods Hole, Mass. Editors: J. W. Lash and M. M. Burger. Raven Press, New York.
Le Lièvre, C. S. (1978): *J. Embryol. exp. Morphol.*, in press.
Le Lièvre, C. S. and Le Douarin, N. (1975): *J. Embryol. exp. Morphol., 34*, 124.
Moscona, A. A. (1962): *J. cell. comp. Physiol., Suppl. 1, 60*, 65.
Pratt, R. M., Larsen, M. A. and Johnston, M. C. (1975): *Develop. Biol., 44*, 298.
Roth, S. (1968): *Develop. Biol., 18*, 602.
Roth, S. (1973): *Quart. Rev. Biol., 48*, 541.
Smith, J., Cochard, P. and Le Douarin, N. (1977): *Cell Diff., 6*, 199.
Steinberg, M. S. (1970): *J. exp. Zool., 173*, 395.
Toole, B. P. (1974): *Amer. Zool., 13*, 1061.
Weston, J. A. (1963): *Develop. Biol., 6*, 279.
Weston, J. A. (1970): *Advanc. Morphogenesis, 8*, 41.
Zwilling, E. (1968): In: *The Emergence of Order in Developing Systems, Develop. Biol., Suppl. 2*, p. 184. Editor: M. Locke. Academic Press, New York.

Developmental potency of normal and neoplastic cells of the early mouse embryo *

R. L. GARDNER

Department of Zoology, University of Oxford, United Kingdom

Differentiation in multicellular organisms seems to be attributable principally to differences in gene activity rather than gene content of somatic cells (Davidson, 1976). Furthermore, the potential for expressing specific programs of gene activity tends to be a heritable cellular trait. This has been deduced from studies on the potency of cells in a variety of abnormal situations (Weiss, 1939; Ursprung, 1968; Bernhard, 1977). The purpose of this article is to summarize recent studies on the potency of normal cells of the early mammalian embryo and their neoplastic counterparts, and to consider some of the implications of this work. Unless indicated otherwise, all experiments and observations relate to the mouse since it has proved the species of choice for most of this research.

Several factors need to be taken into account in attempting to design critical tests of the developmental potentialities of embryonic cells. First, particularly before they become overtly differentiated, cells that are alike in morphology may differ strikingly in potency (e.g. Hadorn, 1966). Hence, unequivocal results can only be obtained by testing single cells. This approach also ensures that the cells are effectively exposed to the particular environment in which they are placed, which may not be the case in the more traditional approach of re-locating relatively large undissociated tissue fragments (Gardner and Papaioannou, 1975). In principle, the simplest way of investigating single cells is by plating them individually or at very low density in culture (Kruse and Patterson, 1973). This has been widely adopted to study the differentiation of a variety of plant and animal cells. However, with exception of cleavage blastomeres, cells of the early mammalian embryo have so far proved refractory to cloning in vitro (Cole and Paul, 1965; Sherman, 1975). Even if cells can be cloned thus, a simple culture system may not be able to support expression of the full range of differentiated cell types that they are capable of forming. Therefore, it is important to also carry out experiments in vivo, and this poses other problems. Above all one must be able to distinguish donor from host cells. Genetic polymorphism provides the only source of cell markers with the stability and heritability essential for clonal analysis in vivo. Marker genes must be cell-limited in their sphere

* Financially supported by The Medical Research Council and The Cancer Research Campaign.

154

of action and expressed in all types of cell. The nature and limitations of genetic markers that are currently available in the mouse are discussed elsewhere (Gardner and Johnson, 1975; McLaren, 1976a).

Potency testing of single cells has been undertaken in adult hosts (Kleinsmith and Pierce, 1964). However, the cloning efficiency was very low. Such tests are further complicated by the need to ensure either that the donor and host are histocompatible, or that the latter is tolerant to cells of the former (Burnet, 1969). Finally, one is again confronted with the problem of adequacy of the environment, particularly for enabling realization of the potency of early embryonic cells. Fertilized eggs, for example, tend to develop only extra-embryonic membranes and trophoblastic tissue when 'cloned' ectopically in adult mice (Kirby, 1970).

The author was prompted by the above considerations to seek a means of cloning single cells of early embryonic origin in vivo in embryos of appropriate gestational age. The possibility of achieving this aim was encouraged by the success with which chimeric mice could be produced by aggregating cleaving eggs (Tarkowski, 1961; Mintz, 1965). However, although embryo aggregation has many applications (see Mintz, 1974; McLaren, 1976a), injection of cells into the more advanced blastocyst stage (Gardner, 1968, 1971) proved the method of choice for clonal analysis (Gardner, 1977a,b). The technique is described in detail elsewhere (Gardner, 1977a). It is important when cloning cells in the early embryo to ensure that their contribution to the resulting chimeras is as large as possible; otherwise, failure to differentiate into certain types of cell may be due to restriction in spatial distribution rather than potency of the clone. Judicious choice of the genotypes of donor and host embryos (Mullen and Whitten, 1971; Kelly, 1977), or experimental reduction in cell number of the host embryos (Lin, 1969; Kelly, 1975; 1977), are 2 ways of imposing a favorable bias.

POTENCY OF NORMAL CELLS IN THE EARLY EMBRYO

Totipotency at the 2-cell stage in the mouse has been demonstrated unequivocally by the production of viable young following destruction of one of the blastomeres (Tarkowski, 1959; Hoppe and Whitten, 1972). Although single blastomeres from 4- and 8-cell embryos can form blastocysts in vitro (Tarkowski and Wroblewska, 1967; Sherman, 1975), and undergo implantation in utero (Rossant, 1976a), they are apparently incapable of normal postimplantation development. When examined at the blastocyst stage they show a greater deficiency of inner cell mass (ICM) than trophectoderm cells, and may be altogether devoid of the former. The magnitude of this effect, and hence the frequency of trophectodermal vesicles, is greater with 1/8 than with 1/4 blastomeres. However, experiments in which isolated blastomeres were combined with 'carrier' blastomeres of a different genotype established that all 4 cells are able to undergo both trophectodermal and ICM differentiation following isolation at the 4-cell stage (Hillman et al., 1972), as are the 2 daughters of a 1/4 blastomere at the 8-cell stage (Kelly, 1975, 1977). Hence, failure of such blastomeres to develop normally in isolation seems to be due to a deficiency of cells rather than to loss of totipotency. Several experimental manipulations have been used to examine cellular potency in later cleavage. While these studies suggest that totipotency is retained throughout cleavage until the late morula or early blastocyst stage, none is unequivocal because clonal techniques were not used. Also, cell position in the blastocyst was the only assay of cell potency that was employed (see Gardner, 1975a, for more detailed discussion).

By 3.5 days post-coitum (p.c.) the embryo is an expanded blastocyst composed of nearly 60 cells from which isolation of pure trophectoderm and ICM tissue can be achieved microsurgically (Gardner, 1971; Gardner and Johnson, 1972). A variety of experimental tests have been carried out on these 2 classes of cells which provide no evidence for persisting lability (Gardner, 1971, 1975a,b, 1977b; Gardner and Johnson, 1972; Rossant, 1975a,b, 1976b). The strongest support for the conclusion that ICM and trophectoderm cells are determined by this stage comes from cloning single cells of both tissues in early morulae of a different genotype (Rossant and Gardner, 1977; R. L. Gardner, unpublished data). Clearly, therefore, the period of development between approximately 2.5 and 3.5 days p.c. merits close investigation by clonal techniques, since it almost certainly spans the stage when the first restrictions in cellular potency occur.

Further differentiation of cells is evident morphologically within both the trophectoderm and ICM by 4.5 days p.c. when the blastocyst has begun to implant. Mural trophectoderm cells have started to enlarge relative to polar (Fig. 1; also Dickson, 1966), a process that is accompanied by endoreduplication of their genomes (Barlow and Sherman, 1972; Sherman et al., 1972). Polar trophectoderm cells continue to divide, though those displaced by growth from the ICM region also undergo giant cell formation (Gardner, 1975a). The contrasting behavior of mural and polar cells is therefore not autonomous, but seems to depend on the ICM and its later derivatives. This impression has been substantiated by studying the

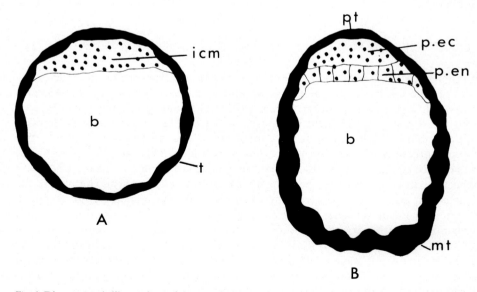

Fig. 1. Diagrammatic illustrations of the morphology of (A) 3.5 day, and (B) 4.5 day p.c. mouse blastocysts. b = blastocoelic cavity; icm = inner cell mass; mt = mural trophectoderm; p.ec = primitive ectoderm; p.en = primitive endoderm; pt = polar trophectoderm.

development in utero of trophectodermal vesicles (Gardner, 1971; Gardner and Johnson, 1972) and blastocyst reconstituted from genetically dissimilar trophectoderm and ICM tissue (Gardner et al., 1973). The former yield only giant cells and the latter normal conceptuses whose extensive trophoblast expresses the genetic marker characterising the trophectoderm donor embryos. As well as highlighting a vital indirect role for the ICM in trophoblast proliferation, the reconstitution experiments demonstrated that mural trophectoderm cells can form polar cells at 3.5 day p.c. (Gardner et al., 1973). Since polar cells form giant cells among their progeny and, indeed, growth of mural trophectoderm in the late blastocyst occurs by recruitment of cells from the polar region (A. J. Copp, personal communication of unpublished data), it would appear likely that all trophectodermal cells are equipotential at 3.5 days p.c. Mitotic activity in diploid derivatives of the polar trophectoderm continues to exhibit dependence on ICM derivatives until at least day 9 of gestation (Rossant and Ofer, 1977). So far, the nature of the interaction has remained elusive. It merits further investigation both from the point of view of understanding how growth of the trophoblast is linked to that of the embryo, and also elucidating control mechanisms in the eukaryotic cell cycle.

The 4.5-day p.c. ICM consists of nearly equal numbers of primitive endoderm and primitive ectoderm cells (McLaren, 1976b). The former are arranged in a monolayer on the blastocoelic surface of the ICM (Fig. 1), and can be distinguished from the latter in suspensions of enzymatically dissociated ICMs. Injection of primitive endoderm cells, either singly or in small groups, into host blastocysts leads to chimerism in only the extra-embryonic derivatives of later conceptuses (Gardner and Papaioannou, 1975). Similar transplantations using primitive ectoderm cells consistenly yield both extra-embryonic and fetal chimerism. The distribution of progeny of the 2 categories of cell was consistent with commitment of primitive endoderm to extra-embryonic endodermal differentiation, and primitive ectoderm cells to formation of the entire fetus plus extra-embryonic mesoderm (Gardner and Papaioannou, 1975). Further support for this conclusion comes from recent experiments in which the visceral yolk sacs of presumptive chimeras were separated into endoderm and mesoderm prior to analysis. Mesoderm was exclusively host type in all conceptuses developing from blastocysts receiving primitive endoderm cells, despite up to 50 % or more donor cells in the adjacent endoderm. Conversely, in those injected with primitive ectoderm cells at the blastocyst stage, the donor cell contribution was confined to the mesodermal component of the visceral yolk sac (Gardner and Rossant, 1977). Since single 3.5-day p.c. ICM cell clones, though not conspicuously larger, can embrace both territories, determination of primitive endoderm versus primitive ectoderm cells must occur subsequent to determination of trophectoderm versus ICM (Rossant and Gardner, 1977).

The potency of 4.5-day primitive ectoderm cells has been investigated more closely by studying postnatal chimeras. More than 20 % of mice obtained from blastocysts injected with single cells are overt chimeras (R. L. Gardner and M. F. Lyon, unpublished data). Detailed analysis of a series of these mice in which the donor clone carried chromosomal markers revealed that chimerism was extensive in a wide variety of organs and tissues originating from all 3 definitive germ layers (C. E. Ford, E. P. Evans, R. L. Gardner and M. F. Lyon, unpublished data). So far no restrictions have been found in the spectrum of adult cell types that single primitive ectodermal clones can form. Formation of functional gametes in addition to somatic cells has been proved by breeding tests (R. L. Gardner and M. F. Lyon, unpublished data).

Nevertheless, one cannot assume at present that all primitive ectoderm cells possess such wide potency at this stage of development, because only a proportion of them yield detectable clones following injection into blastocysts. The cloning efficiency in a representative series of experiments is presented in Table 1. Several factors probably contribute to the unavoidable losses encountered in transplanting blastocysts to the uteri of recipient mice (McLaren and Michie, 1956). There is no evidence that the viability of blastocysts can be affected by the type of embryonic cell injected into them. Indeed, the rate of development of blastocysts injected with a variety of types of cells is comparable to that of 'sham-operated' and uninjected ones (Gardner, 1968, and unpublished observations; Moustafa and Brinster, 1972). However, even assuming absence of pre-natal selection, one still has to explain why roughly three-quarters of the offspring obtained from blastocysts injected with single primitive ectoderm cells appear to be non-chimeric. Several non-specific factors may play a part, but their significance is hard to evaluate. For example, although morphological and dye exclusion criteria are used to select cells for transplantation, these are obviously less stringent tests of cell viability than capacity for massive clonal proliferation in vivo. In some instances the donor cell is clearly not integrated into the host ICM. In addition, recent work by Snow (1977) suggests that later growth of primitive ectoderm derivatives is largely attributable to very rapid cycling within a relatively small focus of cells. The proportion of overt chimeras might therefore reflect the frequency with which the donor clone contributed to the latter. This hypothesis presupposes that the majority of donor cells form much smaller clones that elude detection. This seems unlikely unless the latter only colonize internal tissues since the chimeras were identified primarily on the basis of pigmentation mosaicism in the eyes and coat, where very low levels of donor contribution can be discerned. It is not possible at present to dismiss the possibility that the future proliferative characteristics of primitive ectoderm cells are already determined at the late blastocyst stage.

The conclusion that the entire fetal soma is formed from the primitive ectoderm and that primitive endoderm forms only extra-embryonic endoderm brings the early mouse embryo into line with that of the chick (Bellairs, 1971). It is supported by the results of experiments in which later derivatives of these tissues were grafted to ectopic sites in both the rat and mouse (Skreb et al., 1976; Diwan and Stevens,

TABLE 1

Cloning efficiency of single 4.5-day p.c. primitive ectoderm cells in 3.5-day p.c. blastocysts

Injected blastocysts		Offspring		
Total number transferred	Number transferred to recipients that became pregnant	Number of offspring born	Number of chimeric offspring	Number of chimeras reaching adulthood
138	104	79	18	16

From R. L. Gardner and M. F. Lyon, unpublished data.

1976). What is perhaps more unexpected is the finding that primitive ectoderm cells can give rise to functional gametes, since germ cells have been widely assumed to originate from the extra-embryonic endoderm of the yolk sac (Brambell, 1956; Franchi et al., 1962). The possibility of a dual origin for these cells has been investigated by test-breeding 'primitive endoderm chimeras', none of which has so far transmitted genetic markers of the donor strain (R. L. Gardner, unpublished data). Two points follow from the present findings. First, since single primitive ectoderm cells yield both somatic and germ cell chimerism, the germ cell lineage must segregate later than 4.5 days p.c. Second, although germ cells ultimately express totipotency, they are descended from a cell that does not.

It would be interesting to know whether all primitive ectoderm cells in the late blastocyst are potential germ cell precursors, or whether this property is restricted to a sub-population of them. In attempting to answer this question one is confronted with the problem of cloning efficiency discussed earlier, and with the fact that donor and host cells are of opposite chromosomal sex in approximately half the chimeras (Table 2). Mintz (1969, 1974) asserts that in XX–XY chimeras functional gametes can be formed only by the constituent cell population whose genetic sex accords with the phenotypic sex of the organism. However, while there is considerable evidence that XX germ cells cannot form functional spermatozoa in phenotypic males (e.g. Cattanach, 1975), the capacity for differentiation of XY cells as oocytes in phenotypically female chimeras has not been adequately explored. Recent observations have indeed established that XY oocytes can develop to diakinesis in female chimeras (Evans et al., 1977), and that they can probably support normal development (Ford et al., 1975a).

TABLE 2

Origin of functional germ cells in a series of chimeras obtained by injecting single 4.5-day p.c. primitive ectoderm cells into 3.5-day p.c. host blastocysts

Chimera code No.	Phenotypic sex	Genotypic sex		Germ line
		Donor	Host	
CGL 45	♂	XX	XY	host
GCL 46*	♂	XY	XY	host
CGL 47*	♂	XY	XY	host
CGL 48	♀	XY	XX	sterile
CGL 62	♂	XX	XY	host
CGL 63*	♂	XY	XY	mixed
CGL 64*	♂	XY	XY	mixed
CGL 66	♂	XX	XY	host
CGL 67*	♂	XY	XY	host
CGL 68	♂	XX	XY	host
CGL 69	♀	XY	XX	host
CGL 70	♀	?	XX	host
CGL 71	♀	XY	XX	host
CGL 72*	♀	XX	XX	host
CGL 73*	♂	XY	XY	host
CGL 74	♂	XX	XY	host

* Mice in which the genetic sex of the donor cell accords with that of the host. From C. E. Ford, E. P. Evans, R. L. Gardner and M. F. Lyon, unpublished data.

Breeding data on a series of chimeras obtained by transplanting single primitive ectoderm cells into blastocysts are presented in Table 2. The chromosomal sex of both the donor and host cells was determined in all but one animal. The phenotypic sex of the chimera was the same as the genetic sex of the host in 14 of the remaining 15. The exception was a sterile intersex. Neglecting the very real possibility that XY cells can form functional oocytes in phenotypic females, a donor germ line contribution could be expected in 7 fertile mice in which the genetic sex of both components was the same (Table 2). Two of the latter proved to have such a contribution. Hence, if one assumes that the cloning procedure provides an unbiased sampling of primitive ectoderm cells, it would appear that between one third and one quarter of them (5 to 7 cells, McLaren, 1976b) have germ-line potency. This is necessarily a very tentative estimate.

X-CHROMOSOME INACTIVATION

So far the potency of early embryonic cells has been discussed purely in terms of the spectrum of types of differentiated cells they can produce, and is thus concerned with tissue-specific patterns of differential gene activity. However, in addition, a chromosome-specific type of differential gene activity also occurs in female mammals with inactivation of one or other X-chromosome in somatic cells (Lyon, 1961, 1974), and possibly also in early germ cells (Gartler et al., 1975). Uncertainty persists as to when X-inactivation takes place, though it is clearly later than the 2-cell stage (Hoppe and Whitten, 1972).

Once the feasibility of cloning cells in the blastocyst had been demonstrated (Gardner, 1971), it was adopted as the basis of a functional test for the time of X-inactivation (Gardner and Lyon, 1971). Hitherto, attempts to look for the onset of differential X-chromosome activity were based on criteria such as asynchronous DNA replication in the 2 X-chromosomes, presence or absence of sex chromatin, and analysis of mosaicism in adult females (reviewed in Lyon, 1972). Matings were arranged so that female donor embryos would, as a result of X-inactivation, have one population of melanocytes displaying a pigmented phenotype and the other an albino phenotype. The host blastocysts were of a genotype that gave a coat color distinct from the 2 donor colors (see Gardner and Lyon, 1971 for details). All except 1 chimera obtained by transplanting single 3.5-day p.c. ICM or 4.5-day p.c. primitive ectoderm cells from female embryos showed both donor colors in addition to host color in their coats (Gardner and Lyon, 1971; Gardner, 1974). The conclusion that X-inactivation occurs shortly after implantation is reinforced by preliminary results in a current series of experiments using approximately 4.75-day p.c. donor embryos. To date, 5 out of 10 chimeras known to have received female donor cells exhibit only one or other, and not both, donor colors (R. L. Gardner and M. F. Lyon, unpublished data). The extent of donor contribution to coat pigmentation in these animals is comparable to that in chimeras of the present and previous experiments which displayed both donor colors. Hence, the different behavior of older donor cells is not simply attributable to a lower overall growth rate and consequent increase in likelihood that only one of the 2 classes of cell resulting from random X-inactivation will be represented in the melanocytes.

Deol and Whitten (1972a,b) have argued on the basis of a comparison of pigmentation patterns in mouse chimeras and X-inactivation mosaics for a much later time of inactivation in the CNS-derived melanocytes of the retina and inner ear. While the theoretical basis of this particular study appears to be unsound (West, 1976), the possibility of onset of X-chromosome inactivation at different times in different tissues cannot be dismissed at present. Providing the fraction contributing to the neural crest-derived melanocytes of the coat is representative of the donor cell clone as a whole, the above cell injection experiments give an estimate of the time of X-inactivation in the primitive ectoderm, or at least that part of it forming the fetus. However, as discussed earlier, the trophectoderm and primitive endoderm become established as entirely separate cell populations before the time of implantation. Recent work suggests that these exclusively extra-embryonic tissues may behave rather differently as regards X-inactivation. Thus Takagi and Sasaki (1975) found that the paternally inherited X-chromosome was allocyclic in the majority of metaphases obtained from the visceral yolk sacs of female mouse embryos, and in virtually all those from the trophoblastic chorion. There was much less bias in the allantois (a primitive ectodermal derivative), and approximately equal numbers of metaphases showed an allocyclic maternal X (X^m) and paternal X (X^p) in the embryo proper. A similar distinction between yolk sac and embryo was later found also in the rat (Wake et al., 1976). Very recent work on female mouse embryos that were heterozygous for electrophoretic variants of the X-linked enzyme phosphoglycerate kinase has revealed that the maternal isozyme predominates specifically in the endodermal layer of the yolk sac, and possibly also in trophoblast (West et al., 1977). The same result obtained in heterozygous conceptuses of reciprocal crosses, and when heterozygous blastocysts were transplanted to the uteri of females homozygous for the paternally inherited allele. The data from both the structural and functional studies seem to be more readily explained by preferential inactivation of X^p in primitive endodermal and trophectodermal tissues than by random inactivation followed by selection against cells in which X^p is active (Takagi, 1976; West et al., 1977). If correct, this interpretation reinforces the notion that the random inactivation seen in the primitive ectoderm cannot take place until after segregation of trophectoderm and primitive endoderm. Segregation of the former occurs before 3.5 days and of the latter between 3.5 and 4.5 days p.c. (Gardner and Rossant, 1976; Rossant and Gardner, 1977).

POTENCY OF EMBRYONAL CARCINOMA CELLS

Teratocarcinomas develop from both male and female germ cells in mice, and can also be produced by grafting early embryos ectopically in syngeneic adult hosts (see Sherman and Solter, 1975). The in vitro culture of cells derived from these tumors has been used in recent years to investigate a number of aspects of embryogenesis and cytodifferentiation in mammals (reviewed in Martin, 1975; Sherman and Solter, 1975; Graham, 1977). However, the following discussion is restricted to studies on the potency of the embryonal carcinoma stem cells (EC cells) of these tumors by blastocyst injection. So far, such transplantations have been carried out only with EC cells of embryo-derived teratocarcinomas, both from in vivo passaged tumors (Brinster, 1974; Mintz and Illmensee, 1975; Mintz et al., 1975; Illmensee and Mintz, 1976) and in vitro cultures (Papaioannou et al., 1975, 1977a). The results demonstrate that EC cells from both sources can participate in embryogenesis and exhibit normal differentiation in a wide variety of organs and tissues of the conceptus and post-natal mouse.

In general, donor cells seem to be distributed somewhat erratically in these chimeras (Mintz and Illmensee, 1975; Papaioannou et al., 1975, 1977a) compared with those produced by transplanting ICM cells (Ford et al., 1975b), notwithstanding the injection of several or many EC cells into each blastocyst. This may be due, at least in part, to delayed integration of the tumor-derived cells (Papaioannou et al., 1977a). Nevertheless, the range of normal cell types formed by EC cells in chimeras exceeds that found in both the tumors and in culture, and has included functional spermatozoa in one instance (Mintz and Illmensee, 1975).

The majority of chimeras produced by injecting groups of cultured EC cells into blastocysts also developed tumors which invariably contained cells of donor origin. These tumors tended to fall into one of two categories. Those in the first, prevalent in experiments using cells with a modal chromosome number of 41 (see Papaioannou et al., 1975, for details), appeared around the time of birth. They typically displayed the histological features of primitive teratocarcinomas, and were mainly sub-cutaneous (Papaioannou et al., 1977a). Those in the second category first became evident in adulthood (at 11 to 24 weeks of age), were principally fibrosarcomas, and were associated usually with the skeletal system (Papaioannou et al., 1977a). Interestingly, several mice developing tumors of the second category showed no other evidence of chimerism despite extensive analysis following autopsy.

No tumors were reported in a series of fetuses and young obtained from blastocysts which had each received 5 EC cells from an in vivo passaged tumor (Mintz and Illmensee, 1975; Mintz et al., 1975). However, all except one of the chimeras were killed soon after birth; even the exception was only 11 weeks old at the time of the most recent report (Mintz and Illmensee, 1975). In a subsequent study, single EC cells from the same tumor were injected into each blastocyst. One of the resulting mice was ill and retarded from birth, and was found to have a donor cell-derived tumor associated with the pancreas when autopsied at 2 weeks of age (Illmensee and Mintz, 1976). The only other structures to which the clone had made a detectable contribution were the intestine and stomach, but it was not clear whether these were normal or neoplastic contributions. Hence, further single cell injection experiments, using both cultured and non-cultured EC cells, are needed to resolve the question whether individual clones exhibit only normal or neoplastic growth, or both types of behavior.

Nevertheless, the single cell injection experiments of Illmensee and Mintz (1976) provide the most informative study of the potency of EC cells. In one animal autopsied at 4 weeks post-partum, the EC cell clone had colonized every somatic organ and tissue tested. Five chimeras that were delivered surgically also showed placental chimerism. The significance of the latter is not clear, however, because this organ contains primitive endodermal and ectodermal derivatives as well as trophectodermal ones (Gardner and Papaioannou, 1975). An EC cell contribution to pure trophoblast tissue isolated earlier in development was found by Papaioannou et al. (1975). Colonization of the extra-embryonic endoderm of the visceral yolk sacs of advanced conceptuses has also been established (V. E. Papaioannou and C. F. Graham, personal communication). These data, combined with the one reported case of differentiation of functional male gametes (Mintz and Illmensee, 1975), argue that EC cells can retain totipotency despite in vivo passage for several years, with or without an additional period of months in culture. This finding is particularly surprising because, although EC cells from most sources have a modal chromosome number of 40, their karyotypes are almost invariably aberrant when examined critically by modern chromosome banding techniques (see Graham, 1977, for detailed discussion).

Mintz et al. (1975) suggest that EC cells might correspond to totipotent stem cells persisting in the early post-implantation embryos from which the tumors are derived. However, injection experiments discussed in the first part of this article afford no evidence for persistence of such cells beyond the early blastocyst stage. An alternative possibility would be that they correspond to cells of the germ line which re-acquire totipotency precociously as a consequence of disruption of embryonic organization through ectopic grafting (Papaioannou, 1977b; also see Damjamov and Solter, 1974; Graham, 1977).

Finally, the foregoing studies on injecting EC cells into blastocysts furnish an example of reversal of neoplasia in animal cells (Gardner, 1977c). Earlier work on crown gall teratomas in plants (reviewed by Braun, 1975) clearly established that neoplasia was not necessarily a permanent phenotypic change. However, it remains to be seen whether teratomas and teratocarcinomas represent special cases, or whether conditions can be found that will enable normal growth and differentiation of stem cells from other types of neoplasms. The participation of EC cells in normal embryogenesis seems to depend on their interacting with ICM cells of the host embryo; clumps of EC cells injected into trophectodermal vesicles fail to exhibit normal behavior (R. L. Gardner and M. J. Evans, unpublished results).

CONCLUSIONS

The technique of injecting genetically marked cells into blastocysts has proved to be an extremely valuable way of studying cell lineage and cell commitment in early mammalian development. Knowledge gained from such studies is likely to enhance our understanding of birth defects in a number of ways. Data on cell commitment, for example, may help to identify critical periods in the development of the conceptus which are particularly susceptible to perturbation. Similarly, more precise knowledge of cell lineage relationships in development may enable rationalization of some of the disorders which at present seem to affect a confusing multiplicity of tissues. Finally, there is growing interest in the possibility, suggested by Papaioannou et al. (1975), of harnessing EC cells to obtain animal models of certain heritable biochemical disorders in man. This approach depends on mutating EC cells in culture and then introducing cells carrying selected mutant genes into blastocysts in order to incorporate such genes into mouse stocks via the germ line. However, it is still too early to say whether this will be a viable approach. Formation of functional gametes seems to be an infrequent occurrence with EC cells from in vivo tumors, and has yet to be demonstrated with those taken from culture.

ACKNOWLEDGEMENTS

I wish to thank Mrs. P. Little and Mrs. N. Mann for help in preparing this manuscript.

REFERENCES

Barlow, P. W. and Sherman, M. I. (1972): *J. Embryol. exp. Morph., 27*, 447.
Bellairs, R. (1971): *Developmental Processes in Higher Vertebrates.* Logos Press, London.
Bernhard, H. P. (1977): In: *Report of the Dahlem Workshop on Neoplastic Transformation: Mechanisms and Consequences*, p. 153. Editor: H. Koprowski. Dahlem Konferenzen, Berlin.
Brambell, F. W. R. (1956): In: *Marshall's Physiology of Reproduction, 3rd Ed., Vol. I, part 1.* Chapter 5, p. 397. Longmans, London.
Braun, A. C. (1975): In: *Cell Cycle and Cell Differentiation*, p. 177. Editors: J. Reinert and H. Holtzer. Springer-Verlag, Berlin.
Brinster, R. L. (1974): *J. exp. Med., 140*, 1049.
Burnet, F. M. (1969): *Cellular Immunology.* Cambridge University Press, London.
Cattanach, B. M. (1975): In: *The Early Development of Mammals*, p. 305. Editors: M. Balls and A. E. Wild. Cambridge University Press, Cambridge.
Cole, R. J. and Paul, J. (1965): In: *Preimplantation Stages of Pregnancy: A Ciba Foundation Symposium*, p. 82. Editors: G. E. W. Wolstenholme and M. O'Connor. Churchill, London.
Damjanov, I. and Solter, D. (1974): *Curr. Top. Path., 59*, 69.
Davidson, E. H. (1976): *Gene Activity in Early Development, 2nd Ed.* Academic Press, New York.
Deol, M. S. and Whitten, W. K. (1972a): *Nature New Biol., 238*, 159.
Deol, M. S. and Whitten, W. K. (1972b): *Nature New Biol., 240*, 277.
Dickson, A. D. (1966): *J. Anat. (Lond.), 100*, 335.
Diwan, S. B. and Stevens, L. C. (1976): *J. nat. Cancer Inst., 57*, 937.
Evans, E. P., Ford, C. E. and Lyon, M. F. (1977): *Nature (Lond.), 267*, 430.
Ford, C. E., Evans, E. P., Burtenshaw, M. D., Clegg, H. M., Tuffrey, M. and Barnes, R. D. (1975a): *Proc. roy. Soc. B, 190*, 187.
Ford, C. E., Evans, E. P. and Gardner, R. L. (1975b): *J. Embryol. exp. Morph., 33*, 447.
Franchi, L. L., Mandl, A. M. and Zuckerman, S. (1962): In: *The Ovary, Vol. I*, Chapter 1, p. 1. Editor: S. Zuckerman. Academic Press, New York.
Gardner, R. L. (1968): *Nature (Lond.), 220*, 596.
Gardner, R. L. (1971): *Advanc. Biosci., 6*, 279.
Gardner, R. L. (1974): In: *Birth Defects and Fetal Development: Endocrine and Metabolic Factors*, p. 212. Editor: K. S. Moghissi. Charles C Thomas, Springfield, Ill.
Gardner, R. L. (1975a): In: *Immunobiology of Trophoblast*, p. 43. Editors: R. G. Edwards, C. W. S. Howe and M. H. Johnson. Cambridge University Press, Cambridge.
Gardner, R. L. (1975b): In: *The Developmental Biology of Reproduction*, p. 207. Editors: C. L. Markert and J. Papaconstantinou. Academic Press, New York.
Gardner, R. L. (1977a): In: *Methods in Mammalian Reproduction.* Editor: J. C. Daniel. Academic Press, New York. In press.
Gardner, R. L. (1977b): In: *Genetic Mosaics and Differentiation.* Editor: W. Gehring. Springer-Verlag, Berlin. In press.
Gardner, R. L. (1977c): In: *Report of the Dahlem Workshop on Neoplastic Transformation: Mechanisms and Consequences*, p. 111. Editor: H. Koprowski. Dahlem Konferenzen, Berlin.
Gardner, R. L. and Johnson, M. H. (1972): *J. Embryol. exp. Morph., 28*, 279.
Gardner, R. L. and Johnson, M. H. (1975): In: *Cell patterning: Ciba Foundation Symposium 29 (New Series)*, p. 183. Editors: R. Porter and J. Rivers. Elsevier–Excerpta Medica–North-Holland, Amsterdam –Oxford–New York.
Gardner, R. L. and Lyon, M. F. (1971): *Nature (Lond.), 231*, 385.
Gardner, R. L. and Papaioannou, V. E. (1975): In: *The Early Development of Mammals*, p. 107. Editors: M. Balls and A. E. Wild. Cambridge University Press, Cambridge.
Gardner, R. L., Papaioannou, V. E. and Barton, S. C. (1973): *J. Embryol. exp. Morph., 30*, 561.
Gardner, R. L. and Rossant, J. (1976): In: *Embryogenesis in Mammals: Ciba Foundation Symposium 40 (New Series)*, p. 5. Editors: K. Elliott and M. O'Connor. Elsevier–Excerpta Medica–North-Holland, Amsterdam–Oxford–New York.

Gardner, R. L. and Rossant, J. (1977): Manuscript in preparation.

Gartler, S. M., Andina, R. and Gant, N. (1975): *Exp. Cell Res., 91*, 454.

Graham, C. F. (1977): In: *Concepts in Mammalian Embryogenesis*, p. 315. Editor: M. I. Sherman. MIT Press, Cambridge, Mass.

Hadorn, E. (1966): In: *Major Problems in Developmental Biology*, p. 85. Editor: M. Locke. Academic Press, New York.

Hillman, N., Sherman, M. I. and Graham, C. F. (1972): *J. Embryol. exp. Morph., 28*, 263.

Hoppe, P. C. and Whitten, W. K. (1972): *Nature (Lond.), 239*, 520.

Illmensee, K. and Mintz, B. (1976): *Proc. nat. Acad. Sci. (Wash.), 73*, 549.

Kelly, S. J. (1975): In: *The Early Development of Mammals*, p. 97. Editors: M. Balls and A. E. Wild. Cambridge University Press, Cambridge.

Kelly, S. J. (1977): *J. exp. Zool., 200*, 365.

Kirby, D. R. S. (1970): *Advanc. Biosci., 4*, 255.

Kleinsmith, L. J. and Pierce, G. B. (1964): *Cancer Res., 24*, 1544.

Kruse, P. F. and Patterson, M. K. (1973): *Tissue Culture: Methods and Applications*. Academic Press, New York.

Lin, T. P. (1969): *Nature (Lond.), 222*, 480.

Lyon, M. F. (1961): *Nature (Lond.), 190*, 372.

Lyon, M. F. (1972): *Biol. Rev., 47*, 1.

Lyon, M. F. (1974): *Proc. roy. Soc. B, 187*, 243.

Martin, G. R. (1975): *Cell, 5*, 229.

McLaren, A. (1976a): *Mammalian Chimaeras*. Cambridge University Press, London.

McLaren, A. (1976b): In: *Embryogenesis in Mammals: Ciba Foundation Symposium 40 (New Series)* p. 47. Editors: K. Elliott and M. O'Connor. Elsevier–Excerpta Medica–North-Holland, Amsterdam–Oxford–New York.

McLaren, A. and Michie, D. (1956): *J. exp. Biol., 33*, 394.

Mintz, B. (1965): In: *Preimplantation Stages of Pregnancy: A Ciba Foundation Symposium*, p. 194. Editors: G. E. W. Wolstenholme and M. O'Connor. Churchill, London.

Mintz, B. (1969): In: *Birth Defects: Original Article Series 5*, p. 11. Editors: D. Bergsma and V. McKusick. National Foundation, New York.

Mintz, B. (1974): *Ann. Rev. Genet., 8*, 411.

Mintz, B. and Illmensee, K. (1975): *Proc. nat. Acad. Sci. (Wash.), 72*, 3585.

Mintz, B., Illmensee, K. and Gearhart, J. D. (1975): In: *Teratomas and Differentiation*, p. 59. Editors: M. I. Sherman and D. Solter. Academic Press, New York.

Moustafa, L. A. and Brinster, R. L. (1972): *J. exp. Zool., 181*, 193.

Mullen, R. J. and Whitten, W. K. (1971): *J. exp. Zool., 178*, 165.

Papaioannou, V. E., Gardner, R. L., McBurney, M. W., Babinet, C. and Evans, M. J. (1977a): *J. Embryol. exp. Morph.*, in press.

Papaioannou, V. E., McBurney, M. W., Gardner, R. L. and Evans, M. J., (1975): *Nature (Lond.), 258*, 70.

Papaioannou, V. E., Rossant, J. and Gardner, R. L. (1977b): In: *Stem Cells and Tissue Homeostasis*. Editors: B. I. Lord, C. S. Potten and R. J. Cole. Cambridge University Press, Cambridge. In press.

Rossant, J. (1975a): *J. Embryol. exp. Morph., 33*, 979.

Rossant, J. (1975b): *J. Embryol. exp. Morph., 33*, 991.

Rossant, J. (1976a): *J. Embryol. exp. Morph., 36*, 283.

Rossant, J. (1976b): *J. Embryol. exp. Morph., 36*, 163.

Rossant, J. and Gardner, R. L. (1977): Manuscript in preparation.

Rossant, J. and Ofer, L. (1977): *J. Embryol. exp. Morph., 39*, 183.

Sherman, M. I. (1975): In: *The Early Development of Mammals*, p. 145. Editors: M. Bals and A. E. Wild. Cambridge University Press, Cambridge.

Sherman, M. I., McLaren, A. and Walker, P. M. B. (1972): *Nature New Biol., 238*, 175.

Sherman, M. I. and Solter, D. (Eds.) (1975): *Teratomas and Differentiation*. Academic Press, New York.

Skreb, N., Svajgar, A. and Levak-Svajger, B. (1976): In: *Embryogenesis in Mammals: Ciba Foundation Symposium 40 (New Series)*, p. 27. Editors: K. Elliott and M. O'Connor. Elsevier–Excerpta Medica–North-Holland, Amsterdam–Oxford–New York.

Snow, M. H. L. (1977): *J. Embryol. exp. Morph.*, in press.

Tagaki, N. (1976): *Human Genet., 34*, 207.

Takagi, N. and Sasaki, M. (1975): *Nature (Lond.), 256*, 640.

Tarkowski, A. K. (1959): *Nature (Lond.)*, *184*, 1286.
Tarkowski, A. K. (1961): *Nature (Lond.)*, *190*, 857.
Tarkowski, A. K. and Wroblewska, J. (1967): *J. Embryol. exp. Morph.*, *18*, 155.
Ursprung, H. (Editor) (1968): *The Stability of The Differentiated State*. Springer-Verlag, Berlin.
Wake, N., Takagi, N. and Sasaki, M. (1976): *Nature (Lond.)*, *262*, 580.
Weiss, P. (1939): *Principles of Development*. Holt, New York.
West, J. D. (1976): *J. Embryol. exp. Morph.*, *35*, 445.
West, J. D., Frels, W. I., Chapman, V. M. and Papaioannou, V. E. (1977): *Cell*, *12*, 873.

DEVELOPMENTAL SYSTEMS

Chairman: Widukind Lenz, Münster

Developmental antigens and differentiation

Do T/t locus mutations occur in species other than the mouse?

DOROTHEA BENNETT*

Sloan-Kettering Institute for Cancer Research, New York, N.Y., U.S.A.

The T/t locus in the mouse has been studied for the last 50 years, and has provided a never-ending series of puzzles that tantalizingly promise to tell us something about genetic organization and the control of differentiation in mammals. There are many mutations defined in this genetically complex region of chromosome 17; with respect to morphological effects some are dominant *(T)* and some are recessive *(t)*. These mutations have bizarre and paradoxical properties and break rules that other genetic systems in mammals seem to follow (Bennett, 1975; Klein and Hammerberg, 1977).

For example, many *t*-mutations are lethal or semilethal when homozygous, yet almost all wild populations of mice are polymorphic for just such genes. Heterozygote frequencies are high and range from 15–50%. The maintenance of these lethal genes in wild populations is at least partly achieved by another unorthodox effect of *t*-mutations which results in males preferentially transmitting their lethal gene to the vast majority of their progeny. The transmission ratio advantage of wild *t*-mutations is apparently generated by haploid gene action after meiosis, and usually produces a ratio at fertilization of more than 95:5 in favor of the mutant gene. The selective advantage thus gained by the abrogation of Mendel's rules serves to counterbalance the selective disadvantage of homozygous lethality.

The presence of *t*-mutations in wild populations must also have profound effects on genome structure, since they interfere with genetic recombination in their vicinity. The recombination suppression caused by wild *t*-haplotypes extends over a distance of 15 centimorgans that includes the linked H-2 locus, so that in wild populations a large segment of chromosome containing the MHC must often segregate as an effectively intact unit or 'supergene' (Snell, 1968).

Approximately 35 *t*-haplotypes independently extracted from wild mouse populations have been studied in detail. About 30 of these proved to be lethal when homozygous, but fell into only 4 groups on the basis of embryonic lethal phenotype and genetic complementation. The great majority, almost two-thirds, were of the t^{w5} type, another 6 belonged to the t^{w1} group, and t^0 and t^{w73} were represented only once. Also found were 6 instances of semi-lethal *t*-factors. The heavy representation of t^{w5} haplotypes both in European and American populations, as well as its

---

* The author's work reported here was supported by grants and contracts from NIH, NSF, ERDA and the National Foundation–March of Dimes.

169

occurrence in 2 different subspecies of *Mus* (domesticus and musculus) has led to speculation that t^{w5} is perhaps the original or primordial *t*-mutation of which all the others are mutational descendants (Klein and Hammerberg, 1977). As might be expected, all of these *t*-haplotypes conferred high transmission ratio to *t*-bearing sperm from heterozygous males; without exception all were also recombination suppressors. It is worth noting that no dominant *T*-mutations have ever been found in wild populations, although spontaneous mutations to *T* have frequently been found in laboratory mice.

Although the role that *t*-factors may play, either in population dynamics or with respect to MHC polymorphism, is by no means understood, it must be concluded that they are a normal part of the mouse genome. One of the questions to be addressed in this paper is whether similar sets of mutations may not also be a normal genetic constituent in other species, including man. If such mutations do exist, and it seems likely that this may be the case, they may have so far gone unrecognized because of the unavailability of adequate means and experiments to detect them.

It seems quite likely that the T/t system may have been recognized quite fortuitously because of an unusually effective mechanism for detection and analysis in the mouse. There, the T/t locus is identified and marked by the dominant mutation *T*; heterozygotes are short-tailed and homozygotes die before birth. This dominant mutation provided an essential diagnostic agent for revealing the presence of recessive *t*-mutations. These have no morphological effect in heterozygous combination with wild-type alleles (e.g., $+/t$), but interact with *T* to produce the striking new phenotype of taillessness. Thus, recessive lethal genes that would have otherwise been difficult or impossible to detect were made available for study. Furthermore, since *T* and all recessive *t*-mutations that have been studied behave as genetic alleles to one another, the genetic system has some special features that are not only interesting, but were again crucial in defining many of the peculiar effects of *t*-mutations. Matings between *T/t* animals that carry identical lethal *t*-factors behave as a balanced lethal system; that is, only doubly heterozygous progeny are produced at birth, since both homozygous classes die as embryos. This aspect has permitted the discrimination of the many lethal variants, since matings between double heterozygotes that carry different recessive lethal mutations (e.g., $T/t^x \times T/t^g$) reveal that difference by producing a viable class of offspring (e.g., t^x/t^y) that is normal tailed.

It is this simple way of detecting recessive lethal mutations and testing them for complementation that has made it possible to identify and characterize the large number that has so far been studied. Without the dominant marker, this task would have been virtually impossible.

The study of these mutations has been rewarding. Eleven different mutations that impair early embryonic development have been identified. Each of these produces a distinguishably different syndrome of abnormalities in homozygous embryos during the first 9 days of gestation, the period when the mouse embryo develops from a morula to a definitive embryo with 3 germ layers and important axial structures. The recessive mutations also affect the differentiation of spermatozoa since, as mentioned above, male heterozygotes transmit their deleterious gene to an abnormally large proportion of their progeny, and also, males that carry 2 recessive genes are sterile. Dominant mutations, on the other hand, appear not to affect the function of spermatozoa in any way.

Morphological evidence obtained by electron microscopy implicates the cell membrane in the disorders of differentiation produced by T/t locus mutations. In developing spermatids both the inner and the outer face of the plasma membrane appear to be abnormal. In mutant embryos, membrane-dependent phenomena such as cell junction formation, pseudopod extension, and subsurface microfilament organization are deranged in abnormal cells. These interpretations of membrane abnormalities have been bolstered by serological evidence that abnormal cell surface antigens are specified by T/t locus mutations. These antigens exist only on germ-line cells in the adult, but are also found to be present on preimplantation embryos of appropriate genotype. Thus, the hypothesis can be made that the abnormalities of spermatogenesis and sperm function as well as the many different abnormalities of embryonic differentiation caused by T/t locus genes are due to specific alterations in components of the cell surface. A corollary of this is of course that during development in genetically normal embryos, particular constellations of cell surface molecules control specific steps in early differentiation, and that the genes specifying these molecules function only in the embryo and not in the adult. We tested the general notion of the existence of embryonic stage-specific antigens by using embryonal carcinoma cells as a model, since these stem cells of teratocarcinoma have many similarities to the uncommitted multipotential cells of the preimplantation embryo. We therefore asked as a first question whether immunization of syngeneic recipients with a nullipotential and therefore homogeneous line of embryonal carcinoma (F9) would evoke an immune response. This was indeed the case and antibody of high titer and narrow specificity was produced (Artzt et al., 1973). Anti-F9 antiserum was found to react with F9 cells, and with all other mouse embryonal carcinoma lines, but not with differentiated derivatives of teratocarcinoma nor with a variety of other tumors. When normal cells were examined, the F9 antigen(s) was found to be present only on pre-implantation mouse embryos and germ-line cells in the adult.

Further work on the F9 antigen(s) has established several points of considerable interest.

First, the F9 antigen appears to be specified by a wild-type T/t locus gene(s). The evidence for this rests partly on the results of quantitative absorption experiments, where it was shown that sperm from males of a particular T/t locus genotype ($+/t^{12}$) were only half as effective at removing activity from anti-F9 antiserum as were sperm from $+/+$ males, thus suggesting that the t^{12} gene precluded F9 expression (Artzt et al., 1974). Likewise, indirect immunofluorescence observations on litters of embryos obtained from mating between $+/t^{12}$ parents or from matings of $+/t^{w5}$ parents showed that a portion of the embryos failed to stain with anti-F9 antiserum. It was concluded that t^{12}/t^{12} and t^{w5}/t^{w5} homozygotes did not have detectable amounts of F9 on their surface, and therefore that the mutations t^{12} and t^{w5} both acted as alleles to the F9 gene (Kemler et al., 1976).

Second, the expression of F9 is not confined to the mouse. The same antigen, or one strongly cross-reactive, is found on sperm of all mammalian species examined (Jacob, 1977), as well as on human teratocarcinoma cell lines (Holden et al., 1977; Hogan et al., 1977).

Third, the association of F9 with the genetic complex identified by T/t mutations has made it possible to begin to examine the biochemistry of the cell surface molecules produced. Biochemical studies of mutant antigens have so far been technically impossible because of the weak serological system involved. But the relative robustness of the F9 antibody and the availability of large number of F9 cells has permitted immunoprecipitation studies of F9 antigens. Interestingly, these studies have shown that in molecular weight and subunit structure, F9 is similar to the MHC D and K products (Vitetta et al., 1975). This has in turn led to speculation (Artzt and Bennett, 1975), considered unwarranted by some (Munro and Bright, 1976), that T/t and H-2 are evolutionarily related loci. Genes at the T/t locus perhaps originated early in the evolution of metazoans to govern the relatively simple cell–cell interactions required for early embryonic development. Subsequently one might imagine that duplication of that chromosome segment occurred, leaving one partner free to evolve into the MHC region with its perhaps complicated role in lymphocyte interactions. On the other hand, the widespread distribution of the F9 antigen among mammalian species suggests that this complex region has been strongly conserved during evolution. The question of a relationship between T/t locus and MHC genes has become even more interesting with the finding (Hammerberg and Klein, 1975) of strong linkage disequilibrium between mutant t and H-2 haplotypes in wild populations of mice. With a couple of exceptions, members of the same complementation group, even though independently isolated from geographically remote areas, were found to have identical H-2 types. The simplest explanation for this is that t-factors in the same complementation group represent the same chromosome, spread about the world by migration. Another possibility is that certain t-H-2 combinations are particularly advantageous and therefore are positively selected for in wild populations.

So the question now is not whether there is a T/t *region* in man or other species, because there seems to be good evidence that representatives of wild-type genes do exist in all mammalian species examined. The real question is whether sets of mutations with the same complex characteristics of t-mutations occur in other species and also play some role that may be relevant to the MHC.

If we assume, for the sake of simplicity, that such mutations will have characteristics comparable to those in the mouse, what then will we be looking for — or, just as importantly, not looking for? To assess this properly, it should be remembered that T/t mutations came in 2 classes, whose survival value and genetic complexity is vastly different.

Dominant mutations, although of great importance in revealing the presence of other recessive mutations, are probably purely deleterious genes that appear to have neither redeeming features of selective advantage nor any structural or functional relationships to the MHC other than that of linkage, with free recombination over the intervening distance. Thus, although we might expect to find such mutations occurring, it would be unlikely that they would be at all widespread in natural populations of man or other animals, although they may be maintained by selection in laboratory or domestic animals. Several candidates for this sort of mutation have emerged. In the rat, a number of now extinct short-tailed dominant mutations have been reported (Dunn, 1942) but none were studied for homozygous effects and the possibility of linkage with H-1 was not examined. A new short-tailed dominant in the rat has recently been described (K. Hoshino, personal communication); in homozygous condition the effects of this mutation closely resemble that of those of the mouse mutant T^{Or1}. Experiments to test this mutation for linkage with H-1 are now underway. In cats, the short-tailed 'Manx' condition has many resemblances to the T/t system of mutants, but again the lethal syndrome has not been studied in detail (Kitchen et al., 1972). Furthermore, the MHC in cats is not yet well enough defined to permit linkage studies. In man, spina bifida is frequently considered as a possible counterpart to the short-tailed syndrome seen in T/+ mice, especially since background genetic modifiers may frequently produce spina bifida in short-tailed or tailless mice. Amos et al. (1975) have reported a study of about 100 members of a 4-generation family in which spina bifida and associated disorders appeared to segregate with particular HL-A haplotypes. Although this provides statistical evidence for linkage between the HLA locus and the locus of a genetic factor predisposing to spina bifida, the authors quite rightly point out that uncertainties concerning penetrance and the polygenic inheritance of spina bifida and associated defects render the data less than substantial. In a study with a similar purpose, Bobrow et al. (1975) classified HL-A types in families with more than one case of spina bifida, and found no association of a particular HL-A type with the condition, nor any evidence for linkage. Nevertheless, in spite of the obvious drawbacks, this kind of extensive family study is probably the only way of attempting to reveal the existence and HL-A linkage of putative T-mutations in man.

Recessive *t*-mutations are far more interesting and far more likely to have counterparts in other species, but, in the absence of an interactive marker gene like *T*, far more difficult to detect. Again drawing on the mouse system as a model, some characteristics can be outlined by which *t*-mutations in other species might be detected. They would be expected to be lethal very early in gestation or semilethal when homozygous, to be transmitted in a highly preferential way through males, to show complete linkage with the MHC, and finally to produce sterility in males that carry 2 different lethal '*t*'-haplotypes, or the same semi-lethal haplotype. Since morphological traits may well not be associated with any of these characteristics, it is obvious that special circumstances would be necessary to reveal genes with the above characteristics. Nevertheless, some evidence for their existence in rat and man can be brought forward.

In the rat, Michie and Anderson (1966) reported on a Wistar substrain designated A2, that in spite of 72 generations of brother–sister matings was not skin graft

TABLE 1*

Results of the first breeding plan

Generation	No. of pairs grafted	Both grafts accepted	One graft rejected	Both grafts rejected	Two-way takes
72 + 1	24	10	9	5	42%
72 + 2	8	4	3	1	50%
72 + 3	11	6	3	2	55%
72 + 4	6	3	2	1	50%
Total	49	23	17	9	47%

Skin grafts exchanged between male and female littermates; mutually compatible pairs chosen as parents of the next generation. 47% of one-way rejections were female-to-male grafts, so Y-antigen is not involved. Mean survival in cases of rejection = 14.6 days.
* After Michie and Anderson (1966).

TABLE 2*

Results of testing 25 rats from the original A2 strain by exchanging skin grafts with known homozygous A2/1 partners

Reaction of tested A2 rats with A2/1 (g_1/g_1) partners		Inferred genotype	Observed numbers
As donor	As host		
Is rejected	Accepts	g_1/g_2	21
Is accepted	Accepts	g_1/g_1	4
Is rejected	Rejects	g_2/g_2	0

* After Michie and Anderson (1966).

compatible. About one-half of all grafts made within the strain were rejected during the third week. The original data are shown in Table 1. Clearly, some major selective advantage was maintaining heterozygosity at an important histocompatibility locus even in the face of stringent and long-continued inbreeding. Michie and Anderson analysed the situation as follows. First, they selected as mates pairs of animals that were capable of 2-way graft acceptance, and assumed to be heterozygous (e.g., g_1/g_2) for alleles at the histocompatibility locus involved. The progeny of such pairs were then grafted with skin from both parents with results as shown in Table 2.

Thus, every offspring either accepted both grafts or rejected both grafts, confirming the idea that the parents were heterozygous. Furthermore, there was a considerable deficiency of the double rejectors, which would of course be the homozygous classes. The authors went on to test the members of both putative homozygous classes by skin grafting, and found, surprisingly, that all grafts were accepted among themselves; the inference had to be that these animals were all homozygous for the *same* histocompatibility allele. These tested animals were bred together to produce a substrain designated $A_2/1$ which appeared to be isogenic, since skin grafts could be made in any direction with complete acceptance. This substrain was then used to measure the relative proportion of both homozygous classes and heterozygotes in the original A2 strain, as seen in Table 3.

These data show quite clearly that the A2 strain is predominantly heterozygous, with a deficiency of both homozygous classes. Although the putative g_2/g_2 class was

TABLE 3*

An experiment to detect homozygotes and measure their frequency

	Two-way takes	
Assumed genotypes of selected parents	$g_1/g_2 \times g_1/g_2$	
	$\downarrow$	
Assumed genotypes of offspring	g_1/g_2	g_1/g_1 or g_2/g_2
Reaction to parents' skin	Accept	Reject
Expected frequency (Mendelian)	50%	50%
Observed frequency	Many (80%)	Few (20%)

* Redone from Michie and Anderson (1966).

not detected here, the existence of at least some 2-way rejections in the initial set of skin grafts (see Table 1) assures that this class does exist.

As a whole, these interesting data are entirely compatible with the existence in the original A2 strain of a semilethal *t*-like mutation, showing complete linkage with the MHC (g_2 allele in this case), and having a high male transmission ratio as well. Such a factor could account for the persistence of heterozygosity over many generations of inbreeding because heterozygous males would transmit g_2 to a preponderance of progeny, but homozygous males would be sterile. The deficiency of homozygotes for g_1 can likewise be explained by the relative deficiency of fertilizing g_1 sperm from heterozygous males, and the deficiency of g_2 homozygotes by lethality. Unfortunately, so far as we can determine, the original A2 strain is extinct, so these ideas cannot be tested. However, a similar but less well analyzed situation has been described in another strain of rats. Dr. Darhl Forman (personal communication) has failed to attain homozygosity for H-1 in the course of inbreeding another Wistar-derived line; these animals were still segregating H-1 alleles after a number of generations of brother–sister matings, and in a small sample also showed deficiencies in both homozygous classes. Rats obtained from Dr. Forman are now being bred and tested in our laboratory for the presence of a *t*-like allele. Mating tests of these animals with those that carry the putative dominant T-like mutation mentioned above will also be done, so it is entirely possible that in the future another T/t complex will be defined.

In man, direct evidence for the existence of *t*-like mutations is obviously not easy to come by, given small family size and extensive H-2 polymorphism. One report however strongly suggests that such a mutation may have been detected. Degos et al. (1974) reported a study of the HL-A types in a tribe, the Kel Kummer Tuareg of the South Sahara, where inbreeding is encouraged by strict rules that require marriages with a mother's brother's daughter. This leads to a very high inbreeding coefficient, about 0.11 on the average (F is 0.25 for sib mating). Thus, the tribe exhibits an unusual homogeneity with respect to HL-A, with only 21 haplotypes detected. Two haplotypes, furthermore, are presented in very high frequency, namely HL-A11/W21 (19%) and W28/HL-A7 (17%), but of 106 individuals tested only one is a possible (not proved) homozygote. This again suggests that some consistent barrier to homozygosity may be operating, which as these authors propose, may be a *t*-factor.

Several attempts have been made to detect segregation distortion or HL-A related selection by analyzing the relative frequency of parental haplotypes among the children, and by scoring the relative frequency of sibships having 1, 2, 3, or all 4 of the parental haplotypes (Albert et al., 1973; Amos et al., 1970; Mattiuz et al., 1970). In no case was any clear departure from random segregation noted. It should be noted, however, that these studies comprise statistical averages summed over many families, with sibship sizes no greater than 6. So, although the evidence for random segregation could be a valid reflection of the absence of t-like genes in these families, it could as well result from extensive polymorphism of '*t*'-mutations associated with a large number of different HL-A haplotypes. If this were in fact the case, one would likely miss evidence for abnormal segregation, since all sibships with comparable HL-A haplotypes are pooled. The most profitable way to use such data to attempt to uncover instances of a '*t*'-mutation driving the abnormal transmission of HL-A haplotypes would be to select those 4- or 5-child sibships in which all, or all but one, had received the same paternal HL-A haplotype. Analysis of the segregation of the same haplotype in the father's sibs and grandchildren could then be used to provide evidence for or against distorted transmission. Unfortunately, this sort of extended study has not to my knowledge been done.

Another approach to detecting selective factors associated with HL-A was tried by Lindblom et al. (1972) who selected infertile couples in which no clinical cause for sterility could be found. Of 569 couples surveyed, only 8 met this criterion. No particularly odd combinations of HL-A haplotypes were noted in these 8 couples, although the proportion with negative delta values for linkage disequilibrium was somewhat higher than expected. Unfortunately, men with low sperm counts or decreased sperm motility were excluded from this sample, so if '*t*'-mutations in man behave as they do in the mouse, both homozygotes and complementing heterozygotes would have been effectively eliminated from consideration. Nevertheless, HL-A typing of infertile males with normal endocrinology but abnormal sperm count or motility might be an efficient approach to detecting the human counterpart of *t*-mutations. Again, if the mouse analogy holds, a higher than normal proportion of such men should either be HL-A homozygotes, or carry a non-random selection of HL-A haplotypes.

In summary, although wild-type genetic material corresponding to the T/t region of the mouse almost certainly exists in all mammals, evidence for mutational sets corresponding to T/t mutants is less secure. Another rodent, the rat, very likely does possess such mutations, but definitive proof is so far lacking. In man there is only the most fragmentary evidence for such mutations, but this may simply reflect the inefficiency of the searches that have so far been made. Extensive family studies of HL-A, especially in families identified by sibships with aberrant HL-A segregation ratios, HL-A typing of infertile men, and families with frequent abortion should provide more effective ways of exploring for their existence.

REFERENCES

Albert, E. D., Mickey, M. R., Ting, A. and Terasaki, P. I. (1973): *Transplant. Proc.*, 5, 215.

Amos, B., Cabrera, G., Bias, W. B., MacQueen, J. M., Lancaster, S. L., Southworth, J. G. and Ward, F. E. (1970): In: *Histocompatibility Testing*, p. 221. Editor: P. I. Terasaki. Munksgaard, Copenhagen.

Amos, B., Johnson, A. H., Ruderman, R. J., Mendell, N. and Yunis, E. J. (1975): In: *New Concepts in Transplantation Immunity – M. D. Anderson Symposium.* Editor: R. W. Cumly. University of Texas, Houston.

Artzt, K. and Bennett, D. (1975): *Nature (Lond.)*, 256, 545.

Artzt, K., Bennett, D. and Jacob, F. (1974): *Proc. nat. Acad. Sci. (Wash.)*, 71, 811.

Artzt, K., Dubois, P., Bennett, D., Condamine, H., Babinet, C. and Jacob, F. (1973): *Proc. nat. Acad. Sci. (Wash.)*, 70, 2988.

Bennett, D. (1975): *Cell*, 6, 441.

Bobrow, M., Bodmer, J. G., Bodmer, W. F., McDevitt, H. O., Lorber, J. and Swift P. (1975): *Tissue Antigens*, 5, 234.

Degos, L., Colombani, J., Chaventre, A., Bengtson, B. and Jacquard, A. (1974): *Nature (Lond.)*, 249, 62.

Dunn, L. C. (1942): *Amer. Naturalist*, 76, 552.

Hammerberg, C. and Klein, J. (1975): *Nature (Lond.)*, 258, 296.

Hogan, B., Fellous, M., Avner, P. and Jacob, F. (1977): *Nature (Lond.)*, in press.

Holden, S., Bernard, O., Artzt, K., Whitmore, W. F. and Bennett, D. (1977): *Nature (Lond.)*, in press.

Jacob, F. (1977): *Immunol. Rev.*, 33, 3.

Kemler, R., Babinet, C., Condamine, H., Gachelin, G., Guenet, J. L. and Jacob, F. (1976): *Proc. nat. Acad. Sci. (Wash.)*, *73*, 4080.

Kitchen, H., Murray, R. E. and Cockrell, B. (1972): *Amer. J. Path.*, *68*, 203.

Klein, J. and Hammerberg, C. (1977): *Immunol. Rev.*, *33*, 70.

Lindblom, J. B., Friberg, J., Hagman, C. F. and Gemzel, C. (1972): *Tissue Antigens*, *2*, 352.

Mattiuz, P. L., Ihde, D., Piazza, A., Ceppellini, R. and Bodmer, W. (1970): In: *Histocompatibility Testing*, p. 193. Editor: P. I. Terasaki. Munksgaard, Copenhagen.

Michie, D. and Anderson, N. F. (1966): *Ann. N.Y. Acad. Sci.*, *129(1)*, 88.

Munro, A. and Bright, S. (1976): *Nature (Lond.)*, *264*, 145.

Snell, G. D. (1968): *Folia biol. (Praha)*, *14*, 335.

Vitetta, E., Artzt, K., Bennett, D., Boyse, E. A. and Jacob, F. (1975): *Proc. nat. Acad. Sci. (Wash.)*, *72*, 3215.

The life history of antibody-producing B cells*

M. D. COOPER, J. F. KEARNEY and A. R. LAWTON, III**

Departments of Pediatrics and Microbiology and The Comprehensive Cancer Center, University of Alabama in Birmingham, Birmingham, Ala., U.S.A.

Normal body defense or immunity depends upon the integrated development and function of a number of cell lines, each of which becomes specialized for the production of a finite number of molecular products having distinct biological activities. Some of these cell products are carried as receptors on the external plasma membrane, and may also be secreted on demand into the body fluids. Members of 2 of these cell lines, B and T cells, are specifically immunocompetent (reviewed by Greaves et al., 1973). That is, they are capable of selectively recognizing foreign invaders such as pathogenic microorganisms, toxins and even transformed body cells with the potential for malignant growth. Moreover, B and T cells are capable of discriminating between the chemical configurations or antigens present on normal self elements and those on non-self or altered self. In order to initiate and terminate useful immune responses, B and T cells coordinate their responses through an intricate genetically controlled system of communication. For this they require the help of 'non-specific' cells such as macrophages, other antigen trapping or phagocytic cells, an interacting group of proenzymes belonging to the complement system and a diverse array of other biologically active cell products involved in the inflammatory response. When all of the components of the immune system are normally developed and working in harmony, potentially harmful invaders and altered body cells are inactivated and eliminated.

Immune recognition is primarily mediated by complementary antigen binding sites on antibody molecules that are integrally attached to the plasma membrane surface of B and T cells. Each B and T lymphocyte, of which there are millions, bears antibody receptors whose specificity is determined by V genes. V genes code for the aminoterminal 'variable' sequence of the light V_L and heavy V_H chains of immunoglobulin molecules. The receptors on the membrane of B lymphocytes are immunoglobulin molecules like those in serum. The entire chemical structure of the T cell receptor is not known, but it now seems clear that one of its component chains is similar, if not identical, to the immunoglobulin V_H region (Rajewsky et al.,

*Studies performed in the authors' laboratories were supported by National Foundation–March of Dimes grant 1-354 and by USPHS NIH grants CA 16673, CA 13148, AI 11502 and RR 32.
**A. R. Lawton is recipient of a Research Career Development Award, AI 70780.

1976; Binz and Wigzell, 1977). The regulation of immune function is accomplished by complex interactions among B cells, T cells and macrophages (reviewed by Paul and Benacerraf, 1977). Both initiation and suppression of immune responses are controlled in part by genes within the major histocompatibility complex. The products of these genes are distinct from antibodies, may be expressed on the cell surface or secreted, and carry out the dual functions of mediating communication among the cells of 'self' and distinguishing 'non-self' (e.g. in rejection of allografts). In addition, antibodies themselves play a role in regulation of immune responses both by removal of antigens and by inducing anti-idiotype antibodies which recognize and react with the receptors of other lymphocytes (see Raff, 1977). It is easy to appreciate that failure of one of the components to develop or function normally may alter the balance of the entire system and result in disastrous effects on the health of the individual. For example, the clinical consequences of defective development of B cells and their production of antibodies can include damage to any organ system of the body as a result of a variety of infections, autoimmune syndromes, certain of the leukemias and other lymphoid malignancies.

In this essay, we will focus on what is known about some of the sequential events occurring during normal development of B cells, and attempt to illustrate the relevance of this information to the analysis of clinical disorders involving antibody-producing cells.

GENERAL STATEMENT OF THE PROBLEM OF B CELL DIFFERENTIATION AND DIVERSIFICATION

In order to respond by producing antibodies with binding sites complementary to the diverse array of antigenic determinants present on all potentially harmful invaders or altered self, the genetic capacity to produce an enormous variety of antibodies has evolved in higher vertebrates. It is estimated that mature individuals have developed the genes necessary to code for the production of between 10^6 and 10^8 antibodies having different specificities. Since each B cell produces antibodies having a single antigenic specificity, this means that the precursor hemopoietic stem cells must give rise to at least the same number of different B cells. The actual number of B cells needed is further amplified by the fact that many, if not all, of the different sets of light and heavy chain variable regions (V_L and V_H), which determine antibody specificity, are combined with each of the different heavy chains characteristic of the different immunoglobulin classes, IgM, IgG, IgA, IgE and IgD and their multiple subclasses. Each B cell also produces only 1 of the 2 light chain types, kappa or lambda, and analysis of multiple alleles on different light and heavy chain regions indicates that each B cell expresses the heavy or light chain genes of only 1 parental set of the homologous pairs of chromosomes. A detailed review of the available knowledge on the families of immunoglobulin genes and their products is beyond the scope of this presentation, but it is readily apparent that a large number of genetic decisions occur during the generation of B cell diversity.

In addition, a variety of non-immunoglobulin genes can be expressed during B cell differentiation (Table 1). Such gene products displayed on the surface of B cells include histocompatibility antigens, B cell alloantigens, and receptors for mitogenic

TABLE 1

Non-immunoglobulin gene products expressed by human B cells

A. Surface determinants of the major histocompatibility complex (MHC) of genes located on chromosome 6
   1. HLA-A, B (& C)
      a. Multiple alleles at each gene locus.
      b. Expressed on all nucleated cells.
      c. Important in immune cell recognition and destruction of virus infected cells.
   2. HLA-D
      a. Multiple alleles.
      b. Closely linked or identical to genes coding for B cell alloantigens.
      c. Detected so far only on B cells and cells of monocyte–macrophage series.
      d. Syngeny at this locus is important in collaborative interactions between macrophages, T cells and B cells.

B. Non-MHC gene products on B cells
   1. Fc receptors
      a. B cell receptors for IgG may differ from those expressed on other cell types such as phagocytes, a subset of T cells, 'null' or K cells and virus transformed cells.
      b. Receptors for IgM are present on malignant B cells and on a subpopulation of normal B cells found mainly in the tonsils, but these receptors have characteristics different from those for IgM on helper T cells.
   2. C3 receptors
      (1) Present on a subpopulation of B lymphocytes, monocytes, macrophages and other phagocytic cells.
      (2) May play a significant role in T cell help of B cell responses to certain antigens.
   3. Mitogen receptors
      (1) Allow the stimulation of B cells by mitogenic extracts of bacteria (e.g., lipopolysaccharide), fungi (e.g., nocardia extracts), plants (e.g., pokeweed extract), etc.
   4. Epstein-Barr virus receptors
      (1) Apparently present on all sIg$^+$ B lymphocytes.
      (2) Biologic significance is unknown but could relate to the susceptibility of B lymphocytes to transformation by EBV infection.

substances, the Fc portion of IgG, C3b and C3d fragments of the 3rd complement component and the Epstein-Barr virus.

The factors which determine the selection and expression of genes encoding these B cell products during differentiation of B cell sublines are incompletely understood as is their functional significance. By necessity, therefore, we will present a simplified overview of this process. The emphasis will be placed on the earlier events in B cell differentiation for several reasons: (1) Most of the important genetic decisions are apparently made during early B cell differentiation; (2) currently this is one of the most productive areas of immunological research; and (3) recent data suggest that most of the currently recognized B cell defects occur during the earliest phases of differentiation of this cell line.

STEM CELL DIFFERENTIATION ALONG B CELL LINES

A pool of primitive hemopoietic stem cells capable of giving rise to the progenitor cells for each of the cell lines in blood exists from very early stages in embryonic development throughout the life of normal individuals (Metcalf and Moore, 1971). Such cells can be found in the blood islands of the yolk sac in very young embryos. Later in development they are present in abundance in the fetal liver of mammals when this becomes a hemopoietic tissue. When hemopoiesis later shifts to the bone marrow, this becomes the primary repository for multipotent stem cells, and some can be demonstrated in the circulation. There is now clear evidence that the particular pathway of cellular differentiation which hemopoietic stem cells may take (see Fig. 1) is determined by their migration to specialized inductive microenvironments (see Le Dourain, and Hay, *This Volume*). These commitments are reflected by expression of cell surface determinants termed differentiation antigens as was discussed in the preceding paper by Bennett.

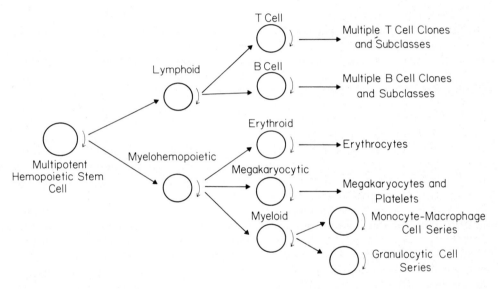

Fig. 1. Schematic representation of how multipotent hemopoietic stem cells may become sequentially committed to different pathways of differentiation.

The definition of congenital immunodeficiency syndromes in which affected infants did not form either T or B cells but who exhibited normal development of the other blood cell lines suggested the existence of a common stem cell for both T and B cells (reviewed by Good, 1973). Evidence for a separate lymphoid stem cell was recently provided by studies in women with polycythemia vera who were also heterozygous for X-linked isoenzymes of glucose-6-phosphate dehydrogenase (Adamson et al., 1976). Cells of the myeloid, megakaryocytic and erythroid cell lines expressed only one allele indicating a common origin from an aberrant stem cell. Lymphoid populations from these patients, as in normal heterozygous women, expressed both isoenzymes.

Convincing evidence now exists that lymphoid stem cells differentiate into T and B cells under the influence of specific inducer molecules produced respectively by thymic epithelial cells in mammals and birds and by epithelial cells of the bursa of birds (Pyke and Gelfand, 1974; Papiernik et al., 1975; Goldstein et al., 1976; Kruisbeek et al., 1977). Whether the basic genetic decisions for commitment to the 2 separate pathways of lymphoid differentiation are made before or after migration of lymphoid stem cells into these specific inductive sites has not been resolved (reviewed by Stutman, 1977). If the first alternative is correct, inducer hormones may merely trigger the execution of the subsequent differentiation events (Scheid et al., 1975).

GENERATION OF PRE-B CELLS AND B LYMPHOCYTES IN FETAL LIVER AND BONE MARROW OF MAMMALS

The first recognizable cells of the B cell lineage in humans are found in the liver by the 7th week of gestation (Gathings et al., 1977). These cells, presently termed pre-B cells (Raff et al., 1976), have the following characteristics: they are heterogeneous in size, although most are larger than typical small lymphocytes. Pre-B cells synthesize small amounts of IgM that can be detected by immunofluorescence within the cytoplasm, lack surface immunoglobulin receptors detectable by the same sensitive technique. The nucleus of the larger pre-B cells has a characteristic cerebriform contour. Large pre-B cells in fetal liver and those later found in bone marrow are rapidly dividing, as shown by the fact that approximately 90% of such cells incorporate radiolabeled thymidine following a brief exposure to this DNA precursor (Okos and Gathings, 1977; Owen et al., 1977). Such studies also indicate that large pre-B cells give rise to smaller infrequently dividing, pre-B cells in fetal liver and bone marrow, and that they in turn develop into immature sIgM$^+$ B lymphocytes (Osmond and Nossal, 1974). During fetal life, pre-B cells may be rarely found in spleen, lymph nodes, and blood, although they are vastly more abundant in liver and bone marrow. In adults these cells are normally confined to the bone marrow. The confinement of pre-B cells within fetal liver and fetal and adult marrow of all mammals thus far studied provides evidence that these sites are the mammalian homologue of the avian bursa of Fabricius.

Large and small pre-B cells share interesting and biologically significant characteristics. In all of the mammalian species in which they have been analyzed, mice (see Owen et al., 1974; Raff et al., 1976; Melchers et al., 1976), rabbits (Hayward et al., 1977) and humans (Gathings et al., 1977), they lack (1) stable surface immunoglobulin receptors, (2) IgG Fc receptors, and (3) C3 receptors. Thus, their development cannot be influenced in any specific way by antigens, antibodies to immunoglobulins, immune complexes, aggregates of maternally derived antibodies, complement activation or probably the normal influence exerted by T cells on B lymphocytes. In addition, they appear to be unresponsive to lymphocyte mitogens (Kearney and Lawton, 1975; Melchers et al., 1976). During this protected early phase in the life history of cells of this lineage, several important differentiation events occur. Besides the selection and activation of the genes coding for heavy chains of IgM, the genetic decision is made as to whether κ or λ chains are to be expressed by an individual pre-B cell and its progeny. Studies of light chain allotypes expressed by pre-B cells in rabbits indicate that the immunoglobulin genes on only one of the paired parental chromosomes is selected for expression (Hayward et al., 1977).

The rapid proliferation of large pre-B cells, along with other considerations, lead us to believe that diversity of germ line V-region genes may be expressed during the pre-B cell stage of differentiation. Results of ongoing studies by Kubagawa and Vogler in our laboratory indeed suggest that the specificity determinants of IgM antibodies are expressed by pre-B cells. The potential survival advantage of the ability to generate clonal diversity without the opportunity of undesirable 'abortion' of potentially useful clones is apparent (see also section on generation of clonal diversity).

IMMATURE AND MATURE B LYMPHOCYTES

Convincing, albeit indirect, evidence in mice and humans indicates that small pre-B cells give rise directly to immature B lymphocytes, which are then disseminated through the blood stream into lymphoid tissues throughout the body (see Burrows et al., 1977; Gathings et al., 1977). In contrast to pre-B cells, immature B lymphocytes bear relatively large amounts of sIgM (Sidman and Unanue, 1975a), while most lack detectable intracytoplasmic IgM. Immature B cells in mice, rabbits and humans do not express sIg of classes other than IgM or C3 receptors (see Abney et al., 1977; Gelfand et al., 1974; Hayward et al., 1977; Gathings et al., 1977). In mice, expression of histocompatibility antigens, including those encoded by the K and I regions of the major histocompatibility complex (MHC), is delayed relative to expression of sIgM (Kearney et al., 1977). Immature B lymphocytes express few if any Fc receptors (B. Pernis, personal communication). Because the development of B lymphocytes occurs so rapidly in mice, the correlation of acquisition of various surface markers with function has been difficult. The least mature B lymphocytes have receptors which permit them to respond to bacterial lipopolysaccharide (Kearney and Lawton, 1975; Melchers et al., 1976), a mitogen which drives these cells to differentiate to plasma cells. If given the help of adult T cells and macrophages, immature B cells are also capable of being triggered by antigens (reviewed by Klinman, 1976; Blaese and Lawrence, 1977). Thus it may be concluded that expression of receptors for T cell factors is an early differentiation event.

Immature B lymphocytes are functionally distinct in at least one important respect; they are much more easily tolerable than are mature B lymphocytes (Nossal and Pike, 1975; Metcalf and Klinman, 1976; Cambier et al., 1976), and this apparently relates to differences in the way that immature B lymphocytes respond to cross-linkage of their sIgM antibodies (Raff et al., 1975; Sidman and Unanue, 1975b; Grossi et al., 1977; Gathings et al., 1977). Mature B lymphocytes, when treated with bivalent antibodies, lose detectable sIgM for a period of time. This phenomenon, called antigenic modulation, involves the formation of complexes of receptor IgM and anti-IgM aggregates (patch formation) which are drawn to one pole of the cell (cap formation) and are then internalized by pinocytosis (Taylor et al., 1971). Modulation of sIgM on immature B lymphocytes differs in at least 2 important respects. First, it occurs at much lower concentrations of cross-linking antibodies than are needed to cause equivalent modulation of sIgM on adult cells; secondly, following such treatment, immature B lymphocytes fail to re-express sIgM, while mature B cells do so within 24 hours in culture. Similarly, in vitro development of mouse and chicken B lymphocytes and their plasma cell progeny can be aborted by injections of anti-IgM antibodies, but only if the treatment is begun very early in development (Kincade et al., 1970; reviewed by Lawton and Cooper, 1974). Moreover, antibodies to the antigen binding sites of the surface antibodies (anti-idiotype) and multivalent antigens have the same effects but act only on members of the particular clone(s) of immature B cells which bear specific antibody receptors for the cross-linking ligand (Cosenza and Köhler, 1972; Metcalf and Klinman, 1976). Thus an important mechanism exists for the 'abortion' of the development of self-reactive clones or in other words B cell tolerance to self antigens.

The initial development of a large population of mature B lymphocytes does not appear to be influenced by external antigens or by T cells, since development of relatively mature B cells occurs normally in congenitally athymic mice raised in a germ-free environment and by mid-gestation in the antigen-sheltered human fetus (Abney et al., 1977; Lawton et al., 1972). Thus 1–2 weeks postnatally in mice and by mid-term in human fetuses, the majority of B lymphocytes in blood and peripheral lymphoid tissues express C3 receptors, Fc receptors, Ia determinants (may be an earlier marker of B cell commitment in humans) and more than one class of surface Ig. These mature B lymphocytes are also more resistant to antigenic modulation and to clonal abortion by antigen.

GENERATION OF CLONAL DIVERSITY

It became apparent in the early 1960's that the specificity of antibodies was determined by the aminoacid sequence of their variable regions, and was therefore based on genetic information. Two theories were advanced to account for the immense diversity of different antibodies (see Hood and Prahl, 1971). The germ line theory held that each specificity which could be expressed in a mature individual was encoded in inherited germ line genes. The opposing somatic mutation theory postulated the inheritance of a few germ line genes which were then expanded, by selection of useful mutations occurring in proliferating lymphocytes, to form the much larger repertoire of the adult individual. The crux of the genetic argument is whether the development of diversity of V region genes occurred during evolutionary time or whether much of it occurs in each individual's lifetime. The major theoretical argument against the germ line theory has been that a substantial amount of total DNA would be required to encode all the different specificities. Somatic mutation theories, on the other hand, needed to postulate special mutational mechanisms to account for the facts that the observed differences among V region sequences of myeloma proteins were largely confined to 3 or 4 hypervariable regions, which are now known to be involved in formation of the antigen binding site.

After more than a decade of argument and experimentation, neither theory has been disproven. The accumulation of larger numbers of fully sequenced antibody V regions has led to an increase in the numbers of genes accepted as germ line by proponents of somatic theories and a corresponding reduction in numbers postulated by germ line theory adherents. It seems likely that the solution to this problem will only come from direct gene counting using newer techniques of nucleic acid chemistry (Hood et al., 1977).

Whatever the mechanism of development of genetic diversity of antibody combining regions, the function of the immune system requires that specificity information be expressed on the surface of individual lymphocytes in the form of receptors for antigens. Figure 2 outlines a scheme by which this may occur.

In 1965 Dreyer and Bennett proposed that immunoglobulin light and heavy chains were each encoded by 2 separate genes: V (variable) genes, which coded for the aminoterminal end of each chain contained specificity information, while C (constant) genes specified the remainder of the molecule and determined heavy chain class or light chain type. Their hypothesis, already widely accepted on the basis of sequence data, has recently been directly confirmed by the demonstration that κ light chain V and C genes in embryonic cells are found on different fragments of DNA, while the 2 genes are integrated in plasma cells (Tonegawa et al., 1977).

Immunoglobulin genes exist in 3 unlinked families which may be on different chromosomes. One family codes for heavy chains, one for κ light chains, and one for λ light chains. Within each family, V and C genes are closely linked, and presumably are arrayed sequentially along a single stretch of chromosome. As indicated above, the number of V genes in each family is unknown. In the heavy chain linkage group any of the V_H genes may become associated with any of the C_H genes (μ, δ, γ, α, ε and known subclasses of $C\gamma$, and $C\alpha$). A less complex situation occurs with light chains, where there are only 1 or 2 C genes, depending upon species.

In men, mice, and rabbits there are codominant allelic variants of several of the C_H and C_L genes. In distinction to other autosomal allelic genes, mature immunoglobulin-producing cells of heterozygotes express only one of the alternative alleles (Pernis et al., 1965; Mage, 1971). In rabbits heterozygous for both C_H and C_κ markers, individual immunoglobulin molecules may express the paternal C_H allotype with the maternal C_κ allotype. Finally, individual immunocytes express either κ or λ light chains, but never both (Bernier and Cebra, 1964). These observations define the following genetic events occurring in the course of B cell differentiation as outlined in Figure 2: first, the permanent selection of either the κ or λ light chain family and corresponding repression of the alternate family and, second, the repression of either the maternal or paternal heavy chain and selected light chain family, a phenomenon called allelic exclusion.

The next genetic events are the integration of the unique V_H and V_L genes which will define the specificity of each developing clone of B cells. A physical translocation of the V gene to a new site on the chromosome adjacent to C genes is involved (Tonegawa et al., 1977). This process is considerably more complex for the heavy chain linkage group than for light chains, since in the former, the selected V_H gene must ultimately be expressed with each of an array of C_H genes. On the basis of evidence to be discussed later that single B lymphocytes may simultaneously synthesize immunoglobulin molecules of 3 classes, each having the same V_H region, we favor the simultaneous insertion model depicted in Figure 2. In this model the selected V_H gene is replicated, perhaps in the form of episomal DNA fragments, and the identical V_H copies are inserted in front of each C_H gene.

There is some evidence that all of these genetic events occur during the pre-B cell stage of differentiation. Pre-B cells synthesize both μ and light chains (Raff et al., 1976; Melchers et al., 1976). In rabbits these cells exhibit allelic exclusion with regard to κ chain allotypes (Hayward et al., 1977). Finally, there are sound theoretical

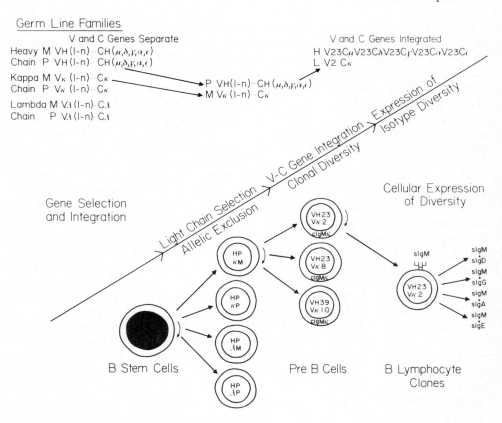

Fig. 2. Model of sequential genetic decisions involved in generation of clonal diversity of B cells. Immuno-globulin molecules are encoded by 3 unlinked gene families: heavy chains and κ and λ light chains. Each family consists of a number of V (variable) genes, coding for the specificity of antibody molecules, which are closely linked to, but separate from, the C (constant) genes specifying antibody class or light chain type. Both structural rearrangements of genetic information and regulation of gene expression are involved in the generation of diverse clones of B cells. Genetic decisions occurring at the pre-B stage of differentiation include the permanent repression of one of the light chain families (κ or λ), and of either the maternal (M) or paternal (P) genes for the selected light chain family and the heavy chain family. The latter process is called allelic exclusion, since it results in the expression of only one of alternative C_H or C_L allelic markers by individual B cells in a heterozygous animal. Probably also at the pre-B cell stage, a single V_H and a V_L gene are selected and physically integrated with C_H and C_L genes respectively. In the case of the heavy chain family, there is evidence that copies of the selected V gene are simultaneously integrated with each of the C genes ($c\mu$, $C\delta$, $C\gamma$, $C\alpha$, $C\varepsilon$). By these processes the specificity information present in germ line V and C genes comes to be expressed in a large number of independent clones of B cells. Assuming that each combination of a V_H and V_L gene confers a unique specificity for antigen, the total number of different specificities is the product of n V_H genes and n V_L genes.

A second level of diversification, occurring at the B lymphocyte stage of differentiation, concerns the expression of antibodies having the same specificity (determined by a unique combination of V_H and V_L gene products) but belonging to different classes (IgM, IgG and so forth). As indicated, the pivotal cell in this process is the immature sIgM⁺ B lymphocyte. Apparently by regulation of expression of already integrated V_H C_H genes, this cell gives rise to sublines which are committed to synthesis of IgM, IgG, IgA, IgE, or IgD antibodies. The unique specificity information encoded by V genes thereby becomes expressed in antibody molecules having widely different biological activities which are determined by C_H information.

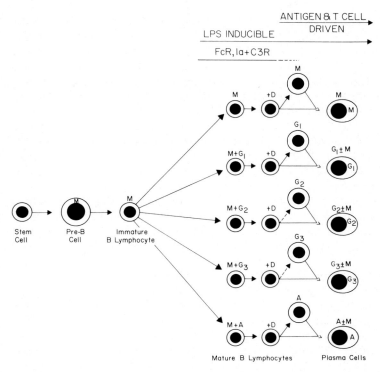

Fig. 3. Model of the intraclonal generation of immunoglobulin isotype diversity. The easily tolerizable, immature sIgM⁺ B lymphocyte is the pivotal cell in the development of multiple B cell sublines ultimately committed to differentiation into plasma cells producing a single immunoglobulin isotype. During development of the clone, cells of the IgG and IgA sublines express their isotype commitment by incorporation of the selected antibody isotype into the plasma membrane in addition to sIgM. Members of each of these sublines later acquire sIgD as a third isotype. Development to this point apparently can occur without antigen or T cell influences. With stimulation by antigen or mitogens, there is a preferential loss of sIgD and, following sufficient proliferation, of sIgM leading to the restriction of synthesis to IgG or IgA by members of these sublines. Work presented by Dr. K. Ishizaka at the Third International Congress of Immunology, Australia, 1977, suggests that IgE-secreting cells also differentiate in accordance with this general scheme. (See text for further details and for references.) (Modified from Abney et al., 1977.)

progeny which will eventually secrete antibodies of a different class, but of the same specificity and light chain type. The pivotal cell in this process is the immature sIgM⁺ B lymphocyte discussed earlier. As was indicated in the preceding section, the genetic rearrangements required for expression of isotype diversity, that is integration of copies of the selected V_H gene with each of the C_H genes, may well occur during the pre-B cell stage. Clearly though it is among the emerging population of B lymphocytes that surface expression of different isotypes begins to reflect the final isotype commitment of individual cells and their progeny. Although expression of isotype diversity may be hastened by exposure of B lymphocytes to an inducing agent such as bacterial lipopolysaccharide (Pernis et al., 1976; Kearney et al., 1977b), it appears normally to be an internally regulated differentiation process that does not require the help of T cells or of exogenous antigens.

The first B lymphocytes to emerge express sIgM exclusively. These rapidly increase in number before a few of the sIgM$^+$ B lymphocytes begin to express a second isotype: sIgD, one of the IgG subclasses, or IgA. At this developmental stage in mice and humans (Abney et al., 1977; Gathings et al., 1977), all B lymphocytes that bear sIgG or sIgA also express sIgM but virtually none express sIgD. With further development, sIgG$^+$.sIgM$^+$ doubles, sIgA$^+$.sIgM$^+$ cells, and sIgM$^+$ cells lacking sIgG or sIgA all acquire sIgD. Treatment with anti-μ antibodies, if begun early enough, prevents development of B cells of all classes. These findings suggest that immature sIgM$^+$ B lymphocytes are the pivotal cells in the generation of the different sublines of B cells, and that sIgD is acquired as a third isotype on B lymphocytes already committed to the eventual synthesis of IgG or IgA or IgM antibodies.

As depicted in the model, there is evidence indicating that, during antigen- or mitogen-driven proliferation and plasma cell differentiation, cells committed to the synthesis of IgG or IgA lose their capacity to synthesize IgM and IgD. Similarly, sIgD is lost or drastically decreased during the proliferation and terminal differentiation of IgM-producing plasma cells (Cooper et al., 1976; Bourgois et al., 1977; Preud'homme, 1977).

The occurrence of sIgD on a large portion of B lymphocytes and its paucity or absence in serum has long suggested that its biological role is primarily one of a surface receptor (Van Boxel et al., 1972; Rowe et al., 1973; Knapp et al., 1973). Recent evidence suggests that the acquisition of sIgD may be an important determinant of the resistance of mature B lymphocytes to tolerance induction or clonal abortion (Cambier et al., 1977; Scott et al., 1977). At the very least, it seems clear that sIgD will prove to be intimately involved in the fine tuning of the type of response to antigen which a virgin B lymphocyte, and possibly memory cells, will make (discussed by Parkhouse and Cooper, 1977).

B LYMPHOCYTE PROLIFERATION AND TERMINAL DIFFERENTIATION

We have repeatedly emphasized the ideas that B cell development, up to and including expression of clonal diversity and of isotype diversity within each clone, occurs in a programmed manner, is probably genetically regulated, and does not depend upon random contact with environmental antigens or on factors provided by T cells. In contrast, the differentiation of B lymphocytes to plasma cells depends upon contact of members of B cell clones with the antigens to which they have complementary immunoglobulin receptors. These differentiation steps are regulated via communications among B cells, macrophages, and T cells. They result in formation of plasma cells which produce thousands of antibody molecules per second having identical specificity to those on the precursor B lymphocyte. Further, through proliferation of the selected B lymphocyte clones, the animal is left with an expanded population of memory cells which permit a more rapid, sustained, and greater response on re-introduction of the same antigen.

The induction of specific antibody responses to most protein antigens requires collaborative interactions with T cells and macrophages (see Paul and Benaceraff, 1977). T cells play a dual role in regulation of antibody responses. One T cell population is involved in positive collaboration, while a distinct subpopulation of T cells indirectly suppresses antibody responses by inhibiting the activity of helper cells (Gershon, 1974; Cantor et al., 1976; Tada, 1977; Moretta et al., 1977b). The requirement for T cell help is greatest for antibody responses of the IgA class and least for IgM responses. Macrophages are clearly involved in T cell–B cell collaboration, in part through their role in presentation of antigen (see Rosenthal et al., 1977; Feldman et al., 1976).

While it is not feasible to undertake a detailed discussion of this important area, some aspects of the regulation of the production of antibody-forming cells will be mentioned briefly. Firstly, optimal cooperation between T cells, macrophages, and B cells in the response to antigen occurs when the interacting cells are genetically identical at the I region of the major histocompatibility complex (MHC) genes (reviewed by Katz and Benacerraf, 1975; Feldman et al., 1976; Tada, 1977) and presumably the same is true for humans. Similarly, it has also been shown that suppressor activity by T cells on antibody production requires genetic identity but at a different sub-region of the I region gene complex (Murphy et al., 1976; Tada, 1977). The interactions between suppressor and helper T cells and of helper T cells with B cells are mediated by biologically active soluble factors released by the appropriate antigen (see Taussig et al., 1975; Tada, 1977). These factors, which may be antigen specific, are incompletely characterized in biochemical terms. However, they contain Ia determinants which are products of I region genes within the MHC (see Tada, 1977). It appears that 2 signals, one provided by the binding of T cell helper factor, and a second mediated by the combination of the B cell's surface antibody with complementary antigen, are required for induction of plasma cell differentiation. The molecular mechanisms of this activation process have not yet been elucidated.

DEFECTS IN B CELL DIFFERENTIATION

The complexity of the sequential steps of B cell differentiation ensure that the occurrence of a great variety of inherited gene defects and of appropriately timed environmental insults will result in a large spectrum of birth defects characterized by abnormal antibody production. Since by necessity the process of B cell differentiation continues throughout life, some inherited abnormalities and spontaneous mutations of genes used by B cells will result in antibody deficiencies of late onset. So far, defects at each major step in B cell differentiation have been identified at a cellular level. We have already mentioned that some infants are born with combined deficiencies of T and B cells, and healthy lymphoid stem cells from the bone marrow of histocompatible siblings have been used to correct these deficiencies. Older hypogammaglobulinemic patients (e.g., those with thymomas) and probably some hypogammaglobulinemic children may show selective failure of stem cell differentiation along B cell lines, as shown by the absence of pre-B cells (Vogler et al., 1976; Pearl et al., 1977). The cellular defect in boys with infantile hypogammaglobulinemia is characterized by normal numbers of bone marrow pre-B cells, few of which are capable of further B-cell differentiation (see Pearl et al., 1978). Many individuals with panhypogammaglobulinemia and with selective isotype deficiencies (e.g., selective IgA deficiency and combined IgG and IgA deficiencies) have normal numbers of circulating B lymphocytes (reviewed by Cooper et al., 1975). Moreover, normal diversity of surface immunoglobulin isotypes can usually be demonstrated in this group of antibody-deficient patients, and evidence for clonal diversity of their antigen-binding B lymphocytes has been presented (Dwyer and Hosking, 1972). Already it is evident that each of these phenotypic forms of 'arrested' B lymphocyte differentiation can be due to a variety of primary defects. For example, the same antibody deficiency syndrome could be due to (1) an inherent B cell defect which prevents induction of terminal plasma cell differentiation of one or all B cell sublines (Wu et al., 1973; Geha et al., 1974; De La Concha et al., 1977), (2) abnormalities of MHC gene products (cites by Van Rood, 1977) or (3) of other cellular products necessary for antigen induction of B cell differentiation (Wu et al., 1973), or (4) primary abnormalities in helper T cells (see Cooper et al., 1975; Moretta et al., 1977a) or their inhibition by suppressor T cells (reviewed by Waldmann and Broder, 1977). In a few antibody-deficient patients, B cell differentiation may even advance to plasma cells which have faulty mechanisms for secretion of the antibodies they produce (Geha et al., 1974). Rare patients have been shown to have deficiencies in the development of sublines of B cells committed to the synthesis of different subclasses of IgG (Yount et al., 1969). B cells in a few immunodeficient individuals fail to espress the κ chain family of immunoglobulin genes (Bernier et al., 1972; Zegers et al., 1976). These examples of B cell defects provide only a brief preview of the many errors in B cell differentiation that remain to be recognized and defined.

The interplay between normal pathways of B cell differentiation and the occurrence of malignancy is equally fascinating. In a virus-induced malignancy of chicken B cells, avian lymphoid leukosis, the target of the oncogenic event is a bursal lymphocyte at a particular stage in its differentiation, and a characteristic of the transformed cells is their failure to undergo further differentiation (Cooper et al., 1974). The B cell malignancies of man and other mammals represent excessive accumulations of single clones of B cells which may involve each of the stages of differentiation briefly covered in this review (see Cooper and Seligmann, 1977). For example, Vogler et al. (1978) have discovered that approximately 20 % of acute lymphoblastic leukemias of childhood may represent clonal overgrowths of pre-B cells. Even for plasma cell myelomas, the oncogenic event apparently can affect the clone at the pre-B cell stage in differentiation (unpublished observations by Preud'homme and Seligmann; and Kubagawa, Vogler et al.).

We conclude that a large spectrum of birth defects that may easily escape detection at birth involve defective differentiation of B cells and their cohort cells of the immune system. A more precise definition of the complex processes involved in B cell differentiation is needed to understand, prevent and successfully treat both congenital and acquired defects in antibody production and their often disastrous consequences. Moreover, knowledge about the basic principles involved in normal and abnormal B cell differentiation may contribute to the eventual understanding of the normal and abnormal development of other cell lines.

ACKNOWLEDGMENTS

We are grateful to our colleagues for sharing their ideas and experimental observations with us, and we thank Mrs. Helen Robison and Mrs. Tina Chaffin for their help in preparation of the manuscript.

REFERENCES

Abney, E. R., Cooper, M. D., Kearney, J. F., Lawton, A. R. and Parkhouse, R. M. E. (1977): In: *ICN-UCLA Symposium Proceedings, Immune System. Genetics and Regulation, Vol. 6*, pp. 309–311. Editors: E. Sercarz, L. A. Herzenberg and C. F. Fox, Academic Press, New York.

Adamson, J. W., Fialkow, P. J., Murphy, S., Prahl, J. F. and Steinman, L. (1976): *New Engl. J. Med., 295*, 913.

Bernier, G. and Cebra, J. J. (1964): *Science, 144*, 1590.

Bernier, G. M., Gunderman, J. R. and Ruymann, F. B. (1972): *Blood, 40*, 795.

Binz, H. and Wigzell, H. (1976): *Cold Spr. Harb. Symp. quant. Biol., 41*, 275.

Blaese, R. M. and Lawrence, E. C. (1977): In: *Development of Host Defenses*, p. 201. Editors: M. D. Cooper and D. H. Dayton. Raven Press, New York.

Bourgois, A., Kitajima, K., Hunter, I. R. and Askonas, B. A. (1977): *Europ. J. Immunol., 7*, 151.

Burrows, P. D., Kearney, J. F., Lawton, A. R. and Cooper, M. D. (1978): *J. Immunol.*, in press.

Cambier, J. C., Kettman, J. R., Vitetta, E. S. and Uhr, J. W. (1976): *J. exp. Med., 142*, 1254.

Cambier, J. C., Vitetta, E. S., Kettman, J. R., Werzel, G. M. and Uhr, J. W. (1977): *J. exp. Med., 146*, 107.

Cantor, H., Shen, F. W. and Boyse, E. A. (1976): *J. exp. Med., 143*, 1391.

Ciccimarra, F., Rosen, F. S., Schneeburger, E. and Merler, E. (1976): *J. clin. Invest., 57*, 1386.

Cohen, J. E., D'Eustachio, P. and Edelman, G. M. (1977): *J. exp. Med., 146*, 394.

Cooper, M. D., Kearney, J. F., Lawton, A. R., Abney, E. R., Parkhouse, R. M. E., Preud'homme, J. L. and Seligmann, M. (1976): *Ann. Immunol. (Inst. Pasteur), 127C*, 573.

Cooper, M. D., Keightley, R. G. and Lawton, A. R. (1975): In: *Membrane Receptors of Lymphocytes*, p. 431. Editors: M. Seligmann, J. L. Preud'homme and F. M. Kourilsky. North-Holland Publishing Company, Amsterdam.

Cooper, M. D., Keightley, R. G., Wu, L. Y. F. and Lawton, A. R. (1973): *Transplant. Rev., 16*, 51.

Cooper, M. D., Purchase, H. G., Bockman, D. E. and Gathings, W. E. (1974): *J. Immunol., 113*, 1210.

Cooper, M. D. and Seligmann, M. (1977): In: *B and T Cells in Immune Recognition*, p. 377. Editors: F. Loor and G. E. Roelants. John Wiley and Sons, Ltd., Chicester, U.K.

Cosenza, H. and Köhler, H. (1972): *Proc. nat. Acad. Sci. (Wash.), 69*, 2701.

Cunningham, A. J. (1976): In: *The Generation of Antibody Diversity*, p. 89. Editor: A. J. Cunningham. Academic Press, New York.

De La Concha, E. G., Oldham, G., Webster, A. D. B., Asherson, G. L. and Platts-Mills, T. A. E. (1977): *Clin. exp. Immunol., 26*, 208.

Dreyer, W. J. and Bennett, J. C. (1965): *Proc. nat. Acad. Sci. (Wash.), 54*, 864.

Dwyer, J. M. and Hosking, C. S. (1972): *Clin. exp. Immunopath., 1*, 84.

Feldman, M., Beverley, P., Erb, P., Howie, S., Kontiainen, S., Maoz, A., Mathies, M., McKenzie, I. and Woody, J. (1976): *Cold Spr. Harb. Symp. quant. Biol., 41*, 165.

Gathings, W. E., Lawton, A. R. and Cooper, M. D. (1977): *Europ. J. Immunol., 7*, 804.

Geha, R. S., Schneeberger, E., Merler, E. and Rosen, F. S. (1974): *New Engl. J. Med., 291*, 1.

Gelfand, M. D., Elfenbein, G. J., Frank, M. M. and Paul, W. E. (1974): *J. exp. Med., 139*, 1128.

Gershon, R. K. (1974): In: *Contemporary Topics in Immunobiology, Vol. 3*, p. 1. Editors: M. D. Cooper and N. L. Warner. Plenum Press, New York–London.

Goidl, E. A. and Siskind, G. W. (1974): *J. exp. Med., 140*, 1285.

Goldstein, G., Scheid, M., Boyse, E. A., Brand, A. and Gilmour, D. G. (1976): *Cold Spr. Harb. Symp. quant. Biol., 41*, 5.

Good, R. A. (1973): *Harvey Lect. Ser., 67*, 1.

Greaves, M. F., Owen, J. J. T. and Raff, M. C. (1973): *T and B Lymphocytes: Origins, Properties and Roles in Immune Responses*. Excerpta Medica, Amsterdam. American Elsevier, New York.

Grossi, C. E., Lydyard, P. M. and Cooper, M. D. (1977): *J. Immunol., 119*, 749.

Hayward, A. R., Simons, M., Lawton, A. R., Cooper, M. D. and Mage, R. G. (1977): *Fed. Proc., 36*, 1295.

Hood, L., Kronenberg, M., Early, P. and Johnson, N. (1977): In: *ICN-UCLA Symposium Proceedings, Immune System. Genetics and Regulation, Vol. 6*, pp. 1–26. Editors: E. Sercarz, L. A. Herzenberg and C. F. Fox. Academic Press, New York.

Hood, L. and Prahl, J. (1971): *Advanc. Immunol., 14*, 291.

Katz, D. H. and Benacerraf, B. (1975): *Transplant. Rev., 22*, 175.

Knapp, W., Boluis, R. L. H., Radl, J. and Hijmans, W. (1973): *J. Immunol., 111*, 1295.

Kearney, J. F., Cooper, M. D., Klein, J., Abney, E. R., Parkhouse, R. M. E. and Lawton, A. R. (1977a): *J. exp. Med., 146*, 297.

Kearney, J. F. and Lawton, A. R. (1975): *J. Immunol., 115*, 677.

Kearney, J. F., Lawton, A. R. and Cooper, M. D. (1977b): In: *ICN-UCLA Symposium Proceedings, Immune System. Genetics and Regulation, Vol. 6*, pp. 313–320. Editors: E. Sercarz, L. A. Herzenberg and C. F. Fox. Academic Press, New York.

Kincade, P. W., Lawton, A. R., Bockman, D. E. and Cooper, M. D. (1970): *Proc. natl. Acad. Sci. (Wash.), 67*, 1918.

Klinman, N. R. (1976): *Amer. J. Path., 69*, 4.

Klinman, N. R., Sigal, N. H., Metcalf, E. S., Pierce, S. K. and Gearhart, P. J. (1976): *Cold Spr. Harb. Symp. quant. Biol., 41*, 165.

Kruisbeek, A. M., Kröse, T. and Zijlstra, C. J. M. (1977): *Europ. J. Immunol., 7*, 375.

Lawton, A. R. and Cooper, M. D. (1974): In: *Contemporary Topics in Immunobiology, Vol. 3*, p. 193. Editors: M. D. Cooper and N. L. Warner. Plenum Press, New York–London.

Lawton, A. R., Self, K. S., Royal, S. A. and Cooper, M. D. (1972): *Clin. Immunol. Immunopath., 1*, 104.

Lydyard, P. M., Grossi, C. E. and Cooper, M. D. (1976): *J. exp. Med., 144*, 79.

Mage, R. G. (1971): In: *Progress in Immunology*, p. 47. Editor: B. Amos. Academic Press, New York.

Melchers, F., Andersson, J. and Phillips, R. A. (1976): *Cold Spr. Harb. Symp. quant. Biol., 41*, 147.

Metcalf, E. S. and Klinman, N. R. (1976): *J. exp. Med., 143*, 1327.

Metcalf, D. and Moore, M. A. S. (1971): *Hemopoietic Cells.* Editors: A. Neuberger and E. L. Tatum. North-Holland Publishing Company, Amsterdam.

Moretta, L., Mingari, M. C., Webb, S. R., Pearl, E. R., Lydyard, P. M., Grossi, C. E., Lawton, A. R. and Cooper, M. D. (1977a): *Europ. J. Immunol.*, in press.

Moretta, L., Webb, S. R., Grossi, C. E., Lydyard, P. M. and Cooper, M. D. (1977b): *J. exp. Med., 146*, 184.

Murphy, D. B., Herzenberg, L. A., Okomura, K., Herzenberg, L. A. and McDevitt, H. O. (1976): *J. exp. Med., 144*, 699.

Nossal, G. J. V. and Pike, B. L. (1975): *J. exp. Med., 141*, 904.

Okos, A. J. and Gathings, W. E. (1977): *Fed. Proc., 36*, 1294A.

Osmond, D. G. and Nossal, G. J. V. (1974): *Cell. Immunol., 13*, 132.

Owen, J. J. T., Cooper, M. D. and Raff, M. C. (1974): *Nature (Lond.), 249*, 361.

Owen, J. J. T., Wright, D. E., Habu, S., Raff, M. C. and Cooper, M. D. (1977): *J. Immunol., 118*, 2067.

Papiernik, M., Nabarra, B. and Back, J.-F. (1975): *Clin. exp. Immunol., 19*, 281.

Parkhouse, R. M. E. and Cooper, M. D. (1977: *Immunol. Rev., 37*, 105.

Paul, W. E. and Benacerraf, B. (1977): *Science, 195*, 1293.

Pearl, E. R., Vogler, L. B., Okos, A. J., Crist, W. M., Lawton, A. R. and Cooper, M. D. (1978): *J. Immunol.*, in press.

Pernis, B., Chiappino, G., Kelus, A. S. and Gell, P. G. H. (1965): *J. exp. Med., 122*, 853.

Pernis, B., Forni, L. and Luzzati, A. L. (1976): *Cold Spr. Harb. Symp. quant. Biol., 41*, 175.

Preud'homme, J. L. (1977): *Europ. J. Immunol., 7*, 191.

Pyke, K. W. and Gelfand, E. W. (1974): *Nature (Lond.), 251*, 421.

Raff, M. C. (1977): *Nature (Lond.), 265*, 205.

Raff, M. C., Feldmann, M. and DePetris, S. (1973): *J. exp. Med., 137*, 1024.

Raff, M. C., Megson, M., Owen, J. J. T. and Cooper, M. D. (1976): *Nature (Lond.), 259*, 224.

Raff, M. C., Owen, J. J. T., Cooper, M. D., Lawton, A. R., Megson, M. and Gathings, W. E. (1975): *J. exp. Med., 142*, 1052.

Rajewsky, K., Hammerling, G. J., Black, S. J., Berek, C. and Eichmann, K. (1976): In: *The Role of Products of the Histocompatibility Gene Complex in Immune Responses*, p. 445. Editors: D. H. Katz and B. Benacerraf. Academic Press, New York.

Rosenthal, A. S., Barcenski, M. A. and Blake, J. T. (1977): *Nature (Lond.), 267*, 156.

Rowe, D. S., Hug, K., Forni, L. and Pernis, B. (1973): *J. exp. Med., 138*, 965.

Scheid, M. P., Goldstein, G., Hammerling, U. and Boyse, E. A. (1975): In: *Membrane Receptors of Lymphocytes*, p. 353. Editors: M. Seligmann, J. L. Preud'homme and F. M. Kourilsky. North-Holland Publishing Company, Amsterdam.

Scott, D. W., Layton, J. E. and Nossal, G. J. V. (1977): *J. exp. Med., 146*, 1473.

Sidman, C. L. and Unanue, E. R. (1975a): *J. Immunol., 114*, 1730.

Sidman, C. L. and Unanue, E. R. (1975b): *Nature (Lond.), 257*, 149.

Stutman, O. (1977): In: *Contemporary Topics in Immunobiology, Vol. 7*, p. 1. Editor: O. Stutman. Plenum Press, New York–London.

Tada, T. (1977): In: *ICN-UCLA Symposium Proceedings, Immune System. Genetics and Regulation, Vol. 6*, pp. 345–361. Editors: E. Sercarz, L. A. Herzenberg and C. F. Fox. Academic Press, New York.

Taylor, R. B., Duffus, W. P. H., Raff, M. C. and de Petris, S. (1971): *Nature New Biol., 233*, 225.

Taussig, M. J., Munro, A. J., Campbell, R., David, C. S. and Staines, N. A. (1975): *J. exp. Med., 142*, 20.

Tonegawa, S., Hozumi, N., Brack, C. and Schuller, R. (1977): In: *ICN-UCLA Symposium Proceedings, Immune System. Genetics and Regulation, Vol. 6*, pp. 43–55. Editors: E. Sercarz, L. A. Herzenberg and C. F. Fox. Academic Press, New York.

Van Boxel, J., Paul, W. E., Terry, W. D. and Green, I. (1972): *J. Immunol., 109*, 649.

Van Rood, J. J. (1977): In: *Progress in Immunology, III*. Editors: T. E. Mandel, C. Cheers, C. S. Hosking, I. F. C. McKenzie and G. J. V. Nossal. Elsevier/North-Holland Inc., New York. In press.

Vogler, L. B., Crist, W. M., Bockman, D. E., Pearl, E. R., Lawton, A. R. and Cooper, M. D. (1978): *New Engl. J. Med.*, in press.

Vogler, L. B., Pearl, E. R., Gathings, W. E., Lawton, A. R. and Cooper, M. D. (1976): *Lancet, 2*, 376.

Waldmann, T. A. and Broder, S. (1977): *Progr. clin. Immunol., 3*, 155.

Wu, L. Y. F., Lawton, A. R. and Cooper, M. D. (1973): *J. clin. Invest., 52*, 3180.

Yount, W. J., Hong, R., Seligmann, M. and Kunkel, H. G. (1969): *J. clin. Invest., 48*, 92a.

Zegers, B. J. M., Maertzdorf, W. J., Van Loghem, E., Mul, N. A. J., Stoop, J. W., Van der Laag, J., Vossen, J. J. and Ballieux, R. E. (1976): *New Engl. J. Med., 294*, 1026.

Molecular analysis of neural recognition

**A potential role for the Tay-Sachs ganglioside (GM$_2$)
in the development of the retino-tectal projection***

STEPHEN ROTH

Department of Biology, The Johns Hopkins University, Baltimore, Md., U.S.A.

This paper will describe an in vitro assay that measures adhesive recognition between retinal cells and tectal surfaces from the developing chick embryo. The differences in cell adhesion are consistent with the physiological map of the retinal ganglion axons on the tectal surfaces in vivo. Enzymatic perturbation of the in vitro assay shows that protease-sensitive elements are important to the recognition and that these are located more heavily on the ventral aspects of the retina and tectum. Experiments with 2 bacterial N-acetylgalactosaminidases show, similarly, that surface moieties sensitive to these enzymes are also important to the recognition but that these elements are distributed, or exposed, more heavily on the dorsal aspects of both retina and tectum.

A number of additional lines of experimentation point to the ganglioside GM$_2$, or a molecule with a similar carbohydrate sequence, as the compound that is more dorsally concentrated. Direct tests of this possibility yield results that are consistent with this proposal.

Therefore, the Tay-Sachs ganglioside, GM$_2$, or a very similar oligosaccharide on a different aglycone, plays a definite role in retino-tectal adhesion in vitro. In vivo experiments will be required to determine the role of this compound in the development, in vivo, of the visual projection.

Anatomy of the retino-tectal projection

The projection of retinal ganglion cell axons onto the optic tecta occurs with remarkable fidelity and, accordingly, this system has become the standard of precision for all of neuromorphogenesis. In the chick embryo, the first retinal ganglion cells appear to undergo their final mitoses in the early days of development (Fujita and Horii, 1963). The last ganglion cells to undergo their final mitosis are those more

*The original research described herein from the author's laboratory has been made possible by research grants and a career development award from the National Institute of Child Health and Human Development, National Institutes of Health of the U.S.A. This is manuscript 915 from the McCollum-Pratt Institute.

196

peripherally located in the retina. By the 8th day of development, all of the ganglion cells are present. Even before the last of the ganglion cells have made their definitive appearances, however, the older ganglion cells, which are more centrally located in the fundus of the retina, have already begun to send their axons over the inner surface of the retina toward the choroid fissure and what will become, eventually, the optic nerve (DeLong and Coulombre, 1965). The ganglionic processes from each retina cross at the chiasm with no mixing and, beginning with the 6th day of chick development, reach the surface of the contralateral tectum. The fibers migrate over the tectal surface in an orderly fashion and create a complete map of the retina on the tectum by about day 11 (Crossland et al., 1974). Histologic and electrophysiologic data show that the visual field is projected onto the tectal surfaces with a reversal in 2 axes (Hamdi and Whitteridge, 1954; McGill et al., 1966; Crossland et al., 1974); that is, ganglion cells from the dorsal retina project to the ventral tectum and vice versa. Ganglion cells from the nasal retina project to the posterior tectum whereas those from the temporal retina project to the anterior tectum. This pattern is identical to those seen in all sub-mammalian vertebrates so far examined (see Jacobson, 1970, for a comprehensive review). Figure 1 shows a dia-

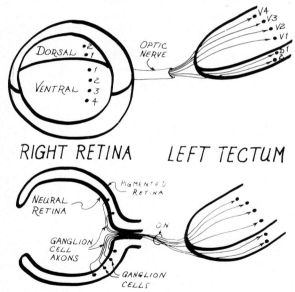

Fig. 1. Highly schematized diagram of tectal innervation by retinal ganglion cells in the chick. In the upper drawing, the view is directly into the right retina through the pupillary opening. Six ganglion cells are indicated by points, 4 of these are located in the ventral half of the retina and 2 in the dorsal half. The ultimate position of the axon tips of these 6 ganglion cells on the surface of the tectum is depicted at the right in both the upper and lower drawings. If the ganglion cell soma is situated more ventrally in the retina, then its axon tip becomes situated more dorsally on the tectal surface by the 12th day of development. For example, ganglion cell V4 is more ventral in the retina than V1. Accordingly, its process terminates more dorsally on the tectum than does the process of V1. Similarly, approximately 10^6 ganglion cells in the retina form a continuous map of the retina on the tectum, although the axes of the tectal map are reversed with respect to those of the retina. The lower drawing shows the retina in sagittal section and illustrates the path of the ganglionic axons along the inner surface of the retina and top of the ganglion cells to the optic nerve. The vast majority of the cells of the neural retina are not ganglion cells but may serve as substrates for the ganglionic axons.

grammatic representation of the retino-tectal projection only for the dorso-ventral axis.

Sperry's hypotheses

In 1925, Matthey showed that newts could regain vision after their optic nerves were sectioned; Roger Sperry duplicated these results (1943) and, further, demonstrated that if the eye were rotated 180° on an anterior-posterior axis after the optic nerve was cut, the newt's regained vision was forever inverted (1945). From a variety of experiments along these lines, Sperry concluded that axons of the optic nerve were chemically different from one another and that the differences increased as the distance between the ganglionic cell bodies increased in the retina. In one model (1963), he suggested that at least 2 perpendicular gradients of complementary molecules could give rise to the retino-tectal projection in the sub-mammalian vertebrates. One version of this kind of model is taken from Marchase et al. (1975) and shows a lock-and-key complementarity with the 'keys' concentrated dorsally and the 'locks' more prevalent ventrally (Fig. 2). Here, a quantitative variation in molecular species could insure that incoming fibers from the dorsal retina tend to migrate ventrally on the tectum because of the firmer adhesions, i.e. more molecular complexes possible, in that direction. Of course, incoming fibers from the ventral

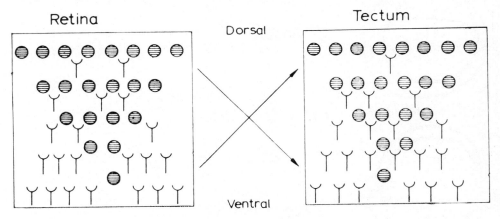

Results in dorsal-to-ventral affinity

Fig. 2. Retino-tectal specificity as a result of gradients of complementary molecules. A simple model that could account, in part, for the retino-tectal projection. Complementary molecules are distributed in 2 gradients of opposite polarity across the surfaces of both the retina and tectum. The molecules are capable of serving as recognition and adhesion components when a lock-and-key fit occurs. For example, ganglion cells that are dorsally located in the retina would have many ⊖'s and fewer Ψ's. Assuming that this molecular composition is shared by the ganglionic axons, the axons would migrate on the tectum in the direction of more stable adhesions, i.e., toward the ventral surface of the tectum where Ψ's are plentiful and ○'s are relatively rare. Given another set of complementary molecules in the naso-temporal axis, and given the inevitable competition for appropriate sites on the tectal surface as 10^6 axons impinge on it, an accurate but inverted map of the retina would result on the tectal surface. Data obtained to date imply that the dorsally located molecules are resistant to proteases and contain oligosaccharide sequences very similar to those found in the Tay-Sachs ganglioside (GM_2).

retina would migrate dorsally for the same reason. Although not diagrammed in Figure 2, a gradient of different lock-and-key components could exist in the naso-temporal axis. Conceivably, 2 gradients like these would specify the information required for the visual projection. The precision of such a projection could be increased by such factors as competition for sites among the million or so incoming retinal axons or the presence of additional gradients (Sperry, 1963; Marchase et al., 1975).

There are other mechanisms postulated for the development of the retinal map on the tectum. Gaze et al. (1963) have suggested that the optic axons always maintain a specific relationship toward one another but that the absolute dimensions of the visual field are plastic and can vary to accommodate tectal fields of different sizes. For this type of model, the retinal axons require a method for judging their own positions relative to the field, but a specific, biochemical label on the tectum is not required.

It is also possible that the incoming fibers take up positions on the surface of the tectum according to the time at which they reach the tectum. For example, the first fibers to arrive might travel the furthest and the last fibers to arrive might take up the more proximal positions, the only positions left at that time. In the vertebrates, many experimental results are inconsistent with temporal models. Most notably, regeneration experiments show that although the usual temporal sequence of arrival of the retinal axons is disturbed compared to that sequence found during embryogenesis, the resulting visual projection is normal. Nevertheless, there is evidence for a temporal mechanism in some lower organisms and, even in the vertebrates, this factor should not be ruled out completely.

The experiments that will be summarized briefly in this report were performed by Drs. Anthony Barbera, Richard Marchase, Michael Pierce and many of their co-workers in our laboratory beginning in 1971. The data obtained are most consistent with Sperry's ideas of biochemical labels on the retina and the tectum, and, specifically, with the model illustrated in Figure 2. Chicken embryos were used throughout and the retinal cells were derived from intact, neural retina dissociated with trypsin. That is, the great bulk of the cells are not ganglion cells and, therefore, never send processes to the tectum, nor do they interact directly with the tectum in any known way. Furthermore, the 1–2% of the cells in the retina suspensions that are, in fact, ganglion cells are devoid of their axons since these were removed during the dissection. The implications of these facts will be discussed.

METHODS AND RESULTS

The in vitro assay

In order to detect adhesive preferences between dorsal retinal cells and ventral tectal surfaces, for example, intact tecta are dissected, bisected and pinned to paraffin-coated Petri dishes. Typically, 6 dorsal tectal halves and 6 ventral tectal halves are pinned and subsequently exposed to a single, labeled suspension of either dorsal or ventral retinal cells. After the cells are allowed to interact with both types of tectal halves, the halves are washed free of non-adherent retinal cells. The tectal halves can then be counted individually in a scintillation counter and the number of adherent cells determined from a previous count of the specific activity of the particular cell suspension being tested. The details of this assay have been published elsewhere (Barbera, 1975; Marchase, 1977). One of the advantages of collection assays of this type is that the collecting surfaces, tectal halves in this case, are exposed to identical cell suspensions. Therefore, many potentially confounding variables are controlled internally. Among these are precise cell diameters and concentrations, cell 'recovery' from the dissociation process, medium viscosity and, finally, the mode of shaking the vessel. When a ventral and a dorsal tectal surface is exposed to, say, a suspension of dorsal retinal cells that had been prelabeled with $^{32}P_i$, any significant difference in the number of adherent cells between dorsal and ventral tectal surfaces is likely to be a manifestation of some cellular property and not an in vitro artifact. Whether

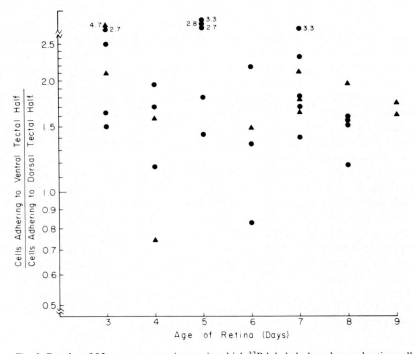

Fig. 3. Results of 35 separate experiments in which ^{32}P-labeled, dorsal neural retina cells were applied to 11–12 day tectal halves. The age of the embryos from which the dorsal retina cells were dissected was varied from 3 to 9 days of development. Each point is a mean of the number of dorsal retina cells collected by ventral tectal halves divided by the number collected by dorsal tectal halves. Each experiment was carried out as described with 6 ventral and 6 dorsal tectal halves pinned to a single dish. The data show that, as early as 3 days of development, dorsal retina cells can distinguish between dorsal and ventral tectal halves and that they adhere preferentially (by a factor of about 2) to the physiologically matching, i.e., ventral tectal half. The solid triangles are experiments in which the tectal halves came from embryos whose eyes were destroyed at day 2. These tectal halves were completely devoid of retinal axons on their surfaces although they are clearly subject to the same adhesive specificity as the innervated tectal halves (solid circles). This control allows the conclusion that the retinal cells are adhering preferentially to tectal tissue and not to retinal processes on tectal surfaces. Furthermore, it is evident that the tectal halves develop their molecular specificities independent of retinal innervation.

or not the differences obtained in vitro are relevant to in vivo neuromorphogenesis is another question, of course, but a question that can be answered.

Results

In brief, the data from over 200 experiments show clearly that cells from dorsal retinal areas adhere preferentially to ventral tectal surfaces by a factor of about 2. The very important reciprocal experiment shows that ventral retinal cells adhere to dorsal tectal surfaces by about the same factor. If tectal age is held constant at 11–12 days while retinal age is varied, the results for dorsal retinal cells is shown in Figure 3 and for ventral retinal cells in Figure 4. In these figures, each point is a ratio of the number of retinal cells adhering to the physiologically matching tectal half

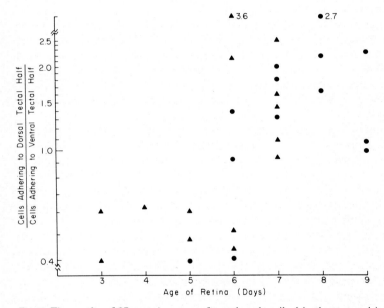

Fig. 4. The results of 27 experiments performed as described in the text and in the legend to Figure 3. Here, however, ^{32}P-labeled, ventral retinal cells were applied to the tectal halves. Each point is a mean ratio obtained by dividing the number of ventral cells collected on dorsal tectal halves by the number collected on ventral tectal halves. Unlike dorsal retinal cells (Fig. 3) which distinguish between 'correct' and 'incorrect' tectal halves throughout development, ventral retinal cells choose 'incorrectly' before day 6. After day 6, they choose correctly. In addition, the ventral retinal cells require 3 to 4 hours of incubation in complete medium after being trypsinized before they can adhere preferentially to dorsal tectal halves. If such an incubation is omitted, or if metabolism is blocked during this incubation, then ventral retinal cells will adhere preferentially to ventral tectal halves – the physiologically 'incorrect' tectal half. Before day 6, no amount of incubation (up to 12 hours) allows ventral retinal cells to adhere preferentially to dorsal tectal halves. Instead, they adhere to ventral tectal halves. These data suggest that, after day 6, ventral retinal cells discriminate between dorsal and ventral tectal halves with protease-sensitive elements. When these are removed by trypsinization, the cells become more like dorsal retinal cells and adhere to ventral tectal halves as dorsal cells do. Only after the proteins are regenerated can the ventral cells adhere to their appropriate, in vivo target, the dorsal tectal surface. Before day 6, either the ventral retina has not elaborated the specific proteins required for adhesive specificity or it is not yet capable of regenerating them once removed.

(e.g., dorsal retina to ventral tectum) divided by the number adhering to the non-matching half (e.g., dorsal retina to dorsal tectum) for a single Petri dish with 6 dorsal tectal halves and 6 ventral halves. It is clear that dorsal retinal cells can adhere preferentially to ventral tectal surfaces before the retina actually does interact with tecta in vivo. In the case of the ventral retina, however, there is an abrupt change in specificity at day 6. Before this time, ventral retinal cells adhere selectively to ventral tectal surfaces, the physiologically non-matching tectal half. Preferential adhesion that correlates with morphogenesis only occurs after day 6. The ventral retinal cells are also different from the dorsal retinal cells in that, after trypsinization, only the ventral cells require a 'recovery' period before they will selectively adhere to dorsal tectal surfaces. If no such incubation is provided, or if it is provided but metabolism is interfered with in any way, then the ventral retinal cells will adhere selectively to ventral tectal surfaces, which are not the surfaces to which the ventral retinal ganglion cells normally project in vivo.

In control experiments with other cell types, non-retinal cells show no preference for either tectal half. Non-innervated tectal halves from embryos that were subjected to early vitrectomy (see Figs. 3 and 4) served as well in these assays as did innervated tectal halves. This shows that retinal cells, in demonstrating this specificity, are not simply adhering to retinal fibers that are already present on the tectal surfaces. All of the data discussed above were taken from the extensive study of this system made by Barbera (1975).

A biochemical analysis of in vitro retino-tectal adhesion assay was undertaken subsequently by Marchase (1977). The data described below come from this work. Marchase (1977) took advantage of the fact that the retino-tectal adhesion system, unlike other in vitro systems for the study of intercellular adhesion, offered the possibility of asymmetric results and, hence, an indication of biological significance. For example, it had already been observed (Barbera et al., 1973; Barbera, 1975) that trypsin affected ventral retinal cells' attachment to dorsal tectal halves much more than it did their attachment to ventral tectal halves. Trypsin did not affect dorsal retinal cells at all. Although it is not news that proteases have adverse affects on intercellular adhesion, the pair-wise comparisons implicit in the system allowed the conclusion that trypsin-sensitive elements necessary for adhesion are more prevalent on ventral retinal cells than on dorsal retinal cells. Treatment of tectal surfaces with trypsin and chymotrypsin showed that only ventral tectal surfaces are protease-sensitive, in a fashion entirely analogous to that found with the retinal cells. Table 1 shows a sample of the type of data obtained when tectal surfaces are treated with proteases, washed extensively and then used as collecting surfaces for labeled, dorsal and ventral retinal cells. Of all the other enzymes tested, only one causes asymmetric and negative results and that enzyme is β-N-acetylgalactosaminidase. Here, however, the enzyme affects dorsal tectal surfaces, not ventral, and dorsal retinal cells, not ventral. Table 2 shows some of these data. Tectal surfaces are treated with the N-acetylgalactosaminidase, washed and used in the collection assay. The attachment of ventral retinal cells to the dorsal tectal surfaces is most severely affected. Enzymes active against β-N-acetylgalactosaminides were purified in our laboratory from 2 different bacterial sources – Diplococcus and Clostridium – and both enzyme preparations have the same effects.

Purified β-galactosidases from these same bacterial supernatants show asymmetric

TABLE 1

Retino-tectal ahhesion following protease treatment of tectal halves

Labeled retinal suspension	Tectal halves	Retinal cells adhering/Tectal half in 30 minutes		
		PBS-treated tecta	Trypsin-treated[a] tecta	Chymotrypsin-treated[b] tecta
Dorsal[c]	Dorsal	1060 ± 190	890 ± 110	910 ± 40
	Ventral	1850 ± 290	620 ± 70*	670 ± 110*
Ventral[d]	Dorsal	920 ± 90	820 ± 100	740 ± 60
	Ventral	1790 ± 150	1530 ± 270	1410 ± 220

*Significantly different from control, $p < 0.01$. [a]0.09% crystalline trypsin, 15 min, 37°. [b]0.17% crystalline chymotrypsin, 15 min, 37°. [c]7 day, 1.0×10^6 cells/ml, 4-hour preincubation. [d]7 day, 1.0×10^6 cells/ml, 4-hour preincubation.

affects but, here, the affect is stimulatory. As can be seen in Table 3, tectal surface treatment with β-galactosidase increases the attachment of ventral retinal cells to ventral tectal halves.

Taken together, these data suggested that an oligosaccharide sequence was prevalent dorsally on both the retina and tectum and important in retinal cell attachment to the appropriate tectal halves. The enzymatic perturbations implied that the oligosaccharide sequence terminated in a β-linked N-acetylgalactosaminide. Further, the results with the galactosidase suggested that this oligosaccharide might be present ventrally, as well, but that on the ventral aspects of the retina and tectum

TABLE 2

Retino-tectal ahhesion following treatment with bacterial β-N-acetylhexosaminidase

Enzyme source	Labeled retinal suspension	Tectal half	Retinal cells adhering/Tectal half in 1 hour		
			Neither tissue treated	Retinal cells treated	Tectal halves treated
Diplococcus pneumoniae[a]	Dorsal[c]	Dorsal	2430 ± 210	1860 ± 90*	2070 ± 260
		Ventral	4560 ± 620	1990 ± 140**	4240 ± 390
	Ventral[d]	Dorsal	6170 ± 390	5850 ± 610	2820 ± 140**
		Ventral	3990 ± 470	3740 ± 210	2810 ± 310*
Clostridium perfringens[b]	Dorsal[e]	Dorsal	2860 ± 350	2450 ± 210	2230 ± 270
		Ventral	5320 ± 390	2730 ± 240**	4820 ± 300
	Ventral[f]	Dorsal	4250 ± 610	3970 ± 390	1960 ± 210**
		Ventral	2290 ± 100	2060 ± 240	1720 ± 260*

*Significantly different from controls, $p < 0.05$. **Significantly different from controls, $p < 0.01$. [a]25 units/ml in PBS pH 6.0, 15 min, 37 ; controls treated with PBS. [b]25 units/ml in PBS pH 6.5, 15 min, 37°; controls treated with PBS. [c]8 day, 1.0×10^6 cells/ml, 0.09 c.p.m./cell, 4 hr preincubation. [d]7 day, 1.0×10^6 cells/ml, 0.24 c.p.m./cell, 4 hr preincubation. [e]7 day, 0.9×10^6 cells/ml, 0.23 c.p.m./cell, 4 hr preincubation. [f]7day, 1.0×10^6 cells/ml, 0.19 c.p.m./cell, 4 hr preincubation.

TABLE 3

Retino-tectal adhesion following treatment with bacterial β-galactosidase

Enzyme source	Labeled retinal suspension	Tectal half	Retinal cells adhering/Tectal half in 1 hour		
			Neither tissue treated	Retinal cells treated	Tectal halves treated
Diplococcus pneumoniae[a]	Dorsal[c]	Dorsal	2850 ± 360	3130 ± 140	3070 ± 290
		Ventral	4640 ± 210	4820 ± 260	4780 ± 410
	Ventral[d]	Dorsal	5190 ± 430	5970 ± 360	5860 ± 610
		Ventral	2860 ± 360	$4640 \pm 190^*$	$5130 \pm 470^*$
Clostridium perfringens[b]	Dorsal[e]	Dorsal	3620 ± 260	3970 ± 380	3920 ± 210
		Ventral	6170 ± 390	6820 ± 850	6350 ± 470
	Ventral[f]	Dorsal	4890 ± 410	5130 ± 290	5470 ± 410
		Ventral	2720 ± 290	$4420 \pm 350^*$	$4430 \pm 280^*$

*Significantly different from controls, $p < 0.01$. [a]25 units/ml in PBS pH 6.5, 15 min, 37°; controls treated with PBS. [b]25 units/ml in PBS pH 6.5, 15 min, 37°; controls treated with PBS. [c]8 day, 1.0×10^6 cells/ml, 0.23 c.p.m./cell, 3 hr preincubation. [d]8 day, 0.9×10^6 cells/ml, 0.19 c.p.m./cell, 3 hr preincubation. [e]7 day, 1.0×10^6 cells/ml, 0.29 c.p.m./cell, 4 hr preincubation. [f]7 day, 1.1×10^6 cells/ml, 0.21 c.p.m./cell, 4 hr preincubation.

it might have a β-linked galactoside terminal to the acetylated galactosamine. The protease-sensitive components situated more ventrally on the retina and tectum would be expected to be complementary to the N-acetylgalactosamine terminus, in the sense conveyed by Figure 2. Attempts to detect gradients of glycoproteins with similar terminal sequences, or to detect inhibition of recognition, failed consistently. In fact, we know of no glycoproteins with a terminal disaccharide sequence of β N-acetylgalactosamine-β-galactose. The ganglioside GM_1, however, has such a terminal disaccharide and, with its terminal galactoside removed, the molecule is GM_2, the Tay-Sachs ganglioside. From the very first, experiments with GM_2, highly purified in our laboratory from Tay-Sachs brains, showed positive results. Table 4, for example, shows the results of an experiment in which GM_2 was incorporated into ^{3}H-dipalmitoyl phosphatidylcholine liposomes by sonicating the unlabeled ganglioside with tritiated lecithin. The resulting vesicles adhere preferentially to ventral tectal surfaces, just as do dorsal retinal cells whose surfaces are postulated to be rich in GM_2 or, at least, the GM_2-like oligosaccharide sequence. Lecithin liposomes prepared with GM_1, GM_3, ceramide lactose or the disialoganglioside GD_{1a} show no adhesive preferences toward either tectal half nor do they adhere to tectal surfaces better than the tritiated vesicles prepared without additions. Finally, if the GM_2 is added to the lecithin vesicles after they have been sonicated, the vesicles, again, show no adhesive preferences nor any tendency to adhere more than simple, ^{3}H-lecithin liposomes.

In a more direct test of the ability of ventral tectal surfaces to bind more GM_2 than dorsal surfaces, Michael Pierce, in our laboratory, has labeled GM_2 by sequential treatments with galactose oxidase and sodium borotritiide. The free ganglioside, also, associates more readily with ventral than with dorsal tectal surfaces.

TABLE 4

The adhesion of lecithin vesicles to tectal halves in 1 hour

Vesicle composition[a]	C.p.m.'s (^{3}H-lecithin) to dorsal half-tecta	Adhering/tectal half to ventral half-tecta
Lecithin	440 ± 30	450 ± 20
Lecithin + 2% GM$_2$	680 ± 60*	780 ± 30*[+]
Lecithin + 2% GM$_3$	410 ± 30	430 ± 20
Lecithin (GM$_2$ added after sonification)	440 ± 30	450 ± 30
Lecithin	560 ± 30	590 ± 40
Lecithin + 2% GM$_2$	630 ± 20	860 ± 60*[+]
Lecithin + 2% cer-glucose	520 ± 10	550 ± 20
Lecithin + 2% GD$_{1b}$	520 ± 40	540 ± 30
Lecithin	420 ± 20	430 ± 40
Lecithin + 2% GM$_2$	580 ± 20*	670 ± 30*[+]
Lecithin + 2% cer-lactose	400 ± 20	390 ± 30
Lecithin + 2% GM$_1$	400 ± 10	420 ± 20

*Significantly greater than the value with lecithin alone, $p < 0.05$. [+]Significantly greater than the corresponding dorsal value, $p < 0.05$. [a]200,000 c.p.m.'s and 4 mg lecithin in 4 ml PBS per assay plate.

The GM$_2$ receptor, which we presume to be more concentrated on ventral than dorsal tectal surfaces and which is protease sensitive, is unknown.

A logical candidate for such a receptor, however, would be the enzyme that transfers a galactose moiety to the terminus of the GM$_2$ – the GM$_1$ synthetase. This protein must be complementary to GM$_2$ and would very likely be sensitive to trypsin and chymotrypsin. In fact, Marchase (1977) has shown that GM$_1$ synthetase is more active in ventral retinal homogenates than in dorsal homogenates and that the increase in GM$_1$ synthetase activity in ventral tissue does not begin until day 6 of development. This is precisely the time (Fig. 4) at which ventral retinal cells acquire the ability to adhere selectively to dorsal tectal surfaces, as shown in 1975 by Barbera. Assays for 18 other enzymes in retinal homogenates, including glycosyltransferases, phosphatases, glycosidases and lactate dehydrogenase, demonstrate that none of these activities is asymmetrically distributed between dorsal or ventral retinal halves.

A recognition function for this enzyme, the GM$_1$ synthetase, is suggested because it is in the right place at the right time, should have the requisite binding activity toward GM$_2$, and would be consistent with a multitude of other studies implicating transferases in recognition phenomena (Roseman, 1970; Shur and Roth, 1976). However, there are, as yet, no data showing that the enzyme is surface-located to any degree and, of course, no direct evidence that it plays any role in the retinal projection onto the tectum.

IMPLICATIONS FOR THE RETINO-TECTAL SYSTEM

Marchase (1977) has shown that far more cells in the labeled retinal cell suspension can discriminate between dorsal and ventral tectal halves than can be accounted for by ganglion cells, assuming that the ganglion cells make up about 1 % of the total. This means that the specificity in question must be shared by non-ganglion cells of the retina and, perhaps, by all of the cells in the retina. In fact, the earliest report of retino-tectal adhesive specificity showed that even pigmented retinal cells could distinguish between tectal halves. One may only guess at the reasons for this ability to distinguish between physiologically appropriate and physiologically inappropriate tectal halves by cells that are, apparently, never faced with this choice. In the case of the pigmented retina cells, it is well known (Stone, 1948) that this tissue can regenerate a neural retina if the neural retina is removed. In some amphibia, if the neural retina is removed and the eye is inverted, the pigmented retina, now upside down, regenerates a neural retina which, in turn, regenerates an optic nerve. However, the animal's regained vision is also upside down. This indicates that the pigmented retina is not only capable of neural retina regeneration but that it also possesses the positional information necessary to allow a normal visual projection. It may also possess the appropriate molecules in the appropriate places.

In the case of the non-ganglionic neural retinal cells, there is an excellent, albeit post hoc, reason for their ability to discriminate between tectal halves. Figure 1 shows that even before the optic axons must find their proper termini on the surface of the tectum, it is necessary for them to find the retinal fundus and exit via the choroid fissure. The same postulated gradient systems, represented in Figure 2, that would allow axons to take up their ultimate positions on the tectum would also allow the axons to migrate toward the retinal fundus if all of the retinal cells shared the molecular labels that the axon tips and tectal surfaces must possess. In other words, all of the retinal cells have the specificities in question; not because all of them use these specificities to migrate over the tectum but because all of them are used as substrates by the ganglionic axons as they exit the retina.

Direct tests of these hypotheses will be possible when extremely low levels of gangliosides may be accurately estimated in fragments of these tissues, when specific antibodies against the various gangliosides can be obtained and labeled with high specific activities and when in vivo perturbation experiments can be accomplished with saturating amounts of the purified ganglioside or with antibodies directed against them.

DISCUSSION

The data summarized here allow a number of conclusions to be made:
1. In vitro assays for intercellular adhesion can yield results that reflect in vivo morphogenesis in the sense that the morphogenetic phenomenon under consideration is explicable in terms of changes in cell adhesion.
2. In vitro assays for intercellular adhesion can be analysed biochemically and enzymatically. The results from such studies should indicate which molecules are important to the recognition being examined and these molecules can be tested directly in the adhesion assays.
3. In the retino-tectal system, specifically, the enzymatic data pointed to the involvement of the ganglioside GM_2 and direct testing of this compound supported a functional role for it in the recognition that can be measured in vitro.

4. The GM_2 receptor may be a galactosyltransferase – GM_1 synthetase. At present, however, the data for this statement are incomplete and indirect.

5. Although it has often been stated that the best systems for the study of inter-cellular adhesion are the simplest (see, for example, statements by Raff on pag 339 of the Ciba Symposium reference (Marchase et al., 1975)), the anatomical complexity of the retino-tectal system was precisely that factor that allowed important enzymatic effects to be separated from trivial effects. The crucial issue is not how complex a structure is, but how well its complexity is understood. I would maintain that we know more about the anatomy of the sub-mammalian visual projection than we do about the anatomy of the slime mold slug. Until our knowledge of the slug and, to take another example, the chick limb bud, are equal, we should not lull ourselves into thinking that the *Dictyostelium* slug is a simple structure whereas the limb bud is hopelessly more complex. Biological complexity can and must be used to the investigators' advantage in the analyses of morphogenesis.

REFERENCES

Barbera, A. J. (1975): *Develop. Biol., 46*, 167.
Barbera, A. J., Marchase, R. B. and Roth, S. (1973): *Proc. nat. Acad. Sci. (Wash.), 70*, 2482
Crossland, W. J., Cowan, W. M., Rogers, L. A. and Kelly, J. (1974): *J. comp. Neurol., 155*, 127.
DeLong, G. R. and Coulombre, A. J. (1965): *Exp. Neurol., 13*, 351.
Fujita, S. and Horii, M. (1963): *Arch. histol. jap., 23*, 359.
Gaze, R. M., Jacobson, M. and Szekely, G. (1963): *J. Physiol. (Lond.), 165*, 484.
Hamdi, F. A. and Whitteridge, D. (1954): *Quant. J. exp. Physiol., 39*, 111.
Jacobson, M. (1970): *Developmental Neurobiology.* Holt, Rhinehart and Winston, Inc., New York.
Marchase, R. B., Barbera, A. J. and Roth, S. (1975): In: *Cell Patterning, Ciba Foundation Symposium 29 (New Series)*, p. 315. Editors: R. Porter and J. Rivers. Elsevier-Excerpta Medica–North-Holland, Amsterdam–Oxford–New York.
Matthey, R. (1925): *C.R. Soc. Biol. (Paris), 93*, 904.
McGill, J. I., Powell, T. P. S. and Cowan, W. M. (1966): *J. Anat. (Lond.), 100*, 5.
Roseman, S. (1970): *Chem. Phys. Lip. 5*, 270.
Shur, B. D. and Roth, S. (1976): *Biochim. biophys. Acta (Amst.), 415*, 473.
Sperry, R. W. (1943): *J. comp. Neurol., 79*, 33.
Sperry, R. W. (1945): *Quart. Rev. Biol., 20*, 311.
Sperry, R. W. (1963): *Proc. nat. Acad. Sci. (Wash.), 50*, 703.
Stone, L. S. (1948): *Ann. N.Y. Acad. Sci., 49*, 856.

The molecular basis for limb morphogenesis*

ARNOLD I. CAPLAN

*Biology and Anatomy Departments, Development Biology Center,
Case Western Reserve University, Cleveland, Ohio, U.S.A.*

The more that we discover, the more we know about the mysteries of how organisms develop, the less we truly understand and the more perplexing and mysterious the developmental process becomes. How is the genetic information handled to allow the fertilized egg to develop into a multicellular complex-tissued organism? In simpler terms, how does an appendage like the limb arise and what controls the size, shape and tissue components and the arrangement of muscle, cartilage and bone of the limb? Even more simply, what controls the differentiation and development of muscle as opposed to cartilage from the cells of the developing limb? Experimentally, answers to these questions are hard to come by. In reality, the molecular biologists have relatively crude tools to excavate the mysteries of information transfer during these complex processes: they are like our ancestors who were in the process of evolving from ape to man and slowly developing the tools to help them better survive. With the models for DNA's structure, Watson and Crick were able to bring us from the dark ages to the 20th century but they also brought us complexities unimagined previously. Rather than dwell on all that we don't know, I would like to share with you some of the facts we do know, especially about aspects of limb development. I would like to take you back to discuss the origins of limb cells, to the many periods of cellular influence, one cell on another and finally to the factors which control muscle, cartilage and bone development. It is here at the end of the developmental process where we know the most and have made the largest gains in our attempt to unravel the details of the control mechanisms governing this complex developmental process. The interesting conclusion from these later studies is that compounds found in all cells have a profound affect on the control apparatus governing developmental events. Furthermore, it is a cell's environment, its positional information which is deterministic in persuading a limb cell to become muscle or cartilage.

What I intend to do here is to briefly describe the history of limb cells before they are committed to a specific phenotypic fate since this history is involved in the programming of the cells to exhibit certain developmental characteristics. Once we

*Supported by grants from National Foundation–March of Dimes, National Institute of Health and Muscular Dystrophy Association of America.

have the cells in the limb per se, I want to describe a tissue culture preparation of limb cells which has helped us to unravel some of the details of muscle and cartilage development. I hope to convince you that we know how the limb architecture sets up 2 distinctly different environments in the limb, how these different external environments communicate with the cell's cytoplasm, and finally how the specific cytoplasmic environment communicates with the cell's genetic material in the cell's nucleus. The description of this intricate molecular communication system allows us to identify various units in the control of normal development and propose the possible molecular origins of some common limb defects.

LIMB CELL HISTORY

The cells destined to become limb cells originate in the mesenchymal layer of the developing embryo. At the primitive streak stage of development of the chick embryo, a single zone of cells destined to form limb structures can be identified (Fig. 1). By day 1, this single area separates into 2 areas, the cells of which will become wing and leg cells. It is during this time that the mesenchymal layer called the somatophore splits into 2 tissues: the group destined to become limb cells and those to be incorporated into somites which eventually give rise to the cartilage and bone of the ribs and the muscles of the back, side and chest area. The mesenchymal cells of both the somite and the limb eventually differentiate into either muscle or cartilage and although back muscle and thigh muscle are indistinguishable in terms of their phenotypic properties, the developmental history and interaction with other tissues is completely different. Thus, the similarities of the end phenotypes is not comparable to the individual developmental histories so that the control of muscle

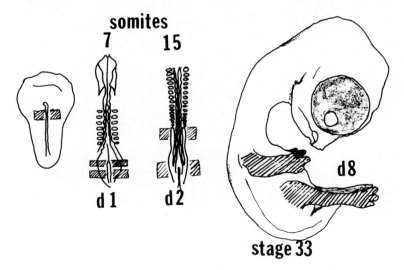

Fig. 1. The relative locations of the 'limb fields' in the developing chick embryo. Embryos at the primitive streak stage, 7 somite stage (day 1), 15 somite stage (day 2), and stage 33 (day 8) are depicted with the shaded area indicating the approximate limb field.

and cartilage development and differentiation is completely different for both groups of mesenchymal cells. Somite cell development is summarized elsewhere (Spratt, 1955, 1957; Lipton and Jacobsen, 1974; Packard and Jacobsen, 1976) and I shall concentrate here on limb mesenchymal cell events.

There are 2 important aspects of pre-limb mesenchymal cells which should be understood prior to discussing muscle and cartilage development. First, the cells of the flank predestined to become either wing or leg are already programmed or committed to fashion their specific structures. For example, the cells from the pre-wing area will *only* make wing structures even if transferred to the leg or other sites. Thus, the *FORM* component of limb development is fixed long before there is a limb bud. Second, the cells of the pre-limb mesenchyme have a powerful and specific

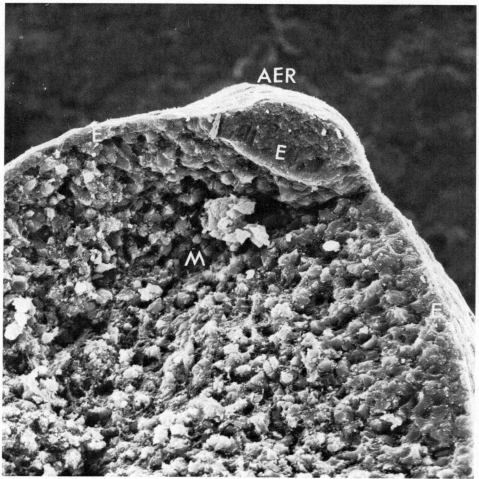

Fig. 2. A scanning electron micrograph of human embryonic limb from stage 15 embryos. The apical ectodermal ridge (AER) is clearly visible as a ridge of cells running along the extremity of the limb with a mass of mesodermal (M) cell beneath the apical ectodermal ridge and the non-ridge ectoderm (E). Electro micrograph kindly supplied by Dr. R. O. Kelly, University of New Mexico.

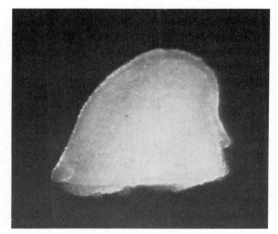

Fig. 3. A recombinant limb. Ectoderm separated in intact form is stuffed with mesoderm and is viewed in this phase contrast micrograph. Such a recombinant can be grafted to the flank or limb stump with the resulting outgrowth appearing normal in morphology and tissue orientation. Micrograph courtesy of Dr. J. MacCabe, University of Tennessee.

inductive effect on the overlaying ectoderm. The limb mesenchymal cells induce the ectoderm to form a ridge of cells (Fig. 2) which are eventually responsible for directing the outgrowth of the limb (Kieny, 1960). Thus, if non-limb ectoderm is placed over pre-limb mesenchyme, the mesenchyme will cause the ectoderm to become specialized and to exhibit properties of limb ectoderm. Interestingly, as the first signs of limb outgrowth can be noticed as a slight bud from the flank, this specific induction capacity is lost and after this time, only limb ectoderm is capable of interacting with mesenchyme to direct outgrowth.

The specific ectodermal-mesenchymal interaction responsible for limb outgrowth has been described by Edgar Zwilling (Zwilling, 1955) and John Saunders (Saunders and Gasseling, 1968) and their students. This interaction is best exemplified by the following experiment: The limb buds from a 3-day-old chick embryo are surgically removed and using techniques developed by Zwilling, the ectodermal coverings are cleanly and completely separated from mesenchymal cells. A wing ectodermal covering is packed with a chunk of leg mesenchyme and this recombinant limb is grafted to the wing or leg stump or the flank of another embryo; Figure 3 pictures a recombinant limb prior to grafting. The resultant outgrowth is normal in every way and is a leg. Thus the conclusion that the mesenchyme codes for limb *form*. If non-limb ectoderm or ectoderm deprived of the special apical ectodermal ridge cells is used to cover the mesenchyme, no outgrowth is observed. Therefore, the interaction between limb ectodermal ridge cells and mesenchyme is necessary for limb outgrowth.

MUSCLE AND CARTILAGE DEVELOPMENT

Using this same type of test system, one can ask questions about 'when do mesenchymal cells commit themselves to a specific phenotypic fate?' The experiments are to take separated ectodermal coverings and pack them with a pellet of separated and centrifugally pelleted mesenchymal cells (Finch and Zwilling, 1971). The separation and centrifugation regime insures that the limb cells are randomly arranged. If the cells of the mesenchyme are obtained before stage 25 of development (day 4), then resulting limb outgrowths are normal in every way especially in the arrangement of the muscle and cartilage units. If the cells are obtained from the limbs of embryos older than stage 25, the limb outgrowths are not normal with misshapened muscle and cartilage units. Two important conclusions can be drawn from this experiment and others. First, before stage 25 the mesenchymal cells are interchangeable one for another and are *NOT* committed to a specific phenotype. If they had been committed to a specific phenotype then randomizing them would have resulted in misshapened limb outgrowth as occurred with the cells from older embryos. Thus, the commitment of chick limb mesenchymal cells to a specific phenotype occurs at about stage 25.

The second conclusion from the randomization experiment is that a single cell prior to stage 25 can become *EITHER* a muscle cell *OR* a cartilage cell. Thus, a choice occurs at the stage of phenotypic commitment and this choice has something to do with the position of the mesenchymal cell in the limb relative to 'pre-muscle' or 'pre-cartilage' area. Zwilling summarized these and other observations in Figure 4

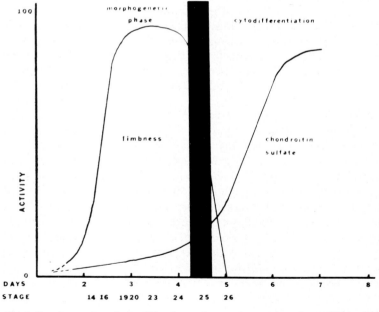

Fig. 4. Development analysis of the change in morphogenetic and cytodifferentiation properties of chick limb cells. (After drawing of Zwilling, 1968.) Developmental time in the horizontal axis is plotted against relative morphogenetic responsiveness or cytodifferentiation. Cellular aspects of limb development involves the morphogenetic phase in which all of the cells of the limb are interchangeable and are responsive to outgrowth signals, especially the stimulus of the apical ectodermal ridge. The cytodifferentiation phase involves the synthesis of large quantities of phenotype specific macromolecule; plotted here is the synthesis of chondroitin sulfate. The vertical bar at stages 24–25 indicates the time period in which limb mesenchymal cells become committed to specific phenotypic compartments.

where the time of commitment is represented by the dark vertical bar at stage 25 which separates the pluripotent 'limbness' stage of development and cytodifferentiation as indicated by the increased production of chondroitin sulfate (Zwilling, 1968).

It is exactly this choice mechanism that interests me and brought me to wonder what might play a role in controlling this choice of limb mesenchymal cell to express muscle or cartilage properties. I was stimulated by the teratogenic studies of Landauer (Landauer, 1957) to suggest that extracellular *NICOTINAMIDE* might play a role in controlling this choice mechanism. Landauer showed that when certain compounds were injected into the yolk sac of 4-day incubated fertile eggs, cartilage malformations resulted; a different group of compounds caused muscle malformations. Interestingly, when nicotinamide was co-injected with either of these groups of compounds, malformations did not develop. Thus, the common link between *NORMAL* muscle and cartilage development seemed to be nicotinamide.

Because of the complications of dealing with the whole embryo, we developed techniques to place pre-stage 24 limb mesenchymal cells into cell cultures (Caplan et al., 1968; Caplan, 1970). The cells in such cultures faithfully mimic the commitment and differentiation pattern seen in vivo. Figure 5 depicts the preparative steps and compares the events seen in vitro with those seen in vivo. Briefly during days 0 to 3, the cells are dividing and are committing to a specific phenotype. By the end of day 3, evidence of both muscle and cartilage development can be noticed. By day 8,

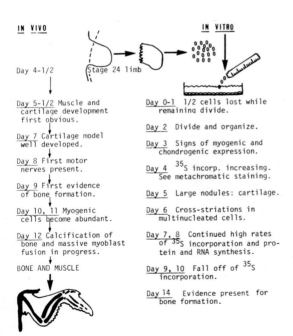

IN VIVO   IN VITRO

Day 4-1/2   (Stage 24 limb

Day 5-1/2 Muscle and   Day 0-1 1/2 cells lost while
cartilage development   remaining divide.
first obvious.
                     Day 2 Divide and organize.
Day 7 Cartilage model
well developed.   Day 3 Signs of myogenic and
                     chondrogenic expression.
Day 8 First motor
nerves present.   Day 4 ^{35}S incorp. increasing.
                     See metachromatic staining.
Day 9 First evidence
of bone formation.   Day 5 Large nodules: cartilage.

Day 10, 11 Myogenic   Day 6 Cross-striations in
cells become abundant.   multinucleated cells.

Day 12 Calcification of   Day 7, 8 Continued high rates
bone and massive myoblast   of ^{35}S incorporation and pro-
fusion in progress.   tein and RNA synthesis.

BONE AND MUSCLE   Day 9, 10 Fall off of ^{35}S
                     incorporation.

Day 14 Evidence present for
bone formation.

Fig. 5. Preparative steps and comparison of in vitro and in vivo limb mesenchymal cell development. Limbs are obtained from stage 24 embryos and the mesenchymal cells freed by the action of trypsin and vigorous vortexing. After counting, the cells are plated at 5–9,000 cell/mm²; day by day comparison of the in vitro and in vivo events are listed.

maximal proteoglycan synthesis is observed. By day 14 evidence for osteogenic phenotypes has been reported.

Detailed studies in my laboratory have shown that when the entrance of nicotin-amide into the cells is severely restricted by the nicotinamide analog 3-acetylpyridine, muscle development cannot be observed while chondrogenic expression is potentiated (Caplan, 1970; Rosenberg and Caplan, 1975). Alternately, by adding high levels of nicotinamide to the culture medium, chondrogenic expression is severely restricted while muscle development is enhanced. Furthermore, restricting nicotinamide's entrance into the cell results in a 10- to 100-fold drop in the intracellular levels of NAD while adding nicotinamide to the culture medium results in the elevation of NAD levels. It is well known that NAD cannot cross the plasma membrane, but that nicotinamide is permeable. Once nicotinamide is inside the cell, it is converted to nicotinamide mononucleotide and with ATP is enzymatically converted to NAD. Thus, changes in the external nicotinamide levels result in changes in the intra-cellular pool sizes of NAD. In addition, *high* NAD pool sizes are correlated with inhibition of chondrogenic development and normal or enhanced myogenic develop-ment while *low* NAD levels are correlated with the potentiation of chondrogenic development and the inhibition of myogenesis. This is diagrammatically summarized in Figure 6.

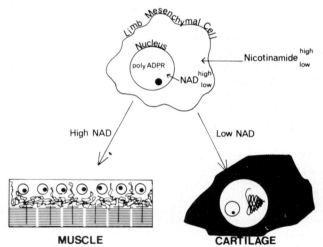

Fig. 6. Limb mesenchymal cell differentiation into cartilage and muscle and the relationship of NAD levels to the decisional process. High or low levels of extracellular nicotinamide regulate the cytoplasmic pool size of NAD. High levels of NAD favor muscle development while low levels of NAD favor cartilage development. The NAD pool size also affects the synthesis of polyADP-ribose, a nuclear restricted chromosomal protein-bound nucleic acid.

Recently, in my laboratory, we have shown that the developing chick limb's vascular system sets up nutrient-rich and nutrient-poor zones in the limb long before stage 25 (Caplan and Koutroupas, 1973). In the nutrient-poor zone, the extracellular level of nicotinamide might be expected to be low while the nutrient-rich zone might be expected to have high extracellular levels of nicotinamide since nicotinamide is stored in the yolk and brought to distant sites by the vascular system. The nutrient-poor zone corresponds to the avascular, pre-chondrogenic zone while the nutrient-rich area is the heavily capillarized premyogenic area. Thus, there exists an anatomical basis for the establishment of a gradient of nicotinamide levels across the limb: low at the pre-chondrogenic core while high at the pre-myogenic periphery.

Since the extracellular nicotinamide is freely permeable to the plasma membrane, the internal pool size of NAD rises and falls as a function of the availability of nicotinamide. Accordingly, cells in the avascular and pre-chondrogenic zone have low NAD pool sizes while those cells found in the pre-myogenic zone have high NAD levels. The quantitative evidence from both the tissue culture system and the studies on in vivo limb development (Rosenberg and Caplan, 1974, 1975) point clearly to the important role of the extracellular environment and the cell's positional information (especially as related to nicotinamide and NAD levels) in the expression of myogenic and chondrogenic phenotypes: changes in the external nicotinamide availability cause changes in the cell's NAD pool size, all of which is correlated with the commitment of the uncommitted limb mesenchymal cell into muscle and cartilage. The question remains as to how cytoplasmic fluctuations in NAD can be related to the genomic events which are controlling the developmental and expressional characteristics of these cells.

Quite recently we have reported the presence of a unique nucleic acid which is formed from the enzymatic conversion of NAD. This nucleic acid is called polyADP-ribose and it is covalently bound to both histone and non-histone chromosomal proteins. The structure and synthetic reactions involved in polyADP-ribose are depicted in Figure 7. Since polyADP-ribose is not degraded by DNAase, RNAase or KOH, labeling intact cells with radioactive adenine or adenosine coupled with the expose of nucleic acids to digestive agents allows the analysis of newly synthesized polyADP-ribose. By assaying the specific RATE of incorporation of labeled adenine into polyADP-ribose on various days of culture of stage 24 limb mesenchymal cells, we have shown that the rate of synthesis increases on days 1 to 3 during the time

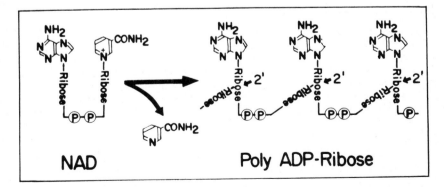

Fig. 7. NAD polymerization in mammalian nucleus. The structure and synthetic reactions involved in the production of polyADP-ribose. PolyADP-ribose forms from the polymerization of NAD with the excision of nicotinamide. More than 95 % of the polyADP-ribose formed in the nuclei of limb mesenchymal cells is bound to chromosomal proteins.

that these cells are committing themselves to a specific phenotype (Fig. 8). On subsequent days when the cells are expressing their committed phenotype, the rate of synthesis falls back to basal levels. When the cells are exposed to the inhibitor of differentiation and development, 5-bromodeoxyuridine, the rate of polyADP-ribose synthesis remains at basal levels as correlated with the lack of phenotypic expression.

Thus, there seems to be a very strong correlation between the synthesis of polyADP-ribose and the commitment of stage 24 limb mesenchymal cells to either muscle or cartilage phenotypes. Furthermore, the intracellular levels of NAD, the substrate for the synthesis of polyADP-ribose, have been correlated with muscle versus cartilage expression; high levels of NAD favor muscle while low levels favor cartilage. These intracellular NAD levels are related to the extracellular availability of nicotinamide. The mesenchymal cells of the limb for reasons of their developmental history (their pre-programming) seem to have an intricate communication system running

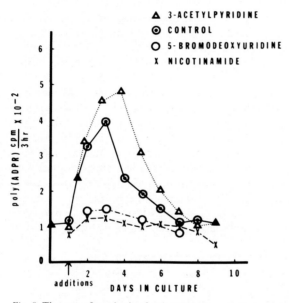

Fig. 8. The rate of synthesis of polyADP-ribose in limb mesenchymal cells as a function of day in culture. Chick limb mesenchymal cells are grown in culture and are exposed to radioactive adenine or adenosine on each day of culture. Subsequently, RNA and DNA are eliminated with the quantitation of the newly synthesized polyADP-ribose. Plotted is the rate of incorporation of adenine into polyADP-ribose as an in vivo measurement. Also shown is the rate of polyADP-ribose synthesis in the presence of nicotinamide, 5-bromodeoxyuridine and 3-acetylpyridine. Differentiation of chick limb cells is inhibited by 5-bromo-deoxyuridine and basal rates of synthesis of polyADP are observed in this case. In cultures structured to produce high levels of chondrogenic development, nicotinamide inhibits this differentiation process and also produces basal levels of polyADP-ribose synthesis. The inclusion of 3-acetylpyridine in the cultures stimulates the differentiation of chondrogenic phenotypes and, in this case, a concomitant increase in the synthesis of polyADP-ribose is noticed during the differentiation and commitment phases of this culture. All of the decisional events are made by the limb mesenchymal cells during the first 3 or 4 days of culture and after these decisional events, the expression of the committed phenotype can be observed. It is clear that the synthesis of polyADP-ribose is correlated with the decisional and early expressive events as opposed to the elaboration of mature phenotypes.

from the cell's molecular environment to the cell's cytoplasm and finally communicating with the cell's genetic material in the nucleus.

The question can now be asked, 'How does the synthesis of polyADP-ribose affect chromatin structure and thus chromatin function as related to the commitment and phenotypic expression of limb mesenchymal cells?' The experimental attempts to answer this question form the basis of the work current in my laboratory. I can assure you that it will be many years before we will be able to answer this question but we are encouraged by the recent advances in chromatin biochemistry. In view of the above, it is of value to briefly review these advances in a simple way with special reference to polyADP-ribosylation and its possible affects on chromatin structure.

Chromatin is made up of 3 major classes of macromolecules: double stranded DNA, histones and non-histone chromosomal protein. For the sake of simplicity I shall only say that the class of non-histone chromosomal proteins represents a diverse and heterogenous group of molecules numbering from 50 to over 300 per nucleus (depending on the cell type and the method for estimating the protein diversity). The specific functions of these proteins are unknown but in all likelihood they are responsible for the control of various aspects of transcription and RNA processing and thus cell function and phenotypic expression.

The DNA found in chromatin is double stranded and is made up of sequences which are found only once per genome interspaced between sequences which are repeated from a few times to many thousands of times (Davidson and Britten, 1973). The unique sequences seem to code for specific proteins as do some of the moderately repeated sequences. Some of the highly repeated sequences are not transcribed and probably play a structural role in chromatin and thus chromosome structure. For example, in some organisms the genes coding for ribosomal RNA are repeated from 10 to 500 times while the mouse AT-rich satellite DNA is not transcribed and is usually found in the chromatid region of interphase chromosomes. It is clear from many studies that the DNA found in most cells contains all of the genetic material to code for a complete organism (Gurdon, 1974). The arrangement of this genetic unit is still an area of active experimentation.

Histones are very basic proteins and are in intimate contact with the double stranded DNA. All cells have at least 5 histones termed H1, H2A, H2B, H3 and H4. The amino acid compositions of these histones are known for a variety of organisms. Surprisingly, the amino acid composition is almost invariant for histones H2A, H2B, H3 and H4, while H1 shows wide variation in amino acid composition and size not only among the various organisms but within the same organism in various tissues. The 4 invariant histones are in intimate contact with each other as well as the double stranded DNA. As a matter of fact, 2 of each of the 4 histones are in a compact assembly called a nucleosome (for a review see Kornberg, 1977). The DNA is wound around each nucleosome like the seams of a baseball and the nucleosomes are situated next to one another with a variable length of DNA between individual nucleosomes. Each nucleosome has a 140 base pair length of DNA tightly associated with itself while the internucleosome piece of DNA varies from 20 to over 100 base pairs in length depending on the organism or the metabolic activity of the cell. The 140 base pair piece of DNA associated with the octamerically arranged histones is further structured into 10 base pair units. All of the DNA lengths have been deduced from studies of the accessibility of these sites to nuclease treatment. The localization of the variable composition and very lysine-rich histone H1 is not completely certain although it is clear that it is situated with the internucleosome lengths of DNA. The above is diagrammatically pictured in Figure 9.

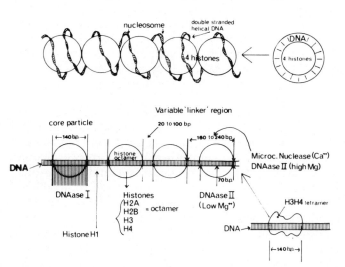

Fig. 9. Chromatin structure. Chromatin is organized into discrete units of protein and DNA. These units are referred to as nucleosomes. The basic unit of the nucleosome is constructed around 4 histones (H2A, H2B, H3 and H4) which are present in equal concentrations with 2 moles of each histone per nucleosome. The octameric structure of the 4 histones is associated with a 140 base pair piece of DNA and individual nucleosomes are spaced apart from one another with variable 'Linker' region of DNA which is 20–100 base pairs in length depending on the cell from which chromatin is isolated. Various nuclease treatments have been used to dissect various structural aspects of this structure. The proposed dissection pattern of nucleases are shown with DNAase I cutting the DNA into 10 base pair pieces: with DNAase II (at low magnesium) cutting at 140 and 70 base pair positions: with DNAase II (high magnesium) cutting at 160 to 240 base pairs and giving the same digestion pattern as micrococcal or staph. nuclease. Independent studies have shown that the H3–H4 tetramer alone can account for the 140 base pair interaction with DNA.

The amino acid composition and sequences for all the histones indicates that the basic amino acids are situated in clusters at the C- and N-terminal regions (Fig. 10). The central region of the amino acid sequence is dominated by the hydrophobic amino acids. Furthermore, it is well known that the histone is substituted (phosphorylated, ADP-ribosylated or acetylated) during various periods of the cell cycle. These substitutions never occur in the hydrophobic region of these histones. Thus, the octameric arrangement of the 4 histones H2A, H2B, H3 and H4 is thought to be dominated by the hydrophobic contacts of the central regions of the polypeptide chains with the N- and C-terminal regions dangling out the sides to make ionic contact with the negatively charged phosphate backbone of the double stranded DNA and to be accessible to the various enzymes which add phosphate, acetate or ADP-ribose groups to the various histones (see Cold Spring Harbor Symposium 42, 1977).

The addition of these various groups to the histones changes their properties considerably. For example, the phosphorylation of H1 seems to be associated with

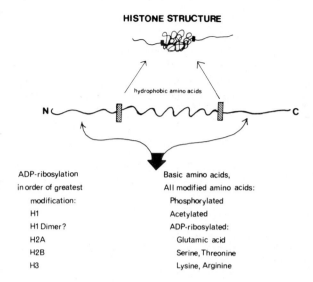

HISTONE STRUCTURE

hydrophobic amino acids

N — — C

ADP-ribosylation	Basic amino acids,
in order of greatest	All modified amino acids:
modification:	Phosphorylated
H1	Acetylated
H1 Dimer?	ADP-ribosylated:
H2A	Glutamic acid
H2B	Serine, Threonine
H3	Lysine, Arginine

Fig. 10. Histone structure. Histones are made up of 2 regions: a hydrophobic cluster of amino acids in the center of the polypeptide chain with adjacent highly basic N- and C-terminal sections. All of the modified amino acids are found in the non-hydrophobic areas with modifications of the amino acids being primarily phosphorylation and acetylation with some ADP-ribosylation. ADP-ribosylation seems to involve all of the histones with the exception of histone H4.

the subsequent condensation of chromatin into chromosomes; this seems to be the case for cells grown in culture as well as for primitive eukaryotes such as the slime mold, *Physarum.* Of special interest to the study of limb development, is the recent report of the isolation of a H1 dimer with each H1 molecule connected to the other by a polyADP-ribose bridge of 15 units in length (Lorimer et al., 1977). Such molecular cross-linking might serve to bring distant sequences of DNA into close proximity to one another. In recent studies completed while I was on sabbatical leave in Professor Pierre Chambon's laboratory, the polyADP-ribosylation of the nucleosomal histones seems to destabilize their interaction with DNA. Such destabilization of nucleosome structure might have a role in the differentiation and development of chick limb mesenchymal cells although a number of technological advancements will be necessary before such analysis can be accomplished in this system.

It seems clear from a variety of studies that the chemical modification of chromosomal proteins, histones and non-histones, has a profound affect on chromatin structure and that such modifications are correlated with transcriptional and functional modulations. In the specific case of polyADP-ribosylation of chromosomal proteins, there seems to be a correlation with the differentiation of limb mesenchymal cells although we are far from determining exactly how these modifications alter chromatin function and phenotypic expression.

In summary, I have tried to quickly take you through selected aspects of limb development, especially the final phases where experimental information is available.

As related to muscle and cartilage development it is clear that the extracellular environment establishes intracellular conditions which affect nuclear reactions and the possible accessibility of genomic information. Limb mesenchymal cells seem to be especially sensitive to nicotinamide and NAD fluctuations which in turn affect the synthesis of chromatin-bound polyADP-ribose. The intimate interaction of histones with DNA is related to normal chromatin structure and presumably function. The description of the exact role of ADP-ribosylation in the control of limb mesenchymal cell development and differentiation provides a stimulating and vital research area and promises to keep us busy for many years to come.

REFERENCES

Caplan, A. I. (1970): *Exp. Cell Res.*, *62*, 341.
Caplan, A. I. and Koutropas, S. (1973): *J. Embryol. exp. Morphol.*, *29*, 571.
Caplan, A. I., Zwilling, E. and Kaplan, N. O. (1968): *Science*, *160*, 1009.
Davidson, E. H. and Britten, R. J. (1973): *Quart. Rev. Biol.*, *48*, 565.
Finch, R. A. and Zwilling, E. (1971): *J. exp. Zool.*, *176*, 397.
Gurdon, J. B. (1974): *The Control of Gene Expression in Animal Development*. Harvard University Press, Cambridge, Mass.
Kieny, M. (1960): *J. Embryol. exp. Morphol.*, *8*, 457.
Kornberg, R. D. (1977): *Ann. Rev. Biochem.*, *46*, 931.
Landauer, W. (1957): *J. exp. Zool.*, *136*, 509.
Lipton, B. H. and Jacobsen, A. G. (1974): *Develop. Biol.*, *38*, 91.
Lorimer III, W., Stone, P. R. and Kidwell, W. R. (1977): *Exp. Cell Res.*, *106*, 261.
Packard, D. S. and Jacobsen, A. G. (1976): *Develop. Biol.*, *53*, 36.
Rosenberg, M. J. and Caplan, A. I. (1974): *Develop. Biol.*, *38*, 157.
Rosenberg, M. J. and Caplan, A. I. (1975): *J. Embryol. exp. Morphol.*, *33*, 947.
Saunders, J. W. and Gasseling, M. T. (1968): In: *Epithelial-Mesenchymal Interactions*, pp. 78–97. Editors: R. Fleischmayer and R. Billingham. The Williams and Wilkins Co., Baltimore, Md.
Spratt Jr, N. T. (1955): *J. exp. Zool.*, *128*, 121.
Spratt Jr, N. T. (1957): *J. exp. Zool.*, *134*, 577.
Zwilling, E. (1955): *J. exp. Zool.*, *128*, 423.
Zwilling, E. (1968): *Develop. Biol.*, *Suppl. 2*, 184.

MECHANISMS OF DISEASE

Chairman: Arno G. Motulsky, Seattle, Wash.

Mechanisms of fetal hemoglobin production*

G. STAMATOYANNOPOULOS and TH. PAPAYANNOPOULOU

Department of Medicine, University of Washington, Seattle, Wash., U.S.A.

A discussion of the mechanism of fetal hemoglobin production is relevant to this symposium on mechanisms of disease in two ways.

First, there are very few biochemical systems in man for which the expression of gene activity during development is as precisely known as in hemoglobin. Many aspects of the genetic control of hemoglobin are well understood, mutants affecting ontogenetic patterns are known as are acquired deviations from the normal developmental pattern, information about the regulation of erythropoiesis is available and, more recently, methods permitting the study of erythroid cell populations in culture have been developed. This background provides excellent opportunities for exploration of the mechanisms that govern the expression of hemoglobin gene activity during development. The information that is obtained from the studies of fetal hemoglobin can be applied to other developmental systems that are less well understood at the biochemical level, and may eventually further our understanding of defects produced by inherited or acquired anomalies in differentiation.

Second, there is excellent evidence that the postnatal continuation of fetal hemoglobin synthesis has therapeutic effects in patients with common hemoglobinopathies, i.e. the β-thalassemia and the Hb S syndromes. Regarding Hb S, the antisickling effect of fetal hemoglobin is supported by the mild clinical course in Hb S homozygotes with high levels of Hb F production (Perrine et al., 1972), studies of the turnover of Hb S and F (Singer and Fisher, 1952), in vitro experiments with irreversibly sickled cells (Bertles and Milner, 1968), and inhibition of sickling (Charache and Conley, 1964). In the β-thalassemias, production of fetal hemoglobin is the only means for compensation of β-chain deficiency and reduction of the α-chain excess of these syndromes (Fessas, 1967); the beneficial effects of efficient Hb F production are supported by clinical observations (Stamatoyannopoulos et al., et al., 1969) and in vitro studies of the turnover of erythrocytes with low or high levels of Hb F (Loukopoulos and Fessas, 1965; Nathan and Gunn, 1966). The synthesis of fetal hemoglobin in these disorders provides a prototypical mechanism by which beneficial effects on the clinical course of genetically determined diseases can be achieved by activation of genes that are normally fully expressed only during fetal development.

*Studies performed in the laboratory of the authors were supported by grants GM 15253 and HL 20899 from the National Institute of Health.

In this brief discussion, the information on developmental patterns of Hb F will be summarized with emphasis on those findings that are relevant to the manner of Hb F regulation. Our studies with erythroid cells in culture, which suggest that cellular mechanisms are operating in Hb F regulation, will subsequently be reviewed. Finally, the data acquired from studies in vitro will be used to construct a model explaining Hb F regulation on the assumption that the differential transcription of the γ- and β-globin genes is achieved during the process of differentiation of erythroid stem cells. This model accounts for several observations on Hb F production in health and disease and provides a conceptual framework for our research aimed at manipulating Hb F synthesis in vitro, and eventually, in vivo.

DEVELOPMENTAL PATTERNS AND MUTATIONS

There are 2 switches in globin gene activity during human development: an early one from embryonic to mostly fetal hemoglobin and a later switch to the almost exclusive production of adult hemoglobin. In contrast to man, most mammalian species undergo only one developmental switch, that from the embryonic to adult hemoglobin, which appears to have been established very early in evolution, since it is also found in amphibia and birds. The mechanism of this switch has been investigated in mice, chickens and frogs and, in these animals, the transition from embryonic to definitive type of hemoglobin formation seems to be accomplished by replacement of cell lines irreversibly committed to fixed patterns of globin gene transcription and associated with specific sites of erythropoiesis (reviewed by Marks and Rifkind, 1972). The regulation of fetal hemoglobin synthesis in man appears more complex. In contrast to embryonic globin formation, there is no relationship between Hb F production and site of erythropoiesis (Wood and Weatherall, 1973). Also, during fetal development there is simultaneous production of fetal and adult hemoglobin in the same red cells. Using fluorescent antibodies for the identification of Hb A in situ, adult hemoglobin has been depicted in liver erythroblasts in fetuses as young as 35 gestational days, i.e. very close to the stage at which the fetal liver erythropoiesis starts; in contrast, no fetal hemoglobin can be detected in erythrocytes of yolk sac origin with the fluorescent antibodies (Papayannopoulou and Stamatoyannopoulos, unpublished data). Thus, the first developmental switch of hemoglobin in man seems to be one from a stage at which there is exclusive formation of embryonic globin to a stage at which 2 hemoglobins, F and A, are synthesized in the erythroid cells, in different proportions.

The second developmental switch, to predominantly adult hemoglobin formation, takes place during the perinatal period. Very little is known about the factors involved in this transition. The switch is independent of birth per se, and is related primarily to gestational age and maturity of the fetus (Bard, 1973). It coincides with a time during which erythropoiesis is suppressed, it follows a surge of steroid hormone production (no direct relationship between the 2 phenomena has yet been established) and may be subject to hormonal influences; suggestive of the latter are findings in sheep which are compatible with a delayed appearance of F to A transition in hypophysectomized fetuses (Wood et al., 1976).

Several mutations associated with continuation of Hb F synthesis in postnatal life, collectively designated as hereditary persistence of fetal hemoglobin, have been observed. In these conditions, the switch-over mechanism from Hb F to Hb A formation appears to fail and various amounts of fetal hemoglobin are synthesized in the adult. It is well documented that more than one γ-chain genes, the $^A\gamma$ and $^G\gamma$ occupying adjacent loci, operate in man, and that they are closely linked to the δ- and β-genes of the adult hemoglobins (Schroeder et al., 1968; Kendall et al., 1973). Analysis of the polypeptide chains synthesized in persons with hereditary persistence of fetal hemoglobin have shown that in most of these mutations there is continuation of postnatal activity of either 1 or 2 γ-chain genes in the absence or presence of β- and δ-gene activity (Huisman et al., 1969, 1970). Hence, mutants with only *cis* $^A\gamma$- and $^G\gamma$-chain synthesis and *cis* absence of β and δ production, or with $^A\gamma,\beta$- and δ-chain synthesis but absence of $^G\gamma$-chain production, or presence of $^G\gamma$-chain synthesis and absence of $^A\gamma,\beta$- and δ-chain production have been noted. Such patterns of globin synthesis are best explained by globin gene deletions (Huisman et al., 1974), and this has been confirmed in the case of the $^A\gamma^G\gamma$ type of hereditary persistence of Hb F, in which a complete deletion of β and δ globin genes has been documented by cDNA/DNA hybridization studies (Kan et al., 1975). Although simultaneous deletions of linked regulator genes have been proposed to explain the persistence of Hb F production (Huisman et al., 1974), the continuation of γ-gene transcription in these conditions may merely reflect position effects and rearrangements in the deletion chromosome that permit transcription of normally inactivated parts of the cistron. Thus, in contrast to other systems in which the study of mutants has been crucial to the understanding of normal mechanisms, the studies of mutations affecting the hemoglobin developmental patterns have provided very few clear insights into the normal mechanism of Hb F regulation.

Data from other forms of hereditary persistence of fetal hemoglobin (HPFH) do not fit the deletion scheme. In the Seattle type of HPFH there is $^A\gamma$- and $^G\gamma$-chain production in *cis* to active β-globin genes (Stamatoyannopoulos et al., 1975). This form of HPFH, recently designated heterocellular (Boyer et al., 1977), may reflect the operation of a gene that alters the process of erythroid stem cell differentiation rather than of genes that directly control γ- and β-gene activities.

POSTNATAL ACTIVATION OF Hb F PRODUCTION

The detailed knowledge of developmental patterns of human hemoglobin has stimulated the formulation of models that explain the regulation of globin activity during development under various assumptions: action of regulatory genes affecting transcription, sequential gene excisions, post-transcriptional regulation, control at the level of mRNA translation, etc. Gene excisions, or translational mechanisms have been tested and appear to be unlikely (Lanyon et al., 1977; Benz et al., 1977; Papayannopoulou et al., 1977b). Most of the clues to the nature of mechanisms of Hb F regulation have come from the in vivo studies of patients with acquired Hb F elevations.

It is well known that traces of fetal hemoglobin are present in every individual's blood; they are restricted to a minority of cells, designated as F cells (Boyer et al., 1975; Wood et al., 1975), each of which contain an average of 20 % fetal hemoglobin.

Immunochemical studies using cellular immunoprecipitation or microcytofluoro-metric analysis show complete bimodality in the Hb F contents of the erythrocytes of the normal adult that suggest that F cells represent a real subpopulation of cells in which the postnatal suppression of Hb F production is incomplete. It is also well established that postnatal activation of Hb F production is not uncommon. It has been observed in normal and pathological conditions (reviewed by Bradley and Ranney, 1973; Weatherall et al., 1974) including pregnancy, anemias of various etiologies, hemopoietic malignancies, non-hemopoietic malignancies, recovery from transient bone marrow aplasia following chemotherapy and during the phase of bone marrow repopulation after marrow transplantation (Alter et al., 1976). In some of these disorders striking Hb F elevations occur. No common denominator is apparent among these acquired Hb F elevations. The only uniform finding is the restriction of Hb F production to a subpopulation of cells. In all situations studied, postnatal activation of Hb F synthesis seems to reflect increased production of F cells rather than the uniform turning on of Hb F genes in all the erythroid cells of the affected individuals.

In addition, certain postnatal reactivations of Hb F synthesis have been associated with the reappearance of other fetal red cell characteristics like little i antigen or a decrease in or absence of erythrocytic carbonic anhydrase, i.e. findings compatible with a reversion to a fetal type of erythropoiesis (Mauer et al., 1972; Weatherall et al., 1976; Alter et al., 1976). Such findings have been explained by postulating that lines of fetal stem cells continue to proliferate in the postnatal hemopoietic tissue and that these lines supply the F cells of the normal adult and the Hb F-synthesizing red cells noted in disorders associated with reactivated Hb F production (Weatherall et al., 1976). This model is, however, unlikely for there is evidence from experiments in culture *(vide infra)* that Hb F synthesizing cells and cells without Hb F production are derived from common *erythroid* stem cell progenitors (Papayannopoulou et al., 1977a). Additional evidence against a pluripotent stem cell model of Hb F regulation has been obtained through immunochemical studies of the peripheral bloods of patients with the clonal disorders paroxysmal nocturnal hemoglobinuria and Philadelphia positive chronic myelogenous leukemia, which suggest, that cells which fail to produce Hb F as well as those that do are found among the erythrocytic progeny of the mutant clone that proliferates in these disorders. It is reasonable, thus, to assume that if the regulation of Hb F production is accomplished at the level of stem cells, the regulatory mechanism becomes operative after the cells have left the pluripotent stem cell compartment and have entered the compartment of stem cells that have been committed to erythropoiesis.

STUDIES OF ERYTHROID CULTURES

The cells of the erythroid stem cell compartment have limited proliferative potentials and very limited (if any) capacity for self renewal; differences among cells in this com-partment are mostly ones of degree of differentiation that are primarily expressed by the ability of these progenitor cells to respond to the growth factor for erythroid cells, the hormone erythropoietin (reviewed by Lajtha and Schofield, 1974). The goals of studies of Hb F in erythroid cultures, summarized below, were to determine if there are differences in commitment to Hb F formation between these progenitors in the erythroid stem cell compartment, and if the option to express the program of Hb F formation is available only in certain stages of differentiation of the erythroid stem cell.

Questions regarding commitment of progenitor cells to a given developmental program arise in all developmental systems; one of the most critical problems met in dealing with them is the difficulty involved in studying progenitor cells directly. In order to do this, the progenitor cells must first be isolated but in most developmental systems, this is currently impossible because cell populations comprise different types of cells at various stages of differentiation and because, in these cell populations, progenitor cells are present in low proportions. However, the commitment of erythroid stem cells to specific developmental programs can be now explored because methods are available that permit the clonal growth of erythroid cells in the form of erythroid colonies each of which originates from a single erythroid stem cell (Stephenson et al., 1971; Tepperman et al., 1974). Through such clonal assays, questions regarding commitment to Hb F production could be answered by studying the synthesis of hemoglobins A and F within each clone. This can be accomplished using fluorescent antibodies specific for Hb F or antibodies specific for Hb A (Papayannopoulou et al., 1976, 1977a).

In our original study of Hb F synthesis in culture, bone marrow cells from adult individuals were used to assess the likelihood that the restricted production of Hb F in adult red cells reflected differences in commitment among erythroid stem cell progenitors. These studies of cells cultured from normal adult marrow donors showed that the production of Hb F in erythroid colonies is clonally distributed, and that a minority of erythroid clones produce Hb F in uniform fashion (Fig. 1). These differences in Hb F production between clones suggest that the progenitor cells, from which the erythroid clones derive, differ in their program for Hb F

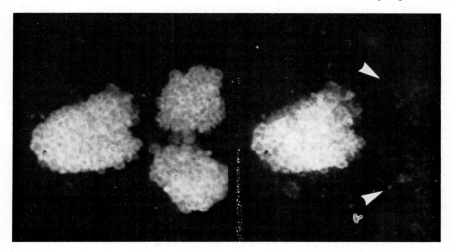

Fig. 1. Expression of fetal and adult hemoglobin in erythroid colonies of an adult bone marrow culture. *Left:* The preparation is labeled with anti-Hb A antibody conjugated to rhodamine. All 3 erythroid colonies produce Hb A. *Right:* The same preparation counter-labeled with anti-Hb F antibody conjugated to fluorescein isothiocyanate. Only 1 of the 3 colonies produces Hb F.

formation and provide direct evidence that regulatory mechanisms determining Hb F production operate at the level of stem cells (Papayannopoulou et al., 1976).

Do these differences in commitment to Hb F formation relate to the differentiative heterogeneity of the erythroid stem cell population? We tried to answer this question by utilizing approaches based on current models of the regulation of erythropoiesis. There is evidence that the differentiative process undergone by the erythroid stem cells in vivo can be partly uncovered in vitro by manipulating culture conditions (Tepperman et al., 1974; Axelrad et al., 1974; Gregory, 1976). The most differentiated type of erythropoietic progenitor cell, operationally defined as the colony-forming unit erythroid (CFUe), proliferates in culture in the presence of low erythropoietin concentrations and forms small erythroid colonies that appear early in culture. Less differentiated stem cells, operationally defined as burst-forming units erythroid (BFUe's), are less sensitive to erythropoietin, requiring higher concentrations of the hormone for their growth; under these conditions, BFUe's also produce waves of erythroid colonies that appear later in culture (Gregory, 1976; Gregory and Eaves, 1977). Thus, it is possible, by manipulating culture conditions and using the fluorescent antibody approach, to learn if the erythroid stem cells capable of F clone formation share the growth characteristics of either of the 2 operational classes of erythroid stem cells. Such studies have shown that there are (a) a positive correlation between erythropoietin concentration and F clone formation, and (b) increases in frequencies and absolute numbers of F clones in late cultures, i.e. growth characteristics that are similar if not identical to those attributed to the less differentiated precursors of the burst-forming unit type (Papayannopoulou et al., 1977a). Hb F production in culture, thus, seems to be associated with the growth of more primitive cells of the adult erythroid stem cell compartment. This interpretation is supported by biosynthetic studies that consistently show activation of Hb F production in erythroid cultures initiated from almost pure populations of burst-forming units recovered from peripheral blood. Induction of γ-gene transcription by components of the culture media, unlikely in any event because of the clonal nature of Hb F production, has been excluded by studying separately the effects on Hb F production of the various components. A direct induction of γ-mRNA production by erythropoietin is also unlikely inasmuch as activation of Hb F synthesis takes place in the erythroid colonies of patients with polycythemia vera that can be raised without added erythropoietin (Papayannopoulou et al., unpublished observations). An additional piece of information which indicates that, in fact, commitment to Hb F formation is a characteristic of the primitive erythroid stem cells of the adult hemopoietic system, has been obtained through studies of Hb F expression in individual subclones initiated from these less differentiated erythroid stem cells.

Under certain culture conditions, the burst-forming units form clusters of colonies, or erythroid bursts; presumably, the parental stem cell divides, producing stem cell progeny that migrate in the culture medium, each initiating its own subcolony. The origin of the subcolonies of each burst from a single burst-forming unit has been demonstrated using genetic markers (Papayannopoulou et al., 1977a). This behavior of the BFUe's in culture provides an unparalleled opportunity for studying the means whereby sister cells exercise their options regarding expression of a program of differentiation. The specific question is whether or not all the progenitor cells that initiate the subcolonies of single erythroid bursts express the same program of fetal hemoglobin production. This question can be answered by checking for the presence of Hb A and Hb F in individual sister subcolonies derived from the same burst-forming unit using the fluorescent anti-Hb A and anti-Hb F antibodies. In well-hemoglobinized bursts, where all subcolonies fully express the Hb A production program, some subcolonies express the Hb F program, others do not and still others show a sectoral expression of Hb F (Papayannopoulou et al., 1977a). This provides a direct demonstration that the progeny of a single BFUe exercises different options regarding expression of the Hb F program.

It is not known if other, more primitive, erythroid stem cells with stable commitments to Hb F production are present in the adult erythroid system. This possibility is currently under investigation. However, information about the types of commitment of erythroid cells of earlier developmental stages has been obtained through studies of neonatal and fetal erythroid cells in culture. Fetal and neonatal cells have higher proliferative potentials than do adult cells, and produce large erythroid colonies early in culture, a pattern suggestive of a considerably shorter cell cycle. Erythroid clones initiated from erythroid stem cells from first and second trimester fetuses show uniformity of Hb A and F expression with production of large amounts of Hb F and reciprocally low amounts of Hb A per clone, suggesting a stable commitment of these cells to the expression of a developmental program that consists of high γ- and low β-globin gene transcription. The study of erythroid clones initiated from neonatal erythroid stem cells reveals, however, a different picture: striking differences in the degree of expression of Hb F and A synthesis among clones, with individual clones showing large, moderate or no Hb F production and a reciprocally related production of Hb A. These findings are of special importance because they suggest that the switch from fetal to adult hemoglobin production in the perinatal period is not accomplished by a gradual increase in levels of β-chain synthesis and a reciprocal gradual decrease in γ-globin gene transcription that occur simultaneously and homogeneously in all erythroid stem cell precursors present in the hemopoietic tissue. It appears more likely that the γ and β switch reflects abrupt changes in commitment that occur within sibling erythroid stem cells. An explanation of these findings is that, in contrast to the situation in the fetus, the stage of differentiation of the erythroid stem cells of the perinatal period is such as to allow the cells to exercise widely different options regarding expression of the program of Hb F or A formation.

SYNTHESIS AND SUMMARY

The data obtained from studies of cultures initiated from adult erythroid progenitors suggest that there is an increase in the ability of the erythroid stem cells to direct Hb F production in their terminally differentiated progeny, as one moves from the more advanced to the less advanced differentiation stages. These findings lead us to postulate that the expression of the developmental program of Hb F formation is dependent upon, and inversely related to, the stage of differentiation of the progenitor cells from which the terminally differentiated erythroblasts derive (Papayannopoulou et al., 1977a). The state of erythroid stem cell differentiation could determine globin gene transcription by directing alternate but specific conformations of chromatin structure. We have also suggested that the pattern of hemoglobin during normal ontogenesis might be explained by a similar mechanism and be attributed to the proliferation of erythroid stem cells that attain successively higher levels of differentiation as development proceeds (Fig. 2).

According to this hypothesis erythroblasts in the fetus are derived from erythroid stem cells that are at the earliest step of the erythroid stem cell differentiative scale and are capable of expressing only the program that specifies production of large excesses of Hb F over Hb A. Drastic changes in erythropoiesis during the perinatal period induce stem cell differentiation to progress to a stage at which the cells can vary in their expression of the programs of Hb A or Hb F formation. Finally, a stage of erythroid stem cell differentiation is reached at which the possibility for expression of the Hb F program is lost (Fig. 2). Thus, the switch from fetal to adult hemoglobin formation is viewed as a reflection of changes in cell kinetics rather than the result of direct action of inducers and repressors on the closely linked γ and β loci.

This view of the mechanism regulating Hb F production can account for several aspects of Hb F synthesis in vivo. The clonal appearance of F cells in the normal adult can be explained by the occasional derivation of erythroblasts from stem cells of the more primitive differentiative state (BFUe). The common denominator, i.e. the effect on the kinetics of erythroid stem cell differentiation, can account for the elevated proportion of F cells found in such diverse situations as rapid marrow regeneration, hemopoietic and non-hemopoietic malignancies and various forms of anemia. This model also implies that those hemopoietic malignancies associated with the appearance of 'fetal red-cell clones' in the bloods of the patients (Mauer et al.,

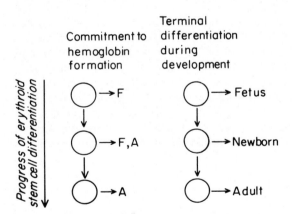

Fig. 2. Diagrammatic presentation of the proposed mechanism of Hb F formation. *Left:* commitment to Hb F formation is considered to be related to the degree of differentiation of erythroid stem cells. *Right:* the normal developmental patterns of hemoglobin are attributed to achievement of more advanced stages of differentiation of the erythroid progenitor cells, as development proceeds. Thus, it is postulated that erythroblasts in the fetus are derived from erythroid stem cells that are still in a 'primitive' stage of differentiation which is associated with chromatin structure that allows for preponderant transcription of the γ-globin genes. On the other hand, erythroid stem cell differentiation in the adult proceeds up to a stage at which chromatin structure is such as to permit only β-gene transcription. This model assumes that earlier stages of erythroid stem cell differentiation exist in the hemopoietic tissue of the adult individual and that the Hb F-containing cells in the normal adult as well as in the person with an acquired Hb F elevation are derived from less differentiated erythroid progenitors.

1972; Weatherall et al., 1976; Pagnier et al., 1977), a typical example of which is the juvenile form of chronic myelogenous leukemia, arise from lesions of primary pluripotent stem cells that also arrest differentiation of the erythroid stem cells at the early stage which normally exists only in the fetus.

This view of the regulatory mechanism of Hb F synthesis also provides a conceptual framework for studies aimed at the manipulation of Hb F production in vitro and, hopefully, in vivo. In the great majority of patients with sickling disorders and β-thalassemia syndromes the levels of fetal hemoglobin produced provide inadequate protection against the consequences of the primary defects in hemoglobin structure or synthesis. Stimulation of fetal hemoglobin production will be required for modifying the clinical courses of these disorders. According to the model just presented, this goal might be achieved, should it become possible to manipulate in vivo the kinetics of differentiation of erythroid stem cells and trigger production of erythroblasts from earlier precursors that have an active program of Hb F expression.

REFERENCES

Alter, B. P., Rappeport, J. M., Huisman, T. H. J., Schroeder, W. A. and Nathan, D. (1976): *Blood, 48*, 843.
Axelrad, A. A., McLeod, D. L., Shreeve, M. M. and Heath, D. S. (1974): In: *Hemopoiesis in Culture*, p. 226. Editor: W. A. Robinson. U.S. Government Printing Office, Washington, D.C.
Bard, H. (1973): *J. clin. Invest., 52*, 1789.
Benz, E., Turner, P., Barker, J. and Nienhuis, A. (1977): *Science, 196*, 1213.
Bertles, J. F. and Milner, P. F. A. (1968): *J. clin. Invest., 47*, 1731.
Boyer, S. H., Belding, T. K., Margolet, L. and Noyes, A. N. (1975): *Science, 188*, 361.
Boyer, S. H., Margolet, L., Boyer, M. L., Huisman, T. H. J., Schroeder, W. A., Wood, W. G., Weatherall, D. J., Clegg, J. B. and Cartner, R. (1977): *Amer. J. hum. Genet., 29*, 256.
Bradley, T. B. and Ranney, H. M. (1973): *Progr. Hematol., 8*, 77.
Charache, S. and Conley, C. L. (1964): *Blood, 24*, 25.
Fessas, Ph. (1967): *Trans. roy. Soc. trop. Med. Hyg., 61*, 164.
Gregory, C. J. (1976): *J. Cell Physiol., 89*, 289.
Gregory, C. J. and Eaves, A. C. (1977): *Blood, 49*, 855.
Huisman, T. H. J., Schroeder, W. A., Dozy, A. M., Shelton, J. R., Shelton, J. B., Boyd, E. M. and Apell, G. (1969): *Ann. N.Y. Acad. Sci., 165*, 320.
Huisman, T. H. J., Schroeder, W. A., Efremov, G. D., Duma, H., Mladenovski, B., Hyman, C. B., Rachmilewitz, E. A., Bouver, N., Miller, A., Brodie, A., Shelton, J. R., Shelton, J. B. and Apell, G. (1974): *Ann. N.Y. Acad. Sci., 232*, 107.
Huisman, T. H. J., Schroeder, W. A., Stamatoyannopoulos, G., Bouver, N., Shelton, J. R., Shelton, J. B. and Apell, G. (1970): *J. clin. Invest., 49*, 1035.
Kan, Y. W., Holland, J. P., Dozy, A. M., Charache, S. and Kazazian, H. H. (1975): *Nature (Lond.), 258*, 162.
Kendall, A. G., Ojwang, P. J., Schroeder, W. A. and Huisman, T. H. J. (1973): *Amer. J. hum. Genet., 25*, 548.
Lajtha, L. G. and Schofield, R. (1974): *Differentiation, 2*, 313.
Lanyon, W. G., Ottolenghi, S. and Williamson, R. (1977): *Proc. nat. Acad. Sci. (Wash.), 72*, 258.
Loukopoulos, D. and Fessas, Ph. (1965): *J. clin. Invest., 44*, 231.
Marks, P. A. and Rifkind, R. A. (1972): *Science, 175*, 955.
Mauer, H. S., Vida, L. N. and Honig, G. R. (1972): *Blood, 39*, 778.
Nathan, D. G. and Gunn, R. B. (1966): *Amer. J. Med., 41*, 815.
Pagnier, J., Lopez, M., Mathiot, C., Habibi, B., Zamet, P., Varet, B. and Labie, D. (1977): *Blood, 50*, 249.
Papayannopoulou, Th., Brice, M. and Stamatoyannopoulos, G. (1976): *Proc. nat. Acad. Sci. (Wash.), 73*, 2033.
Papayannopoulou, Th., Brice, M. and Stamatoyannopoulos, G. (1977a): *Proc. nat. Acad. Sci. (Wash.), 74*, 2923.

Papayannopoulou, Th., Nute, P. E., Stamatoyannopoulos, G. and McGuire, T. C. (1977b): *Science*, *196*, 1215.
Perrine, R. P., Brown, M. J., Clegg, J. B., Weatherall, D. J. and May, A. (1972): *Lancet*, *2*, 1163.
Schroeder, W. A., Huisman, T. H. J., Shelton, J. R., Shelton, J. B., Kleihauer, E. F., Dozy, A. M. and Robberson, B. (1968): *Proc. nat. Acad. Sci. (Wash.)*, *60*, 537.
Singer, K. and Fisher, B. (1952): *Blood*, *7*, 1216.
Stamatoyannopoulos, G., Fessas, Ph. and Papayannopoulou, Th. (1969): *Amer. J. Med.*, *47*, 194.
Stamatoyannopoulos, G., Wood, W. G., Papayannopoulou, Th. and Nute, P. E. (1975): *Blood*, *46*, 683.
Stephenson, J. R., Axelrad, A. A., McLeod, D. L. and Shreeve, M. M. (1971): *Proc. nat. Acad. Sci. (Wash.)*, *68*, 1542.
Teppermenn, A. D., Curtis, J. E. and McCulloch, E. A. (1974): *Blood*, *44*, 659.
Weatherall, D. J., Clegg, J. B. and Wood, W. G. (1976): *Lancet*, *2*, 660.
Weatherall, D. J., Pembrey, M. E. and Pritchard, J. (1974): *Clin. in Haematol.*, *3*, 467.
Wood, W. G., Pearce, K., Clegg, J. B., Weatherall, D. J., Robinson, J. S., Thorburn, G. D. and Dawes, G. S. (1976): *Nature (Lond.)*, *264*, 799.
Wood, W. G., Stamatoyannopoulos, G., Lim, G. and Nute, P. E. (1975): *Blood*, *46*, 671.
Wood, W. G. and Weatherall, D. J. (1973): *Nature (Lond.)*, *244*, 162.

The effects of the epidermal and fibroblast growth factors upon cell proliferation using vascular and corneal endothelial cells as a model*

D. GOSPODAROWICZ[1,2], I. VLODAVSKY[1], P. FIELDING[3] and C. R. BIRDWELL[4]

[1]Cancer Research Institute, [2]Department of Medicine, and [3]Cardiovascular Research Institute, University of California, Medical Center, San Francisco, Calif. and [4]Scripps Research Clinic, La Jolla, Calif., U.S.A.

Considerable effort has recently been expended in attempts to isolate putative growth factors from tissue or from serum. The study of these growth factors had a special interest, since it was believed that the addition of these factors to a defined medium would allow normal cells to proliferate, thus eliminating the requirement for whole serum as a necessary adjuvant for cell culture and perhaps permitting the establishment of new cell lines.

Parallel to these efforts to identify and purify growth factors, similar efforts were made by developmental biologists involved in the in vivo control of cell proliferation and differentiation. Pathologists involved in the study of the development of atherosclerosis and wound healing started to develop an interest in growth factors and their role in controlling the proliferation of the different cell types in these processes. From the efforts of these different groups the identification and purification of new growth factors and a better understanding of their role in the control of cell proliferation in vitro and in vivo has emerged.

DIFFERENT CLASSES OF GROWTH FACTORS PRODUCED IN VIVO

Until 1970 only a few growth factors had been identified and purified. Among the most prominent were the epidermal growth factor (EGF), nerve growth factor (NGF), erythropoietin, colony-stimulating factor, thymopoietin, and a few postulated serum factors and wound-healing hormones. Since 1971, however, a population explosion has taken place and has led to the discovery and purification of active, not very active, or inactive growth factors, depending on the criteria of mitogenic

*This work was supported by grants HL20197 and HD-11082 from the National Institutes of Health and VC-194 from the American Cancer Society. I. Vlodavsky is a recipient of the Chaim Weizmann Research Training Fellowship.

233

activity one chooses to follow (e.g. initiation of DNA synthesis, a few cycles in subconfluent populations, multiple cycles in sparse cultures or in clonal growth). Included among these new factors are the somatomedins A, B, and C, the non-suppressible insulin-like activity (NSILA-S), multiplication-stimulating activity, the platelet and macrophage factors, the cationic peptide, and fibroblast growth factor (FGF). Soon, some of these growth factors started to breed and led to 'families' such as the family of somatomedins A and B, which themselves were the forerunners of the A_1, A_2, and B_1, B_2, and B_3 subclasses. NSILA-S has split into classes I and II. Since these factors are purified from plasma, the proteolytic activity present in plasma could conceivably have something to do with this breeding phenomenon.

One way to reunite these disparate families could emerge from the innovative approach taken by the group of Sato and his co-workers. Basing their procedures on the observation that most of the serum growth factors are heat-stable, Sato and his group decided to attempt their purification from heat-denatured blood, commonly known as blood meal, a substance also used as a fertilizer. Since the initial heat treatment should denature most of the plasma proteases responsible for the pleio-morphism of serum growth factors, use of this material could conceivably ease the purification of homogenous fractions of serum factors.

The identification of new mitogens can be traced back to 2 different concepts. One is that mitogens have an insulin-like structure and that growth hormones could act indirectly by generating the formation of mitogens with insulin-like activity. Included among the insulin-like compounds are the somatomedins, NSILA, and MSA. If, however, one examines the evidence for the mitogenic activity of these factors in vitro, this type of factor, with the exceptions of MSA and somatomedin C, rarely stimulates mitotic activity to any great extent. Although they have been shown to induce DNA synthesis in serum-starved cultures or to induce 1 or 2 division cycles in subconfluent cultures, the mitotic activity of these compounds is so weak in comparison to serum that they cannot be considered to be true mitogens.

A second concept is that cell proliferation such as that which takes place during atherosclerosis or wound healing could be induced by factors, which are released locally from circulating cells such as platelets or macrophages. The possible presence of mitogenic factors in platelets was first pointed out by Balk, who observed that cells divided at a slow rate when maintained in the presence of plasma, whereas, in the presence of serum, active proliferation took place (1). He reasoned that, when platelets aggregate during coagulation, they could be releasing a mitogenic factor or could activate a mitogenic zymogen present in plasma, since serum is produced from plasma. Evidence that this could be the case has been provided by Ross and Glomset (3) and by Kohler and Lipton (2). These authors have shown that, although vascular smooth muscle or 3T3 cells divide slowly or not at all in the presence of plasma, the addition of a thrombin-treated platelet supernatant or platelet crude extract to plasma restored the mitogenic activity of plasma to a level comparable to that of serum. Possibly related to the platelet factor is the cationic peptide isolated from serum (4), since radioimmunoassay of that factor suggests that it could cross-react immunologically with the platelet factor. Mitogens could also be produced by macrophages (5) as suggested by the following lines of evidence: (a) active prolifera-tion of fibroblasts and vascular endothelial cells takes place in wound healing when macrophages are present; elimination of the macrophages with macrophage antiserum and glucocorticoids results in strong impairment of the wound healing process (5); (b) macrophages activated with endotoxin and implanted in an avascular space, such as the cornea, induce capillary proliferation (6); (c) wound fluid obtained from a subcutaneous wound chamber has a much higher mitotic activity than the plasma or serum of the same donor (7); (d) macrophages derived from wound fluid, when co-cultured with vascular smooth muscle or vascular endothelial cells, maintained under otherwise limiting conditions, induce an increase in the rate of cell proliferation (7). These lines of evidence suggest that macrophages release mitogenic factors and could be a key cellular element involved in the production of mitogenic factors.

Another class of growth factors is represented by the fibroblast growth factor (FGF). Since current techniques have not been entirely adequate to permit the purification of more than tiny amounts of growth factors from serum, investigators have turned their attention to tissue sources. Recent work has focused on 2 promising sources of growth factors: the pituitary (8–11) and neural tissue, since nerves have been shown to be essential for limb regeneration in lower vertebrates (12).

From both these sources, bovine pituitary and bovine brain (13, 14), the mitogen FGF has been isolated. This is a basic polypeptide having a molecular weight of 13,400 (13, 14). First named on the basis of its mitogenic potency for Balb/c 3T3 fibroblasts (15), it has also been shown to stimulate the division of a wide variety of mesoderm-derived cells (Table 1).

The effect of FGF has been compared to that of epidermal growth factor (EGF), an acidic polypeptide with a molecular weight of 6045 (16) that was first isolated by Stanley Cohen from the submaxillary glands of adult male mice (17). Originally shown to stimulate the proliferation of epidermal cells both in vivo (18) and in vitro (19), EGF has also been reported to be a potent mitogen for human diploid fibroblasts (20–22). It is of considerable interest that EGF has recently been shown to be similar in structure to urogastrone in humans (23), a polypeptide that is involved in blocking the release of HCl from the gastric mucosa and that is also considered to play a role in the repair process of the stomach wall.

Since it will be impossible, in a short review, to detail the characteristics of the mitogenic response of mesoderm-derived cells to FGF and EGF, we will here review recent studies in our laboratory regarding the use of these growth factors to establish 2 given cell types, the vascular and corneal endothelial cells, in tissue culture. Using EGF and FGF as tools, we have developed endothelial cell lines from bovine and human origin in order to study the metabolic properties and growth control of these cells, both in vivo and in vitro.

VASCULAR ENDOTHELIAL CELLS

Endothelial cells constitute the inner lining of the blood vascular system. Because of their location at the interface between blood and tissue, they are the chief element involved in the permeability of blood vessels (58, 59). Abnormalities of the endothelial cell structure and function are prominent in the pathology of a number of diseases of the blood vessel walls, such as thromboangitis and microangiopathy (60). Since the continuity of the vascular endothelium is essential for the survival of the organism, the elucidation of the factors involved in the endothelial cell's

TABLE 1

Comparison of the mitogenic effects of FGF and EGF

Cell type	Species	FGF sensitivity	EGF sensitivity	References
Balb/c 3T3	mouse	+++	++	11, 15, 24, 25, 26
Swiss 3T3	mouse	++	++	26, 27
3T3 thermosensitive mutant	permissive temperature	—	NT	28
	unpermissive temperature	+++	NT	28
Foreskin fibroblasts	human	++	++	20–22, 29
Glial cells	human	+	++	30, 31
Kidney fibroblasts	bovine	+	NT	Gospodarowicz, unpublished observations
Amniotic cells (fibroblasts)	human, bovine	+++	+	32
Chondrocytes	rabbit ear and articular chondrocytes	++	+++	14, 33, 34, 35
Myoblasts	bovine fetus	++	—	35, 36, 37
Vascular smooth muscle	primate, bovine	++	+	38, 39
Vascular endothelial cells	bovine umbilical vein	++	—	14, 40
	aortic arch	++	—	39, 40, 41, 42
	fetal heart	++	—	40, 43, 44
Human endothelial cells	umbilical vein	++	+	40, 43, 44
Cornea endothelial cells	bovine	+++	+++	45, 46
Cornea epithelial cells	bovine	+++	—	47
Lens epithelial cells	bovine	+++	—	47
Cornea epithelium in vivo organ culture or with feeder layer	rabbit, human	++	+++	19, 47, 48, 49
Y1 adrenal cortex cells	mouse	++	—	50
Adrenal cortex cells	bovine	++	—	51, 52
Granulosa cells	bovine	++	+++	52, 53
Luteal cells	bovine	++	—	54, 55
Liver cells	rat (endoderm)	—	—	42
Anterior pituitary cells	rat (endoderm)	—	NT	42
Thyroid cells	cow (endoderm)	—	—	Gospodarowicz, unpublished observations
Epidermal cells	human, rabbit, chick (ectoderm)	—	+++	18, 42, 56
Pancreatic cells	rat (endoderm)	—	NT	42
Blastemal cells	frog	++	NT	57
Blastemal cells	*Triturus viridescens*	++	—	36

NT = not tested; — = not active; ++ = active (ng/ml); +++ = very active (pg/fg/ml).

survival and proliferation is important. The survival and proliferation of this cell can be examined most easily in tissue culture.

Two observations have led us to examine the effect of FGF on vascular endothelial cells: (a) FGF is a potent mitogen for Balb/c 3T3 cells (13, 14, 24). Although these cells are commonly referred to as fibroblasts, their morphology and the fact that they can produce vasoformative sarcomas in vivo suggest that they are derived from vascular endothelium (61). (b) Although FGF was named fibroblast growth factor when first isolated, subsequent studies have shown that it is a mitogen for a wide variety of mesoderm-derived cells (36). Since the vascular endothelium is derived from the embryonic mesoderm, one would expect endothelial cells also to be responsive to FGF.

We have examined the possibility that FGF is a survival factor as well as a mitogen for cultured vascular endothelial cells. These studies have demonstrated that FGF can be used to maintain and grow endothelial cells in tissue culture for prolonged periods.

Control of the proliferation of bovine vascular endothelial cells

Our first attempt to look at the effect of FGF on the proliferation of vascular endothelium started with bovine tissue. Bovine tissues, unlike human ones, are readily available, and their use allows the easy examination of the characteristics of endothelial cells derived from different vascular territories, as well as from donors varying in age from fetal to adult.

Since we had intended to study at a later time the effect of FGF on capillary proliferation in vivo, and since capillaries originate from endothelial cells, we first examined the comparative mitogenic effects of FGF and EGF on endothelial cell cultures derived from the bovine aorta. When primary cultures of cells from bovine aortic endothelium are started with relatively few cells (30 cells per cm^2), the develop-

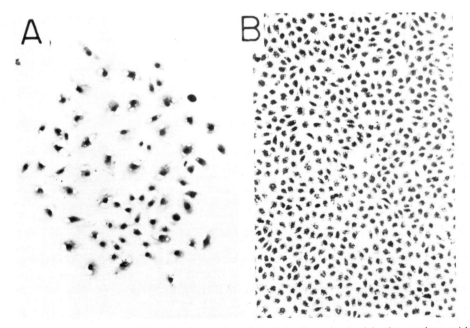

Fig. 1. Primary cultures of fetal bovine aortic endothelial cells maintained in tissue culture with and without FGF. A. Colony of endothelial cells maintained in 10% calf serum for 6 days without FGF. The cells are vacuolated with a broad and thin peripheral cytoplasm (cells were fixed with 10% formalin and stained with 0.1% Giemsa, 60×). B. Monolayer obtained after 6 days in culture in the presence of 100 ng/ml of FGF and 10% calf serum. The cells are polygonal and closely apposed (cells were fixed and stained, as described in 'A', 60×).

ment of a monolayer is dependent on the presence of FGF in the culture medium. In 10% calf serum alone small colonies developed from cell aggregates during the first few days, but the cells appeared unhealthy, soon became heavily vacuolated, and later died (41) (Fig. 1). In contrast, if FGF was added, the cells proliferated vigorously and formed a monolayer (Fig. 1). As little as 1 ng/ml of FGF stimulated the proliferation of vascular endothelial cells, and a maximal effect was seen at 25 to 50 ng/ml (39–42) (Fig. 2). EGF did not stimulate cell proliferation, even at concentrations as high as 1 μg/ml (Fig. 2). Insulin or glucagon were also ineffective. We also looked, in these earlier studies, at the effect of thrombin, a serine protease, which has been shown to potentiate the growth response of other cell types to FGF and EGF (62, 63). Since vascular endothelial cells may be expected to be exposed to high thrombin concentrations following trauma or in any pathological state associated with thrombosis, they are of particular interest with respect to the physiological role of this protease in potentiating cell proliferation. In these initial studies, however, we were unable to detect that thrombin potentiates the mitogenic effects of FGF and EGF when the protease was tested on a cloned cell line derived from the bovine aortic arch (Fig. 2).

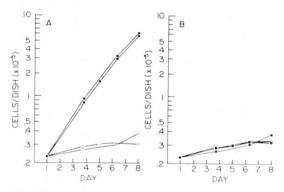

Fig. 2. Growth rate of bovine endothelial cells maintained in the presence of FGF or EGF with or without thrombin. Vascular endothelial cells derived from the adult aortic arch (56 passages, 336 generations) were plated at 740 cells per cm² in 6-cm dishes in DME supplemented with 10% calf serum. A. The cells were maintained in the presence of FGF alone (● + ●), FGF + thrombin (■-■), thrombin alone (□-□), or without addition (○ + ○). FGF was added every other day at a final concentration of 100 ng/ml and thrombin every 4 days at a final concentration of 2 μg/ml. B. Same as 'A' but with EGF (100 ng/ml) instead of FGF.

Since the lack of response of the bovine vascular endothelial cells to EGF and to the potentiating effect of thrombin could be due to their origin (the aortic arch) and to the selection of an unresponsive cell type during the cloning selection, we have compared the mitogenic effects of EGF and FGF on bovine vascular endothelial cells derived from vascular territories as diverse as the bovine heart, the aortic arch, and the umbilical vein, and obtained from tissues as diverse in age as fetal and adult. In no case were we able to obtain a mitogenic effect of EGF, although the cells did respond quite well to FGF (Fig. 3). Likewise, thrombin did not have any potentiating effect on cultures maintained in the presence of either EGF or FGF (40, 43).

Our results with the bovine endothelium thus demonstrate that FGF is a mitogenic

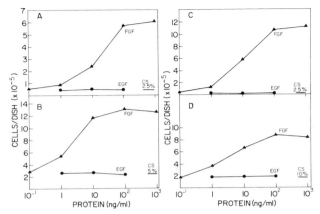

Fig. 3. Effect of increasing concentrations of EGF and FGF on the proliferation of bovine vascular endothelial cells derived from the umbilical vein (A), the fetal aortic arch (B), the fetal heart (C), and the calf aortic arch (D). The cells were plated at 740 cells per cm^2 in a 6-cm dish in DME supplemented with calf serum. The vascular endothelial cells derived from the umbilical vein and the fetal heart (A and C) were maintained in the presence of 2.5% calf serum, while the endothelial cells derived from the fetal aortic arch (B) or the calf aortic arch (D) were maintained in the presence of 5 and 10% calf serum respectively. All cell strains were in their third passage – FGF or EGF was added at 100 ng/ml every other day. Cells from the umbilical vein were counted on day 7, and cells from the fetal heart, fetal aortic arch, and calf aortic arch were counted on day 8. The final cell densities reached in the absence of FGF or EGF for the cells derived from the umbilical vein and the fetal heart were 2036 cells/cm^2 and 1000 cells/cm^2 respectively, indicating a nearly total dependence upon FGF for proliferation. With both fetal and calf aortic arch the densities reached were 8150 cells/cm^2 and 6500 cells/cm^2.

agent for bovine vascular endothelial cells and can be used to develop clonal cell lines, since it acts as a survival agent when those cells are maintained at extremely low density (8 cells/cm^2). Endothelial cells from similar fetal or adult vascular territories respond to FGF in the same way. Moreover, we did not observe any significant differences between cells from venous endothelium and those from aortic endothelium in their response to FGF. We have, by now, been able to develop in tissue culture cloned cell lines derived from the fetal, calf, and adult aortic arch. The adult bovine aortic arch endothelial cell line has been passaged weekly with a split ratio of 1 to 64 for over 65 weeks (390 generations) without loss of differentiated functions as expressed by its contact inhibition pattern at confluency and the presence of AHF-antigen (40).

Each of the cell lines is used as a tool to study different properties of the vascular endothelium. The fetal heart endothelial cell, which shows an absolute requirement for FGF and responds to it even when the cells are maintained in serum concentrations as low as 0.1% (Figs. 4 and 5), is used for the study of metabolic agents which interact with the endothelium and which have a short half-life in high serum concentration. The adult bovine aortic endothelial cell line, which responds to FGF only in high serum concentration (10%) and does not proliferate at all in the absence of FGF, has been used to study the release of mitogens from transformed cells. In such experiments growth of low density cultures of endothelial cells is monitored in the presence and absence of irradiated tumor cells (80). Finally, the fetal aortic endothelial and calf aortic endothelial cell lines can be used to study the synthesis

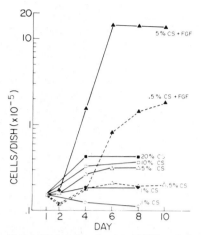

Fig. 4. Correlation between FGF and the serum concentration on the growth of fetal heart endothelial cell cultures. Fetal heart endothelial cells (15 passages, 125 generations) were plated at 14,000 cells per 6-cm dish and maintained in the presence or absence of 100 ng/ml of FGF with different concentrations of calf serum ranging from 0.1% to 20%. FGF (100 ng/ml) was added every other day and the media were changed every 4 days. Eight days later the plates were washed, fixed with formalin, and stained with 0.1% Giemsa.

and secretion of components of the basement membrane such as collagen and LETS protein (67).

Control of in vitro proliferation of human vascular endothelial cells

As mentioned earlier, the use of FGF has permitted the development of clonal endothelial cell lines of bovine origin. The development of human cloned cell lines is, however, more challenging, since it has, in the past, been prevented by the frequent

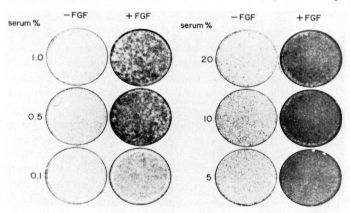

Fig. 5. Effect of FGF on the proliferation of fetal heart endothelial cell cultures. Fetal heart endothelial cells (15 passages, 125 generations) were plated at 15,000 cells per 6-cm dish and maintained in the presence of DME supplemented with 0.1, 0.5, 1.5, 10, and 20% calf serum or 0.5% and 5% calf serum plus 100 ng/ml of FGF. FGF was added every other day, at which time triplicate plates were trypsinized and counted.

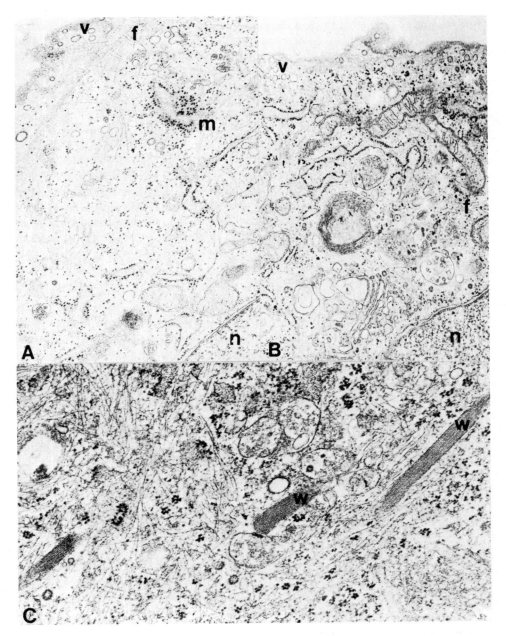

Fig. 6. Electron micrograph of vascular endothelial cells derived from (A) the adult bovine aortic arch, (B) the bovine umbilical vein, and (C) the human umbilical vein. A. Numerous residues are seen near the cell surface. 60–70 Å and 100 Å filaments (f) are evident as are microtubules (m). Numerous ribosomes and polysomes are seen in the cytoplasm, nucleus (n). B. The same structural features can be seen as in 'A'. C. Numerous Weibel-Palade bodies (W) can be seen in the cytoplasm of the cells; other structural features are similar to those seen for adult bovine aortic arch (A) and the bovine umbilical vein (B).

difficulties encountered in obtaining cultures that could be passaged repeatedly
while maintaining a high mitotic index, as well as by an inability to maintain human
vascular endothelial cells at a low enough cell density to permit cloning (65). Our
studies concerning the effects of EGF and FGF on human endothelial cell cultures
obtained by collagenase treatment of human umbilical vein demonstrate that these
cells are responsive to FGF, although at much higher concentrations (1 μg/ml)
than those required for the proliferation of bovine vascular endothelial cells.

These cultures, upon reaching confluency, exhibited the characteristic morphology
of highly contact inhibited cells (40). The presence of Weibel-Palade bodies (Fig. 6)
and of AHF antigen (Factor VIII) (40, 43) conclusively shows that these cells were
derived from the vascular endothelium.

As mentioned earlier, the concentration of FGF required to obtain a mitogenic
effect on human cells was 100-fold higher than it was for bovine endothelial cells.
Since it has been previously observed that thrombin is able to potentiate the response
of cells to FGF, we decided to test the response of human endothelial cells to increasing concentrations of FGF and EGF in the presence or absence of thrombin.
As shown in Figure 7, thrombin acts to potentiate the effect of FGF in such a way
that the log dose response is displaced by greater than 2 orders of magnitude. For
example, the increase in cell number observed when one incubates cells with 1 ng/ml
FGF plus 2 μg/ml thrombin exceeds that observed with 100 ng/ml FGF and no
thrombin. Whereas thrombin alone induces only a 3-fold increase in cell number
after 15 days, cells incubated in the presence of thrombin plus FGF increase more
than 100-fold (Fig. 7A). Although thrombin does potentiate the effect of saturating
concentrations of FGF, the most pronounced effects of thrombin are observed when
sub-saturating doses of FGF are employed (40, 43). Human cells, unlike bovine
vascular endothelial cell cultures, are also responsive to EGF (40, 43). This has been
correlated with the presence of EGF binding sites in human endothelial cell cultures
(43).

EGF effectively stimulates the proliferation of human vascular endothelial cells,
although to a lesser extent than does FGF. Whereas lower doses of EGF are required
to induce a proliferative response (Fig. 7B), the maximal cell numbers obtained are

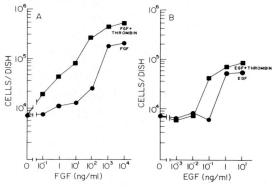

Fig. 7. Effect of thrombin on the response of human endothelial cells to FGF and EGF. Cells were maintained in the presence of (A) FGF or (B) EGF in the presence or absence of thrombin. On day 15 the
cells were trypsinized and counted in triplicate. Controls treated with thrombin alone contained
2.2×10^4 cells.

never as great as with FGF. Thrombin can be seen in Figure 7B to potentiate the response to EGF in much the same way as to FGF, for in both cases it allows the cells to respond to reduced concentrations of the growth factor.

Our finding that thrombin allows cultured human endothelial cells to respond to concentrations of FGF or EGF that by themselves would be insufficient gives an indication of the kind of situation in which thrombin might be expected to play a role in regulating cell proliferation. Normal vascular endothelium represents a slowly renewing population of cells in vivo. However, endothelial cell regeneration can be triggered by a variety of stimuli, especially intimal denudation, during which organization of thrombi takes place. This organization occurs together with the release of the contents of secretory granules from platelets and with the generation of high localized concentrations of thrombin. The thrombin, in turn, could make the human vascular endothelial cells sensitive to plasma growth factors.

The mechanism by which thrombin potentiates the effect of other growth factors is unclear but is probably mediated by action on the cells themselves and not by cleavage of the factors (62). The observation that thrombin can remove specific proteins from cell surfaces (63) suggests that the enzyme could act to expose new binding or transport sites for the other growth-effecting molecules. Whether thrombin is internalized by endothelial cells, as it is by chick embryo fibroblasts, is not yet known (64).

The use of vascular endothelial cells in vitro

Since the continuity of the vascular endothelium is essential for the growth and survival of the organism, the elucidation of the factors involved in endothelial cell survival and proliferation is important (65). The development of endothelial cell lines is one of the first steps toward such an understanding. In addition to the success achieved in developing such cell lines there are further practical implications as well. The elucidation of the functions and mechanisms through which endothelial cells are able to mature and thrive can only be investigated by first establishing the natural requirements for survival and proliferation of this cell type. These requirements are best investigated by long-term maintenance of endothelial cells at low density and by high mitotic index of the cultures (66). Such cell lines should provide an adequate model for the study of the metabolic function of the vascular endothelium.

LETS PROTEIN AND THE VASCULAR ENDOTHELIUM

One of the morphological characteristics of vascular endothelial cells is that they grow as a monolayer (66). Another characteristic is their ability to secrete enormous amounts of extracellular material. Fetal aortic endothelial cells are capable of covering the culture dish with an amorphous material which forms concentric circles 2 to 4 layers deep and can readily be detected by light microscopy (66). This property is not unique to the fetal tissue, since calf aortic endothelial cells also share it. As shown in Figure 8, if one treats the monolayer of calf endothelial cells with detergent, an amorphous material similar to that observed in the case of fetal cells can be discerned (Figs. 8 and 9).

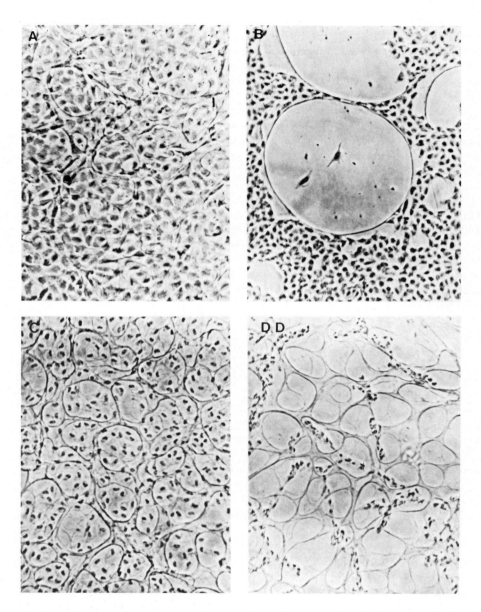

Fig. 8. Configuration of a monolayer of bovine calf aortic arch endothelial cell culture maintained for a long period of time (phase contrast 128 ×). Bovine calf aortic arch endothelial cell cultures were seeded at 100,000 cells per 10-cm dish in the presence of DME, 10% calf serum and 100 ng/ml of FGF. When the cells reached confluency the medium was changed to DME, 10% calf serum and 1 ng/ml of FGF. Two weeks later, an amorphous material appeared under the monolayer (A) and the cells started to retract and to form concentric circles (B) limited on their inside by a membrane. When the monolayer was treated with PBS containing 0.1% Triton X, the monolayer was dissolved, leaving behind the nuclei of the cells and the basement membrane (C, D).

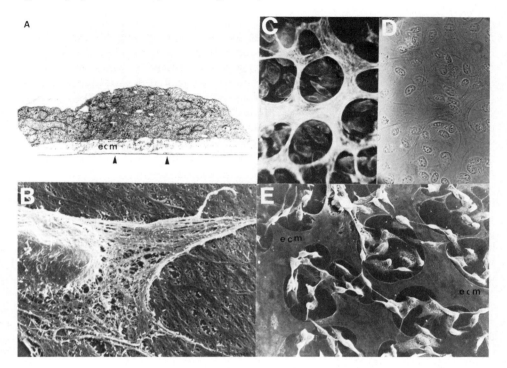

Fig. 9. Electron micrograph of vascular endothelial cells and immunofluorescence of LETS antigen. A clone of adult bovine aortic endothelial (ABAE) cell cultures in their 20th passage (107 generations) was used (A and B). A and B. Electron micrographs of 2-week-old ABAE cultures. A. Transmission electron micrograph of a thin section of an ABAE monolayer cut perpendicular to the monolayer which shows the extracellular matrix (em) underneath the cells. The dark line (arrows) along the bottom of the micrographs is the plastic substrate of the tissue culture dish. B. Scanning electron micrograph of a 2-week-old ABAE culture treated briefly with 0.5% Triton X-100. This micrograph shows a single ABAE cyto-skeleton (cs) and attached nucleus (n) stretched over the extracellular matrix (em). C and D. Indirect immunofluorescence of LETS on ABAE cultures. C. Staining of 2-week-old culture following Triton X-100 treatment shows areas of fluorescence which correspond to the basement membrane. D. Phase contrast micrograph of the same field as in 'C'. E. Scanning electron micrograph of an ABAE monolayer treated very briefly with 0.5% Triton X-100. The extracellular matrix (em) is quite apparent and many ABAE cytoskeletons are still attached to the substrate.

When, using antibodies against LETS protein, we analyzed this material by immunofluorescence, it was found to be LETS protein (Fig. 9). This cell surface glycoprotein was localized on the endothelial surface exposed to the substrate but not on the endothelial surface exposed to the medium (44, 67). This unique polarity in the production of LETS protein by the vascular endothelium could be related to the non-thrombogenic properties of the vascular endothelium and to those of other types of endothelium, such as the corneal, since the cellular side exposed to the bloodstream or to the aqueous humor is not covered by the LETS protein (also called fibronectin). It thus seems that the vascular endothelium produces this cell surface glycoprotein in large quantities, and one might well wonder why vascular endothelial cells produce so much of it.

The LETS protein has been shown to be related to cell adhesion and morphology

(68). Since the endothelial cells grow as a single layer of flattened cells (indeed, one of the most flattened which can exist when seen by scanning electron microscopy), it makes sense that these cells will produce much LETS to help maintain their flattened morphology. Furthermore, the endothelial cells which form the inner lining of the arteries may need to secrete enormous amounts of LETS in order to stay attached to the basal lamina. If one considers the turbulence, the pressure variations, and the speed of the blood flow in the aortic arch, there are few cell types which could form a monolayer and remain attached to the basement membrane unless they developed a special means to stick to it. Such a means could be the production of great amounts of extracellular material, such as LETS, which primarily functions to enforce cell adhesion.

It has recently been observed that cold, insoluble globulin (CIG), a protein found in plasma in concentrations in excess of 300 μg/ml, is antigenically identical to the LETS protein (69). To date no major physiological role has been ascribed to this protein. However, the vascular endothelium, in order to stay attached to the basal lamina, makes great amounts of LETS protein, and it makes sense that part of it will be shed into the bloodstream, where it will appear as CIG. It might, therefore, be concluded that, because of their morphology (monolayer), shape (flattened), and situation (inner layer of the arteries and veins), vascular endothelial cells could be called upon to make a major contribution toward the production of the LETS protein found in the basement membrane of blood vessels as well as that found in plasma as CIG.

THE BINDING, UPTAKE, AND DEGRADATION OF LOW-DENSITY LIPOPROTEIN BY CULTURED VASCULAR ENDOTHELIAL CELLS

Endothelial cells are exposed to various substances at concentrations and proportions far different from those in the extravascular region and are therefore expected to possess unique properties both as a barrier and as a transport system. Among the questions which are raised concerning the metabolism and transport function of the endothelial cells is that of why vascular endothelial cells do not contain a significant amount of cholesterol, although they are continuously exposed to high concentrations of plasma low-density lipoprotein (LDL). It would seem to be a reasonable hypothesis that in the early stage of human atherosclerosis endothelial cells lose their barrier function and that therefore large amounts of cholesterol esters derived from plasma lipoprotein might accumulate within lipid-rich cells in the subendothelial region.

The establishment of clonal endothelial cell lines from different species and origins provides us now with a well-defined and controlled system for the study of the interaction between plasma lipoproteins and the vascular endothelium. Using sparse and subconfluent endothelial cell cultures derived from bovine fetal heart and from calf and adult aortic arch, we have demonstrated the presence on the cell surface of a specific, high-affinity receptor site for the plasma low-density lipoprotein (LDL). Its presence was indicated by the observations that the binding of ^{125}I-LDL was saturable (half-maximal binding obtained at 15 μg protein/ml) (Fig. 10A), showed the expected competition with native LDL and VLDL molecules,

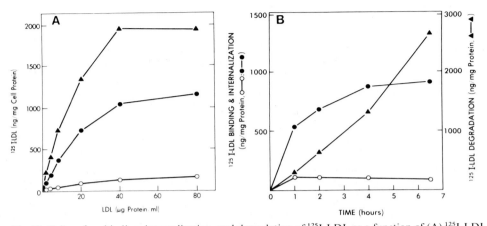

Fig. 10. Cell surface binding, internalization, and degradation of ^{125}I-LDL as a function of (A) ^{125}I-LDL concentration and (B) time of incubation with LDL. Subconfluent cultures of fetal bovine heart endo-thelial cells (FBHE) in 35-mm Petri dishes were first incubated for 48 hours in growth medium containing 5% lipoprotein-deficient serum (LPDS). Monolayers were then washed and incubated (3 hours, 37°C) in a CO_2 incubator with various concentrations of ^{125}I-LDL in 1 ml of the standard growth medium containing 5% lipoprotein-deficient serum (A). For the time-course experiment (B) cells were similarly incubated with ^{125}I-LDL (10 μg/ml) for the indicated time periods. After the appropriate interval the medium was removed and treated with trichloroacetic acid to a final concentration of 12.5% (v/v). The acid-soluble fraction was treated with hydrogen peroxide and then extracted with chloroform to remove free iodine. An aliquot of the aqueous phase was counted to determine the amount of ^{125}I-labeled, acid-soluble material formed by the cells and released to the medium (▲). A blank value was determined by incubation of the ^{125}I-LDL at 37°C in growth medium containing no cells. To determine the amount of ^{125}I-LDL bound to the cell surface (○) and the amount that had entered the cells (●) each cell mono-layer was chilled rapidly to 4°C to stop the uptake process. The monolayers were then washed 12 times at 4°C with phosphate-buffered saline containing 0.2% bovine serum albumin. One ml of solution con-taining 50 mM NaCl, 10 mM HEPES and 10 mg/ml sodium heparin were then added to each dish, the dishes were incubated at 4°C for 1 hour to release the ^{125}I-LDL that had been bound to the cell surface, and the heparin-containing medium was removed and counted in a well-type gamma counter. After the incubation with heparin each monolayer was washed 6 times, dissolved in 0.1 N NaOH, and counted to determine the total amount of ^{125}I-LDL that had entered the cells and was therefore resistant to heparin release. Each value represents the average of duplicate incubations, and the data are expressed as specific ^{125}I-LDL binding and specific receptor-mediated accumulations and degradations of ^{125}I-LDL. The non-specific value at each concentration of ^{125}I-LDL was determined by incubating the monolayer with ^{125}I-LDL in the presence of 400 μg/ml of unlabeled LDL. These values were subtracted from the observed total ^{125}I-LDL values and ranged from 3 to 25% at non-saturating and saturating concentrations of ^{125}I-LDL, respectively. Similar results were obtained with adult bovine aortic endothelial cells (ABAE).

and the amount bound reached a plateau as time proceeded (Fig. 10B). We have also shown that subsequent to this binding the bound material was, as for fibroblasts and smooth muscle cells (70), internalized and degraded to a product that could no longer be precipitated with TCA (Fig. 10).

The sequence of events that underlies the uptake of LDL at 37°C was followed by using the amount of heparin releasable ^{125}I-LDL as a measure of the amount of LDL bound at the cell surface.

LDL is first bound to its cell surface receptor. The bound LDL is then internalized (and thus becomes resistant to heparin) and replaced at the receptor site by a new particle of LDL from the medium. As the amount of LDL within the cells increases with time, the lipoprotein begins to be degraded and the hydrolyzed amino acids appear in the culture medium (Fig. 10B). When the rate of LDL degradation equals its rate of cellular uptake (3–4 hours), a final steady state is reached in which the total cellular content of LDL is constant. The degradation of ^{125}I-LDL was competitively inhibited by native LDL and reached a maximal rate at the same LDL concentration as that required to saturate the high-affinity receptor binding site (Fig. 10A). It seems, therefore, that the high-affinity uptake and degradation of LDL by endothelial cells is, as in other cell systems, dependent upon the prior binding of LDL to its specific cell surface receptor site (70).

Since the vascular endothelium is exposed to large amounts of plasma lipoproteins, a control mechanism must exist to limit the uptake of LDL and to protect against the accumulation of cholesterol esters in both endothelial and smooth muscle cells of the arterial wall. It is therefore possible that the massive accumulation of cholesterol esters within aortic smooth muscle cells in natural or experimentally induced atherosclerosis is due to lesions, already at the endothelial level, in the controlled uptake of LDL.

One of the main characteristics of vascular endothelial cells in vivo is their appearance as a single layer of highly flattened and contact-inhibited cells. It is only by establishing conditions for the long-term maintenance of endothelial cells characterized by their unique morphology and growth properties at confluency that one can avoid misleading conclusions regarding the real capabilities of these cells. Using cells that fulfill this requirement, we have now found that the early stage of the formation of a contact-inhibited cell monolayer was already associated, 24–48 hours after reaching confluency, with a 75–85 % decrease in the capacity of the cells to internalize and degrade LDL particles (Fig. 11). This inhibition was even more dramatic (90–95 %) in cells that were tested 1–2 weeks after reaching confluency (Fig. 11, Table 2). The same cells, following disruption of the confluent monolayer by EDTA dissociation and reseeding the single cell's suspension at a split ratio of 1 to 5, showed within 24 hours a 10- to 20-fold higher LDL uptake and degradation activity (Table 2). Similarly, removal of about 10 % of the cells along an artificial wound in a confluent monolayer gave a 2- to 2.5-fold increase in the uptake and degradation of LDL 24 hours later, although the rest of the cells remained highly contact-inhibited and cell proliferation did not occur. (Calf and adult bovine endothelial cells did not proliferate despite the addition of FGF in 5 % lipoprotein deficient serum even at low cell density.) The formation of cell–cell contacts, rather than the inhibition of cell proliferation, seems, therefore, more likely to induce the inhibition of LDL uptake at confluency (Fig. 11). This may explain why the vascular endothelium, which form a perfect monolayer, does not accumulate cholesterol esters, although it is exposed to high concentrations of LDL, which is the main cholesterol-carrying lipoprotein in blood. Our results may further imply an in vivo situation in which damage to the endothelial layer might stimulate the uptake of LDL and initiate the process of atherosclerosis. When a wound is made in the endothelium, the cells at the periphery of the wound start migrating and proliferating into the wound. Those cells are then released from the restriction imposed by contact inhibition and are again capable of LDL uptake and thus accumulate cholesterol. Cells far away from the wound, on the other hand, remain contact inhibited and do not gain the capacity to internalize LDL. Thus, after each wounding

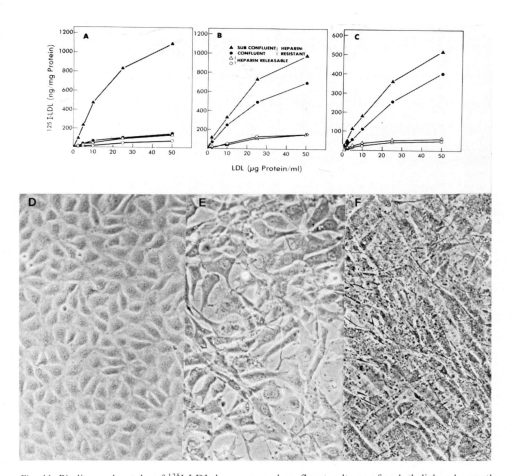

Fig. 11. Binding and uptake of ^{125}I-LDL by sparse and confluent cultures of endothelial and smooth muscle cells (A, B, C). A. Adult bovine aortic endothelial cells. B. Adult bovine aortic endothelial cells that have lost contact inhibition. (This clone was derived from cells that were seeded and maintained in the absence of FGF for 4 passages.) C. Adult bovine aortic smooth muscle cells. D, E and F represent the morphology at confluency of cultures A, B and C respectively at the time of experiment. Endothelial and smooth muscle cells were plated at an initial density of 20,000 cells per 35-mm dish and tested before (△, ▲) and 4–6 days after (○, ●) reaching confluency. Similar results were obtained with cells that were seeded at low and high densities to obtain confluent and sparse cultures on the day of the experiment. To obtain a highly confluent and contact-inhibited monolayer of endothelial cells, cells were seeded at low density (20,000 cells per 35-mm dish), and FGF was added every other day until the cells were nearly confluent (5–7 days). The cultures were then maintained for an additional 8–10 days, at which time they assumed the distinct appearance of flattened, closely apposed, contact inhibited cells (D). These cells gave the regular 90% plating efficiency in subculturing. 32 to 48 hours before the experiment the growth medium was removed and replaced with fresh medium containing 5% LPDS. Monolayers were then washed with various concentrations of ^{125}I-LDL in 1 ml of medium containing 5% LPDS, and incubated. The cell monolayers were then washed and the amounts of heparin releasable ^{125}I-LDL (△, ○), which reflect the amount of bound LDL, and heparin resistant ^{125}I-LDL, which reflect the amount of internalized LDL (▲, ■), were determined.

TABLE 2

Effect of cell density on [125]*I-LDL binding, internalization, and degradation by endothelial and smooth muscle cells*

Cell type	Parameter measured	Cell density	
		High	Low
Calf bovine aortic endothelial cells	protein	216.6	57.1
	^{125}I-LDL internalization	28.8	355.4
EDTA dissociated cells from the			
above confluent monolayer, seeded	protein	216.6	30.3
at low density, and tested 24 hours later	^{125}I-LDL internalization	28.8	606.5
Adult bovine aortic endothelial cells	protein	321.3	64.2
	^{125}I-LDL binding	15.1	41.5
	^{125}I-LDL internalization	21.2	341.8
	^{125}I-LDL degradation	15.7	299.8
	% inhibition by a 24 hour pre-		
	incubation with native LDL		
	(50 μg/ml)	23.6	88.5
Adult bovine aortic endothelial	protein	148.7	90.1
cells – a clone that lost contact	^{125}I-LDL binding	49.0	52.6
inhibition of growth	^{125}I-LDL internalization	252.6	310.0
Bovine aortic smooth muscle cells	protein	406.8	119.0
	^{125}I-LDL binding	43.2	65.9
	^{125}I-LDL internalization	268.3	334.9
	^{125}I-LDL degradation	193.0	188.5
	% inhibition by a 24 hour pre-		
	incubation with LDL (50 μg/ml)	70.0	72.0

Cells were cultured and incubated (2.5 hours, 37°C) with ^{125}I-LDL (10 μg/ml) as described in the legend to Figure 11. The amounts of trichloroacetic soluble material, heparin-releasable material, and heparin resistant ^{125}I-LDL were determined as described in the legend to Figure 10. Data for cell protein are expressed in μg per dish and for the metabolism of ^{125}I-LDL in ng per mg cell protein.

of the endothelium, the wound area will fill up with vascular endothelial cells laden with cholesterol. The accumulated lipids could in turn cause transformation of the cells and, if they are no longer contact inhibited, they could proliferate in a multiple layer and thus produce the initial atherosclerotic plaque. That this could, indeed, be the case was demonstrated by the following experiment. When a monolayer of vascular endothelial cells was wounded and then exposed to a high concentration of LDL, an accumulation of lipids was only observed in the cells migrating into the wound, *but not* in the cells which remain highly contact inhibited (i.e. the cells located far away from the wound) (Fig. 12). In confluent smooth muscle cultures which were wounded and then exposed to high concentrations of LDL, on the other hand, an accumulation of lipids was observed both in the cells migrating into the wound and in cells located *far away* from the wound area (Fig. 13).

We have shown that, as in other cell types, the high-affinity uptake of LDL was 4–7 times lower in sparse cultures of endothelial cells that were cultured in the

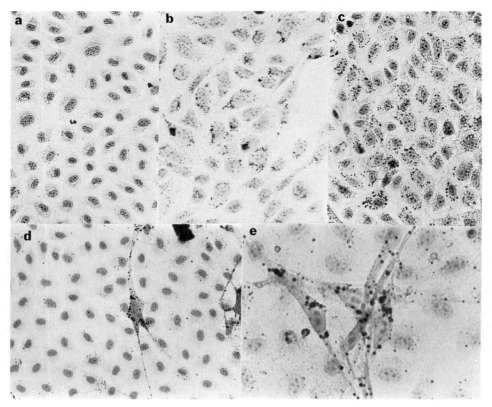

Fig. 12. Confluent monolayer of vascular endothelial cells exposed to high concentration of LDL. Confluent monolayer of bovine vascular endothelial cells were wounded and then exposed for 5 days to high concentrations of LDL (300 μg/ml added every day). The plates were then fixed and stained with oil red O. 'A' shows an area which is far away from the wound. The cells are contact inhibited and do not show any lipids (lack of black dots). 'B' shows the wound area with vascular endothelial cells migrating into the wound and heavily labeled with lipids (black dots). 'C' shows the reestablishment of the monolayer in the wound and cells which now contain lipids (black dots). 'D' shows an endothelial cell which has been transformed and has grown on top of the monolayer. This cell now contains lipids, in contrast with the monolayer, which contains none. 'E' shows cells proliferating on top of the monolayer and heavily labeled with lipids (black dots).

presence of LDL. This lower uptake is due to a diminished synthesis of the LDL receptor itself and is therefore effective relatively late after the exposure of the cells to LDL. This receptor regulation was little or not effective in a contact-inhibited endothelial monolayer as reflected by a lower degree of so-called 'down-regulation' of the LDL receptor sites in confluent, as opposed to sparse, endothelial cell cultures. This might be due to a slower turnover of the endothelial plasma membrane in confluent cultures caused by an increased rigidity of the plasma membrane. In contrast, a similar degree of inhibition was induced by preincubation with LDL of confluent and non-confluent cultures of smooth muscle cells (Table 2).

The results summarized in Table 2 indicate that the binding of LDL (measured at 4°C or as heparin releasable material in cells incubated with LDL at 37°C) was less

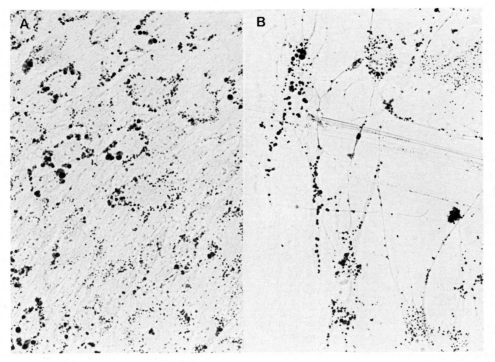

Fig. 13. Confluent cultures of smooth muscle cells exposed to high concentration of LDL. Confluent bovine vascular smooth muscle cultures were wounded and then exposed for 5 days to high concentrations (300 μg/ml) of LDL. The plates were then fixed and stained with oil red O. 'A' shows an area which has not been wounded. The smooth muscle cells are heavily labeled with red particles (black dots) which reflect the accumulated lipids. 'B' shows the wound area with heavily labeled (black dots) smooth muscle cells migrating into the wound.

affected by the formation of cell–cell contacts than the LDL internalization process. In fact, the 2- to 3-fold decrease in LDL binding in confluent monolayers could have resulted from the decrease in surface area available for LDL binding. The higher inhibition of the LDL uptake process at confluency might be due to a change in the cell surface membrane which slowed down the endocytosis of each receptor-bound LDL particle on the surface. Such a change might be induced by the massive production of LETS protein which accumulates at confluency and functions to enforce cell adhesion. Other kinds of experiments on the lateral mobility of cell surface receptors suggest that the surface membrane becomes more rigid in contact-inhibited cells. This rigidity might limit the rate of the LDL receptor-mediated endocytosis and could be caused by the accumulation of LETS protein.

MEMBRANE CHANGES INDUCED BY FGF IN VASCULAR ENDOTHELIAL CELLS

Changes in growth properties and the induction of cell proliferation by various mitogens and enzymes are often associated with structural and functional changes in the cell surface. Since glycoproteins and glycolipids are intimately involved in cell recognition, interaction, and growth control, lectins that bind specifically to these surface components can be used as probes to study the relationship between membrane changes and growth alterations.

The interaction between various lectins and glycoproteins that are capable of lateral diffusion in the plane of the membrane can lead to a selective redistribution of the lectin–receptor complexes in a process which results in so-called 'patch formation' (passive clustering of cross-linked macromolecules) and subsequent 'cap formation' (segregation of the cross-linked patches to one pole of the cell by an active, microfilament-dependent process). The capped complexes may undergo pinocytosis leading to extensive loss of the appropriate membrane receptors, a phenomenon referred to as 'antigenic modulation'. The long-range receptor movement involved in patching and capping can be directly observed by using fluorescein-labeled lectins. Short-range lateral movements like those involved in the lectin-

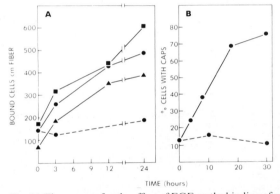

TIME (hours)

Fig. 14. Time course for the effect of FGF on the binding of vascular endothelial cells to nylon fibers coated with con-A and for its effect on the formation of caps by con-A. The cells for these experiments were seeded at high density (10^6 cells/100-mm Petri dish), and FGF (25 ng/ml)(——) or EGF (50 ng/ml)(– – –) was added 36–48 hours later. Cells were dissociated at the appropriate time with 0.03% EDTA solution to prepare a single cell suspension, spun, and washed with PBS before use in the experiments. A. Binding of cells to fibers coated with con-A molecules. Nylon fibers were strung in polyethylene frames, washed successively with petroleum ether and carbon tetrachloride, dried, incubated (30 minutes, 21°C) with con-A solution (500 μg/ml) in PBS, and washed 3 times in PBS. This procedure resulted in strong adsorption to the fiber surface of about 20 ng con-A/cm fiber. In order to obtain fiber coated with lower densities of con-A molecules (2.5 (▲), 5 (●), and 10 (■) ng con-A/cm fiber), the con-A solution was diluted in PBS containing 500 μg BSA/ml to keep the concentration of protein constant (500 μg/ml). There was no binding of cells to fibers coated only with BSA. To measure the binding to fibers, a 4-ml cell suspension in PBS (4×10^5 cells/ml) was incubated with the fibers (30 minutes, 21°C) with gentle shaking. Cells attached along both edges of a 1-cm fiber segment were counted at $100 \times$ magnification. The standard deviation of 3–5 independent cell–fiber binding experiments was $\pm 10\%$ over a range of 400–700 cells/cm. Below 100 cells/cm the standard deviation increased up to $\pm 25\%$. B. Cap formation by con-A. To assay the formation of con-A-induced caps, cells were incubated for 15 minutes at 37°C with 100 μg/ml fluorescein conjugated con-A (F-con-A). Cells were washed with PBS, pipetted to dissociate aggregates, and the percentage of cells with a cap was determined with a Zeiss fluorescence microscope with transmitted ultraviolet light. Similar results were obtained with 10 μg con-A/ml. 200 cells were counted for each point and only single cells were scored. When the percentage of cap-forming cells was below 20%, the reproducibility of the results was ± 20–30%. With higher percentages of cap-forming cells the reproducibility ranged from 10–15%.

mediated receptor clustering and cell agglutination can be indirectly quantified by measuring the ability of cells to bind to nylon fibers coated with different densities of lectin molecules. This binding requires a short-range lateral mobility of the appropriate receptors to allow their alignment with the lectin molecules on the fiber. By using these techniques (fluorescence microscopy and binding of cells to fibers) with bovine endothelial cells and the lectin concanavalin A (con-A), we have demonstrated that both the short- and long-range types of receptor mobility were increased in response to preincubation with FGF (Fig. 14). These changes were not obtained by preincubation with EGF, which does not bind and has no mitogenic effect on the bovine endothelial cells.

A 6–9 hour preincubation with FGF gave a nearly maximal increase (2- to 4-fold) in the binding of cells to con-A molecules on the fibers, and a significant effect was obtained already at 3 hours (Fig. 14). A longer preincubation period (12–24 hours) with FGF was required to induce, in a large proportion (60–80%) of the cells, the ability to form caps upon addition of con-A (Figs. 14 and 15). Redistribution and/or clustering of surface receptors are facilitated by a higher degree of receptor mobility and have been suggested as possible early events in mitogenesis. Our present findings suggest that changes in the cell surface membrane are associated with the mitogenic activity of FGF, but it is not yet clear whether the induced alterations are actually required for and involved in the stimulation of cell division.

There are obvious advantages in obtaining a higher degree of membrane fluidity. It may facilitate the interaction of hormones and mitogens with their appropriate

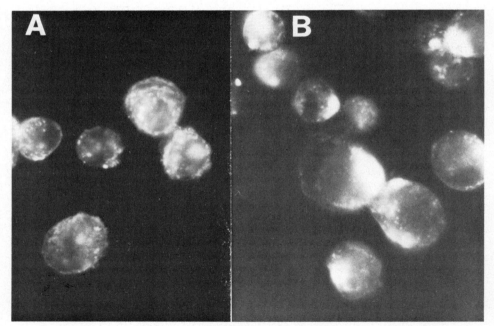

Fig. 15. Fluorescence micrographs of F-con-A binding to FBHE cells with or without preincubation with FGF. A. Cells that were not incubated with FGF. 15% cap-forming cells. B. 18-hour preincubation with FGF (25 ng/ml). A high frequency (about 80%) of cells with con-A-induced caps. Cells were incubated with F-con-A (100 μg/ml) and washed as described in the legend to Figure 14.

surface receptors and enable membrane enzymes and their substrates to come together and interact. A fluid membrane provides a simple means of distributing proteins and lipids to regions of the membrane remote from their point of insertion and for dividing membrane components evenly between daughter cells at the time of cell division. In this regard, it is of interest that the time of preincubation with FGF required to induce a maximal effect on receptor capping is the same as that required for FGF to induce a stimulated synthesis of DNA and, ultimately, cell proliferation.

Endothelial cells are characterized by the ability to form a monolayer of highly flattened and contact-inhibited cells. In this stage neither cell division nor the ability to form caps is induced by FGF. This inability might be due to the massive accumulation of LETS protein which occurs in contact-inhibited monolayers and might have a rigidifying effect on the cell surface membrane. The lateral mobility of surface components is affected by changes in the membrane lipid fluidity and the trans-membrane interaction with cytoskeletal elements. Whether changes in these properties can be induced by FGF requires a further investigation.

VASCULAR ENDOTHELIAL CELLS AND THE PRODUCTION OF MITOGENS BY TUMOR CELLS

Tumors induce vascularization into the neoplasm to provide needed cell nutrients and remove wastes. Vascularization appears to depend, in part, on the proliferation of vascular endothelial cells, which, in turn, are controlled by the secretion of tumor angiogenesis factor (TAF) (71–74). Extracts of tumors (72–75) and certain established cell lines have been shown to possess TAF activity in in vivo assays; however, little is known about the molecular nature and mechanism of action of TAF.

A convenient method to study angiogenesis and endothelial repair would be with an in vitro endothelial cell system, but the lack of uniform, reliable, cultured endothelial cell lines has delayed progress in this area. Most studies (76–78), with some exceptions (79), have utilized uncloned vascular cells, which are often slow growing and heterogenous in cell type. Using a cloned adult bovine endothelial (ABAE) cell line which has maintained its endothelial properties for over 1 year in culture, provided that FGF is present in the growth medium, we have looked at the mitogenic effects of several untransformed and transformed cell lines on cloned ABAE cells and non-vascular endothelial cell controls (80).

Endothelial cell proliferation was monitored by seeding ABAE cells or control non-vascular adult bovine corneal endothelial cells onto γ-irradiated feeder layers of test cell cultures and measuring proliferation of the unirradiated endothelial cells in the absence of FGF. When vascular ABAE cells were seeded onto γ-irradiated feeder layers of MSV-transformed Balb/c 3T3 (MSV3T3) or Balb/c 3T3 (clone A 31) cells, by day 12 ABAE cells grew almost 100 times more than ABAE cells grown in Dulbecco's modified minimal essential medium (DMEM) with 10% calf serum (Fig. 16A). MSV3T3 cells were almost as effective as FGF (100 ng/ml) and more effective than Balb/c 3T3 cells in promoting growth of aortic endothelial cells, while NIH Swiss 3T3 and aortic endothelial feeder cells had little effect (Fig. 16A). When corneal endothelial cells were substituted for vascular endothelial cells, none of the

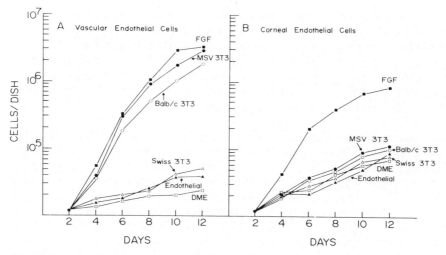

Fig. 16. Growth of adult bovine endothelial cells on γ-irradiated cells. A. Aortic endothelial cells.
B. Corneal endothelial cells. The in vitro assay of endothelial cell proliferation using γ-irradiated cells was
conducted as described in (80). 10,000 test cells were seeded, and, after the cells had attached (4–12 hours),
the dishes were γ-irradiated with a total of 6,000 roentgens from a cobalt-60 irradiator to block cell division.
The medium was then removed and 5,000 endothelial cells were seeded in DME with 10% calf serum
on top of the test cell feeder layer. The following controls were employed: dishes of irradiated test cells
alone, endothelial cells grown on γ-irradiated endothelial cells, and endothelial cells grown alone in the
presence and absence of FGF (100 ng/ml); FGF was added every other day.

cell lines tested induced corneal endothelial cell proliferation, although those cells
respond effectively to FGF (Fig. 16B). Several other γ-irradiated untransformed cell
lines, such as smooth muscle, granulosa, corneal, and lens epithelial cells were tested
for their ability to promote the growth of ABAE cells. Although some of these
cell lines caused a slight increase in ABAE cell growth, none of the lines was significantly mitogenic for ABAE cells. Thus far, every transformed cell line tested has
stimulated vascular but not corneal endothelial cell proliferation.

Conditioned medium from 3T3 and MSV3T3 cells also stimulated growth of
vascular endothelial cells. Endothelial cells grown in 3T3- and MSV3T3-conditioned
media reached a final cell density 20 and 30 times greater, respectively, than cells
grown in DMEM with 10% calf serum. Although this effect was less than the effect
of γ-irradiated Balb/c or MSV3T3 cells on vascular endothelial cell proliferation, it
indicates that the former cell lines release an endothelial cell growth-promoting
factor(s) into the medium.

Our finding that untransformed Balb/c 3T3 (A-31) but not untransformed NIH
Swiss 3T3 cells will significantly stimulate vascular endothelial cell growth (80) may
be related to other observations concerning Balb/c 3T3 cells. When Balb/c 3T3
(A-31) cells adherent to glass or plastic are implanted subcutaneously into Balb/c
mice, hemangioendotheliomas or vasoformative sarcomas are formed, and Boone
has suggested, on the basis of these experiments, that Balb/c 3T3 (A-31) cells may be
preneoplastic (81). These results, together with morphological studies on Balb/c
3T3 cells (82) show that these cells are probably of endothelial, rather than fibroblastic, origin. Balb/c 3T3 cells also possess a nerve growth factor (83) and TAF

activities (75), but it is unclear if the presence of these factors is related to a pre-neoplastic state.

The nature of the factor(s) released by Balb/c 3T3 and MSV3T3 cells in our experiments is not known. It appears to be different from FGF, since FGF, but not Balb/c 3T3 or MSV3T3 cells, stimulated corneal endothelial cells to proliferate (Fig. 16B). As mentioned earlier, Klagsburn et al. (75) have shown that extracts of Balb/c 3T3 cells induce vascularization when placed on the chorioallantoic membrane of the chicken embryo, whereas Balb/c primary mouse embryo fibroblasts have no effect. We have likewise found that Balb/c 3T3 cells, but not Balb/c primary mouse embryo fibroblasts, will stimulate the proliferation of vascular endothelial cells in vitro. Further study will be necessary to ascertain if the same factor responsible for the reported in vivo TAF activity of Balb/c 3T3 cells is responsible for the proliferation of vascular endothelial cells in vitro.

PROLIFERATION OF VASCULAR ENDOTHELIAL CELLS IN VIVO

Cellular proliferation in a tridimensional structure is controlled by the accessibility of nutrients and oxygen to the cells (71, 84). Since nutritional elements as well as oxygen are present in the blood, the capillary density in a given organ (and hence, the amount of nutrients available) is one way of regulating the growth and size of the organ. An increase in the capillary density of a tissue results in increased access to both nutrients and oxygen by the cells and could allow accelerated growth. Since capillaries form as a result of vascular endothelial cell proliferation, mitogenic factors for these cells could indirectly regulate the overall growth of a given tissue.

FGF was found to be such a potent mitogen for endothelial cells in vitro that we tested its ability to induce the proliferation of endothelial cells in vivo. Such growth is most easily observed when capillaries proliferate to vascularize a normally avascular

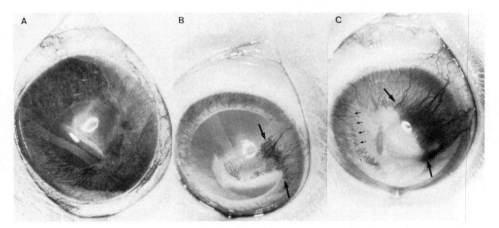

Fig. 17. Proliferation of capillaries induced by FGF or EGF in the rabbit cornea. Angiogenesis induced by a slow release form polymers (acrylamide) containing either 10 μg EGF (B) or 10 μg FGF (C). Strong vascularization (arrows) of the corneas observed by day 12. In the absence of mitogens (A) the acrylamide pellet did not induce vascularization.

space. Using the technique described by Gimbrone et al (84), we found that FGF was capable of inducing neovascularization of the rabbit cornea (Fig. 17). This property was also shared by EGF, which was an even more potent angiogenesis factor than FGF. Since human vascular endothelial cells have been shown to be sensitive to both FGF and EGF, it could be that rabbit vascular endothelial cells have a similar sensitivity, unlike bovine vascular endothelial cells, which are only sensitive to FGF and not to EGF. Moreover, the ability of EGF to stimulate capillary proliferation in rabbit cornea can be related to the observation made by Knighton and Folkman that crude extracts of mouse salivary gland (the main site of synthesis of EGF) stimulated the in vivo proliferation of capillaries (85).

The control of capillary proliferation by rapidly growing tissue such as tumoral tissue has been postulated by others (86), and it is of interest to consider whether the same controls might apply for some normal tissues. It is apparent that the correlation between capillary proliferation and cell proliferation is most applicable to cells maintained in an avascular area where growth is limited by the availability of nutrients and is controlled by the ratio of surface area to volume.

One such example can be found in the ovaries. The ovarian cycle is a 2-part process. The initial phase consists of the growth and maturation of follicles composed of a central cavity surrounded by multiple layers of granulosa cells and 2 external cell layers, the richly vascularized thecae interna and externa (Fig. 18). The second part of the ovarian cycle is the formation, after ovulation, of the corpus luteum.

Following ovulation the basement membrane breaks down, allowing blood vessels

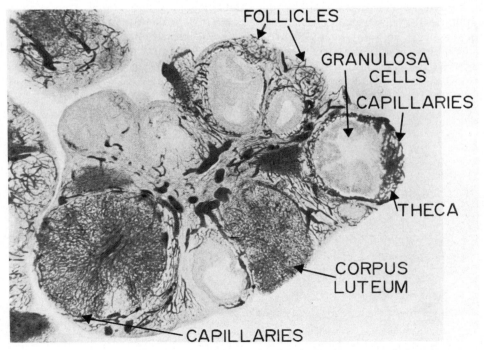

Fig. 18. A thick section of rat ovary in which the blood vessels were perfused with carmine gelatin. Notice the rich vasculature of the corpora lutea, while the granulosa cell layers within the follicles are avascular.

to invade the stratum granulosum. During this period of corpus luteum formation the layers of granulosa cells become vascularized and relieve the nutrient limitation on cell proliferation. Granulosa cells and capillaries proliferate and rapidly fill in the empty space of the follicle (Fig. 18). This rapid invasion of the stratum granulosum by connective tissue elements and sprouts of capillary endothelium, which later form a complex network of capillaries throughout the gland (Fig. 18), is the crucial event in the formation of the corpus luteum, since, besides relieving the nutrient limitation on the luteal cells, it also allows an increased rate of diffusion of steroids from the cells into the bloodstream. In follicles that do not ovulate the basement membrane does not break down, and the follicles consequently undergo atresia characterized by the disaggregation of the granulosa cell layer. Thus, factors, whether physical or biological, which control the proliferation of vascular endothelial cells leading to capillary formation in the corpus luteum are critical for the development of this tissue.

One might wonder what the new situation is that causes the luteal cells to synthesize and release an angiogenic factor. As pointed out by Bassett (87), who made the only known study of the changes of the vascular pattern of the rat ovary during the estrous cycle, one of the main factors dictating the degree of vascularization of the various components of the ovaries is their metabolic requirement. This requirement is not peculiar to the ovaries, however, since capillary proliferation within a tissue seems, in most cases, to be correlative with an increased demand for oxygen by that tissue. There is, for example, direct evidence suggesting that the initial stimulus attracting blood vessels in the fetal retina is an increased demand for O_2 arising from the inner layer of the retina which, in turn, directly or indirectly stimulates capillary proliferation (88). A dramatic example of the modulation of capillary proliferation by O_2 is offered by the pathology of retrolental fibroplasia. This form of blindness is caused by the formation of fibrous tissue behind the lens and appears when premature children are kept in incubators under high O_2 tension. Under these conditions hyperoxia produces vascular spasm, and a total regression of retinal capillaries occurs. When the infant is later exposed to normal O_2 tension, however, there is a wild regrowth of the vessels, which, in some cases, leads to extensive hemorrhage and formation of fibrous scar tissue (89).

Considering the ovary in light of the retinal model, one notes that luteal cells secrete huge amounts of steroids (primarily progesterone) which are synthesized from acetate, a process requiring great amounts of energy and, therefore, of O_2. This high requirement for energy is reflected by the high mitochondrial content observed in luteal cells. Granulosa cells, in contrast, are relatively dormant metabolically, and this dormancy is reflected by their low mitochondrial content. It is, then, reasonable that capillary proliferation should accompany the granulosa–luteal conversion as a response to the increased demand for oxygen by the luteal cells. An increased demand for O_2 could consequently stimulate the production of other factors, such as angiogenic factors, which could, in turn, directly stimulate the proliferation of capillaries, as is observed with tumor or transformed cells. If this is the case, one should be able to demonstrate a lack of angiogenic agents in follicles which have a low O_2 requirement and, conversely, one should find high concentrations of angiogenic factors in early-phase corpora lutea. This possibility has been investigated by implanting corpora lutea into rabbit corneas. As shown in Figures 19

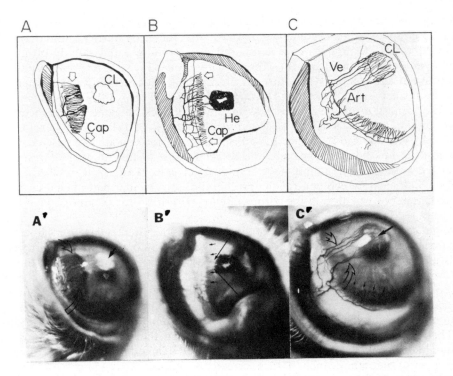

Fig. 19. Proliferation of capillaries induced by implant of rabbit corpus luteum in the rabbit cornea. A. The corpus luteum (CL) has been implanted in the center of the eye. Six days following the implantation capillaries (Cap) proliferate as a brush border from the limbus toward the implant. B. Corpus luteum implanted near the limbus. By day 3 capillaries (Cap) derived from the limbus have connected with the implant and anastomose with luteal capillaries leading to a hemorrhage (He) around the implant. C. By day 14 the capillaries have invaded the corpus luteum and reorganization of the vascularization has taken place. The capillaries connecting with the corpus luteum have differentiated into arterioles (Art) and venules (Ve) forming 3 main vascular trunks. The capillaries not connecting are regressing, thereby leaving ghost vessels. A, B, and C are graphic illustrations of replicate photographs (A', B', C').

and 20, the implanted corpus luteum induces capillary proliferation and neovascularization.

If the corpus luteum was grafted near the limbus (3 mm) within 2 days, capillary proliferation was observed. Capillaries from the host then anastomosed with surviving capillaries from the implant, as shown by the hemorrhage which surrounds the corpus luteum (Fig. 19B). That this revascularization occurred in the host vessel is evident, since they had to proliferate through 3 mm of cornea. If the corpus luteum was far away from the limbus (6 mm), the capillaries from the limbus projected as a brush border (Fig. 19A). Seven to 8 days later, when they reached the corpus luteum, they invaded the tissue, as was already observed with tumors (Fig. 19C). The capillaries present in the initial implant were dead by that time, so that no anastomosis to already preexisting vessels in the implant could take place and no hemorrhage was observed. Only capillaries making a connection with the corpus luteum survive. All others regress and leave 2 or 3 main vascular trunks going from the limbus to

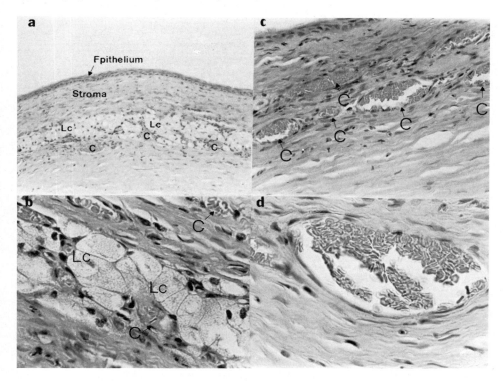

Fig. 20. Corpus luteum 15 days after implantation into the rabbit cornea. A. The luteal cells can be seen to be localized deep in the stroma. Corneal epithelium (Ep), stroma (St), luteal cells (Lc), capillaries (c) (hematoxylin eosin staining 22 ×). B. Capillaries growing deep in the stroma and invading the corpus luteum implant. Luteal cells (Lc), capillaries (c) (55 ×). C. Luteal cells (220 ×). D. Capillaries (arrows) growing deep in the stroma and full of red blood cells.

the graft (Figs. 19C, 20). These results demonstrate that adult tissue can stimulate capillary proliferation. They further demonstrate that a connection with preexisting capillaries present in the implant can take place, provided the graft is near the limbus. This is not an absolute requirement, since invasion of the capillaries from the host into the grafted tissue can also be observed when the site of implantation is far away from the limbus. Of 15 corpus luteum implants, vascularization was observed in 13 cases (90).

In contrast to the corpus luteum, ovarian follicles implanted into the rabbit cornea did not stimulate the proliferation of capillaries. Of 18 follicular implants, 18 failed to stimulate neovascularization. Furthermore, if one compares the mitotic activity of crude extract of corpus luteum to that of follicles, using Balb/c 3T3 as a target cell, the corpus luteum extracts are strongly mitogenic. Crude extracts of follicles or crude extract of the ovaries from which the corpora lutea have been removed, on the other hand, have a low activity (90) (Fig. 21). A similar observation was made when vascular endothelial, instead of 3T3, were used as a target cell.

It has thus been demonstrated that normal adult organs, in which an active phase of capillary proliferation takes place, can secrete angiogenic factors just as tumors do.

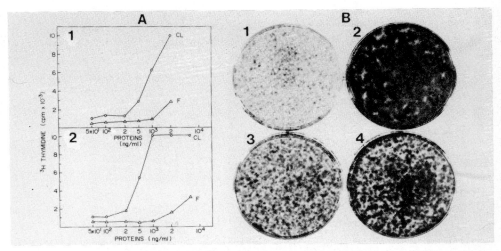

Fig. 21. Effect of crude extract of ovarian follicles and corpus luteum on the initiation of DNA synthesis in resting populations of BALB/c 3T3 cells and on the proliferation of vascular endothelial cells. A. Increasing concentrations of crude extracts of ovarian follicles (△) or corpus luteum (○) were added to resting populations of BALB/c 3T3 cells. [3H]thymidine incorporation into DNA was determined. Graphs 1 and 2 show the results of 2 different experiments. B. Effect of crude extract of corpus luteum on the proliferation of vascular endothelial cells. Bovine vascular endothelial cells (41, 44) were seeded at 20,000 cells per 6-cm dish in 5 ml of Dulbecco's modified Eagle's medium supplemented with 2.5% calf serum. Plate 1. No additive; 2. fibroblast growth factor (100 ng/ml), or corpus luteum crude extract; 3. (1 µg/ml): or 4. (10 µg/ml) was added every other day. On day 7 the plates were fixed and stained with 0.1% crystal violet. The cell number in absence of mitogenic addition was 61,000, while it was 1.2×10^6 cells for the cultures maintained in presence of 100 ng/ml of purified fibroblast growth factor and 550,000 and 860,000 cells, respectively, for cultures maintained in presence of 1 µg and 10 µg/ml of corpus luteum crude extract.

The relationship of those factors to EGF and FGF or to TAF is not yet known but should be a fruitful field of investigation.

CORNEAL ENDOTHELIAL CELLS

The corneal endothelium consists of a single layer of flattened cells on the posterior surface of the cornea and separates the corneal stroma from the aqueous humor. A viable endothelium is of primary importance if transplanted corneas are to remain transparent in the host eye (91), and the regenerative response of the endothelium is necessary for normal healing of penetrating corneal injuries (92). Numerous endothelial dystrophies have been recognized (93). Elucidation of the factors involved in the survival of corneal endothelial cells and their proliferation in response to injury is therefore of interest for several reasons. As pointed out by other workers (94–96), the metabolic properties and proliferative characteristics of these cells can be examined most easily in tissue culture.

Since FGF has been shown to be a survival and a mitogenic agent for vascular endothelial cells, which resemble corneal endothelial cells in several respects, including their in situ morphology as a monolayer and their functional importance in active transport, we have examined the possibility that, as with vascular endothelial cells, FGF could be a mitogenic agent for corneal endothelial cells, and we have compared its effect to that of EGF.

The establishment of corneal endothelial cells in tissue culture

Endothelial cells from bovine corneas can easily be established in tissue culture, and the morphology of the growing colonies closely resembles the description of endothelial cell cultures from rabbit corneas (95, 96) and human corneas (97). The pattern of colony growth and the distribution of mitotic figures were also very similar to the regenerating endothelium following mechanical denudation of Descemet's membrane in vivo (98). Colonies grow as monolayers of polygonal cells in which the apposition of one cell to another is extremely close, as is shown by silver

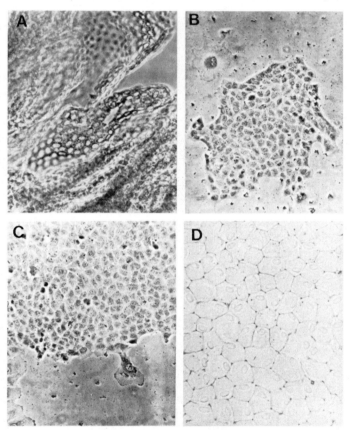

Fig. 22. Bovine corneal endothelial cells in tissue culture. A. Fragments of endothelium/Descemet's membrane immediately after explantation to tissue culture medium (phase contrast 150 ×). B. Colony of endothelial cells arising from a fragment of endothelium. A binucleated cell can be seen at the top (phase contrast 150 ×). C. Monolayer outgrowth from endothelium after 7 days in culture (phase contrast 150 ×). D. Endothelial cell monolayer after fixation and silver nitrate staining (phase contrast 300 ×).

nitrate staining of the cell junction (Fig. 22). As the colonies differentiate, the cells synthesize collagenous material which is deposited extracellularly and which can be visualized both in fixed cultures stained with alcian green and in electron micrographs of cultured cells (46). These findings suggest, therefore, that secretion of the collagenous substance is very likely to be an expression in vitro of a normal corneal endothelial cell function.

Low density, secondary cultures of corneal endothelial cells grow much more rapidly in the presence of EGF or FGF than in their absence (46) (Fig. 23). We have observed a similar effect with FGF on human corneal endothelial cells (unpublished data).

The observation that FGF and EGF are potent mitogens for corneal endothelial cells has found a practical application in the development of cloned cell lines from the corneal endothelium. This was not possible previously because the cells will not survive and divide at low density (less than 100 cells per cm^2). The finding that

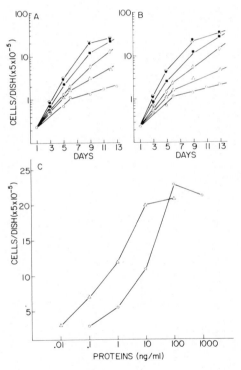

Fig. 23. Effects of FGF and EGF on growth of corneal endothelial cells. Cells were distributed at 5,000 cells/6-cm dish with media changed twice a week. EGF or FGF was added every other day. A. Cells maintained in DME containing 5% bovine plasma alone (○-○) or 5%·plasma plus EGF at 0.01 ng/ml (△-△), 0.1 ng/ml (◇-◇), 1 ng/ml (■-■), 10 ng/ml (●-●), or 100 ng/ml (□-□). B. Cells maintained in DME containing 5% bovine plasma alone (○-○) or 5% plasma plus FGF at 0.1 ng/ml (△-△), 1 ng/ml (◇-◇), 10 ng/ml (■-■), 100 ng/ml (●-●), or 1 µg/ml (△-△). C. Final cell numbers from growth curves shown in 'A' and 'B' at day 9 are given as a function of increasing amounts of EGF (△-△) and FGF (○-○). Cell number in cultures maintained in the absence of EGF or FGF was 65,000. Each point is the mean of triplicate culture, and standard error did not exceed 8% of the mean.

addition of FGF to the medium allowed the cells to divide at a density (about 0.6 cells/cm^2) which permitted cloning (46) has proved to be critical for the isolation of clonal cell strains of corneal endothelium used to study the control of differentiation and proliferation. Clonal cell strains of corneal endothelial cells have been maintained for the past 6 months in our laboratory and have been passaged every week with a split ratio of 1 to 30. The late-passage cultures have consistently shown the same sensitivity to FGF or EGF as secondary passages of endothelial cells and also exhibited the same characteristic differentiation at high density.

LETS protein and the corneal endothelium

One of the morphological characteristics of the corneal endothelium is that it develops as a monolayer. A second characteristic is its ability to secrete enormous amounts of extracellular material which will later form the Descemet membrane.

The LETS protein, as has been pointed out earlier, has been found to be related to cell adhesion and covers the basement membrane. Since the corneal endothelial cells grow as a single layer of flattened cells and produce the Descemet membrane, it makes sense that, if they are to stay attached to that membrane and to maintain a flattened morphology, these cells should secrete the LETS protein. This is, indeed, the case, since, as shown in Figure 24, when examined by immunofluorescence the corneal endothelium is shown to produce considerable amounts of LETS protein.

The production of high concentrations of LETS protein is related to the strict contact inhibition of growth observed with the corneal and vascular endothelium.

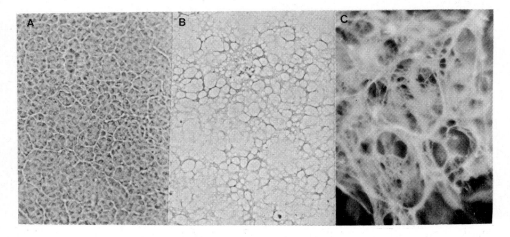

Fig. 24. Production of LETS by cultured corneal endothelial cells. A. Phase contrast micrograph of a culture of corneal endothelial cells maintained at confluence of 14 days ($\times$ 110). B. Amorphous basement membrane-like material visible after treatment of confluent monolayer with 0.5 % Triton X-100 ($\times$ 110). C. Production of LETS protein by cultured bovine corneal endothelial cells. The distribution of the LETS protein can be seen as a fine fibrillar network attached to the substratum as well as a thicker accumulation that follows the polygonal outline of the intercellular spaces.

The repair of the corneal endothelium maintained in tissue culture

It is well known that an intact endothelium of the donor tissue is essential for a successful corneal transplant. If the endothelium of the donor button is destroyed in some manner, the button remains edematous, and although healing of the wound edges may result, the graft does not clear. Experimental studies on the repair of endothelial damage indicate that the small defects in this cellular layer may be covered by a migration of neighboring cells. If the endothelial defect is too great, however, it cannot be covered by migration or replication of the endothelial cell; in this event, edema of the cornea persists.

Since FGF, as well as EGF, is mitogenic for the corneal endothelial cells, we have investigated the effects of both mitogens on large wounds of the cornea maintained in organ culture. We were greatly aided in these studies by the unique structure of the corneal endothelium. Individual endothelial cells are held together by an intercellular cement. This intercellular cement can easily be stained using Alizarin red, and the intercellular lines stand out beautifully in yellow red (clearly emphasizing the polygonal shape of the cells) (Fig. 25A). Areas where denudation takes place and the Descemet membrane is exposed appear as a bright red. Using this staining technique, one can easily evaluate the size of the wound and the degree of daily regeneration.

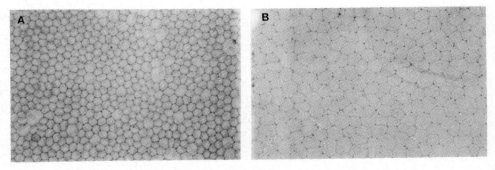

Fig. 25. Organization of corneal endothelial cells in vivo and in vitro. A. Segments of bovine cornea were removed from intact eyes and the endothelial layer stained with Alizarin red. Intercellular boundary areas stain preferentially. B. Cultures of corneal endothelial cells were grown to confluence in medium containing 10% calf serum and 100 ng/ml FGF and maintained for 14 days after reaching confluence. Intercellular boundary areas were stained in vitro with silver nitrate. The cells assume a polygonal shape both in vitro and in vivo.

As shown in Figure 26, corneas which are wounded with a spatula, so that the endothelium is removed on a width of 5 mm (Fig. 26A), do not show complete regeneration by day 4 when maintained in organ culture in the presence of DME supplemented with calf serum (Fig. 26B). By way of contrast, when maintained in organ culture in the presence of EGF (Fig. 26C) or FGF (Fig. 26D), complete healing took place, thus indicating that the cells have migrated and proliferated over the denuded area. When one compares the morphology of the endothelial cells at the edge of the wound at day 0, the endothelium can be seen to have regained its typical honeycomb structure at day 4. With the cornea maintained in absence of

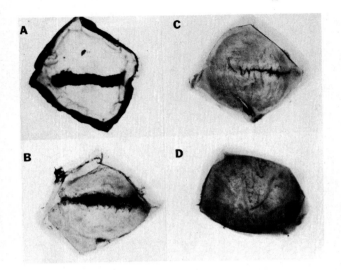

Fig. 26. The repair of the corneal endothelium in cornea maintained in organ culture. Bovine cornea were dissected out and their endothelium was removed using a blunt spatula on a length of 2 cm and a width of 5 mm. The cornea were then maintained in organ culture in the presence or absence of either 100 ng/ml EGF or 1 μg/ml FGF. The cornea were stained with Alizarin red to follow the rate of repair of the corneal endothelium. The area covered by the corneal endothelium appears white, while the wound area is stained in bright red. A. Control at day 0. B. Control at day 4. C. FGF at day 4. D. EGF at day 4. In 'C' the arrows show where the wound was initially made and the migration of the corneal endothelial cells into the wound.

EGF or FGF the cells advanced into the wound but clearly did not cover it (Fig. 27B). While the cells at the edge of the wound are enlarged, the endothelial cells which are located far away from the edges still have kept their typical honeycomb pattern (Fig. 27C). In contrast, endothelial cells of cornea maintained in the presence of EGF or FGF have migrated into the wound and present a disorganized configuration (Fig. 27D and E). In some places small areas of the Descemet membrane are still exposed. When one looks at the configuration of the endothelial cells which are located far away from the edges, they, unlike the cornea maintained in absence of mitogens, present a disorganized configuration that reflects the extent of the endothelial reorganization that occurs following the wound (Fig. 27F).

These studies demonstrate, therefore, that EGF and FGF can accelerate the healing process that occurs following the wounding of the corneal endothelium.

So, in conclusion, the vascular and corneal endothelia have provided a model system for examining the interaction of a specific cell type with the factors that control its proliferation. These interactions can be studied not only in cell culture, but equally well in organ culture or in vivo, as, for example, in the study of capillary proliferation in response to implantation of tissue or growth factors in the rabbit eye. As is the case with all mesoderm-derived cells tested to date, endothelial cells proliferate in response to treatment with fibroblast growth factor, and use of this factor has enabled the establishment of clonal endothelial cell lines from several species including pig, cow, rat, and human. Use of these cultured cells has provided

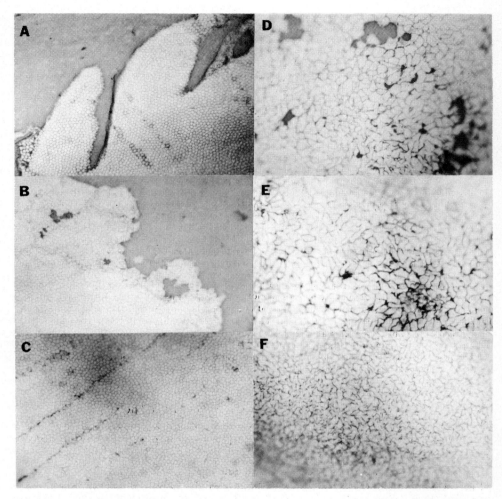

Fig. 27. Repair of bovine corneal endothelium maintained in organ culture in the presence or absence of FGF and EGF. A. Wound border stained with Alizarin red at day 0 (11.4 ×). B. Wound border stained with Alizarin red at 48 hours. The cornea were maintained in absence of mitogens (11.4 ×). C. Endothelium pattern in cornea maintained in absence of mitogens. The area photographed was far away from the site of injury. D. Wound area of cornea maintained in the presence of FGF (22.8 ×). E. Same as 'D' but maintained in the presence of EGF. F. Same as 'C' but the cornea was maintained in the presence of FGF. Similar staining pattern and cellular organization was observed with EGF.

new information regarding the function of these cells in vascular and corneal endo-thelial regeneration, nutrient transport, and the production of materials found in plasma and basement membranes, as well as information regarding their response to growth factors, inhibitors, vasoactive substances, and proteases. It is hoped that further examination of these cells could provide insights into the pathology of heart and blood vessels and that it will be of practical use in corneal preservation and transplantation.

ACKNOWLEDGMENT

We wish to thank Dr. P. Fielding for her generous gift of LDL and radiolabeled LDL.

REFERENCES

1. Balk, S. D. (1971): *Prod. nat. Acad. Sci. (Wash.)*, *68*, 271.
2. Kohler, N. and Lipton, A. (1974): *Exp. Cell Res.*, *87*, 297.
3. Ross, R., Glomset, T., Kariya, B. and Harker, L. (1974): *Proc. nat. Acad. Sci. (Wash.)*, *71*, 1207.
4. Antoniades, H. N., Sthathakos, D. and Scher, C. D. (1975): *Proc. nat. Acad. Sci. (Wash.)*, *72*, 2635.
5. Leibovich, S. J. and Ross, R. (1976): *Amer. J. Path.*, *78*, 71.
6. Fromer, C. H. and Klintworth, G. K. (1975): *Amer. J. Path.*, *79*, 437.
7. Greenburg, G. and Hunt, T. K. (1978): Submitted for publication.
8. Holley, R. W. and Kiernan, J. A. (1968): *Proc. nat. Acad. Sci. (Wash.)*, *60*, 300.
9. Corvol, M., Malemud, C. J. and Sokoloff, L. (1972): *Endocrinology*, *90*, 262.
10. Clarck, J. F., Jones, K. L., Gospodarowicz, D. and Sato, G. (1972): *Nature New Biol.*, *236*, 180.
11. Armelin, H. A. (1973): *Proc. nat. Acad. Sci. (Wash.)*, *70*, 2702.
12. Singer, M. (1974): *Ann. N.Y. Acad. Sci.*, *288*, 308.
13. Gospodarowicz, D. (1975): *J. biol. Chem.*, *250*, 2515.
14. Gospodarowicz, D., Moran, J. and Bialecki, H. (1976): In: *Growth Hormones and Related Peptides*, p. 141. Editors: A. Pecile and E. E. Müller. Excerpta Medica, Amsterdam.
15. Gospodarowicz, D. (1974): *Nature (Lond.)*, *249*, 123.
16. Savage Jr, C. R., Ingami, T. and Cohen, S. (1972): *J. biol. Chem.*, *247*, 7612.
17. Cohen, S. (1962): *J. biol. Chem.*, *237*, 1555.
18. Cohen, S. (1965): *Develop. Biol.*, *12*, 394.
19. Savage, C. R. and Cohen, S. (1973): *Exp. Eye Res.*, *15*, 361.
20. Hollenberg, M. D. and Cuatrecasas, P. (1975): *Proc. nat. Acad. Sci. (Wash.)*, *72*, 3845.
21. Cohen, S. and Carpenter, G. (1975): *Proc. nat. Acad. Sci. (Wash.)*, *72*, 1317.
22. Lembach, K. J. (1976): *Proc. nat. Acad. Sci. (Wash.)*, *73*, 183.
23. Gregory, H. (1975): *Nature (Lond.)*, *257*, 325.
24. Gospodarowicz, D. and Moran, J. S. (1974): *Proc. nat. Acad. Sci. (Wash.)*, *71*, 4584.
25. Gospodarowicz, D. and Moran, J. (1974): *Proc. nat. Acad. Sci. (Wash.)*, *71*, 4648.
26. Rudland, P. S., Seifert, W. and Gospodarowicz, D. (1974): *Proc. nat. Acad. Sci. (Wash.)*, *71*, 2600.
27. Rose, S., Pruss, R. and Herschman, H. (1975): *J. Cell Physiol.*, *86*, 593.
28. Rudland, P. S., Eckhart, W., Gospodarowicz, D. and Seifert, W. (1974): *Nature (Lond.)*, *250*, 337.
29. Gospodarowicz, D. and Moran, J. (1975): *J. Cell Biol.*, *66*, 451.
30. Westermark, B. and Wasteson, A. (1975): *Advanc. metab. Disorders*, *8*, 85.
31. Westermark, B. (1976): *Biochem. biophys. Res. Commun.*, *69*, 304.
32. Gospodarowicz, D., Moran, J. and Owashi, N. (1977): *J. clin. Endocr.*, *44*, 651.
33. Jones, K. S. and Addison, T. (1975): *Endocrinology*, *97*, 359.
34. Gospodarowicz, D. and Moran, J. S. (1977): In: *Cell Culture and its Application*, pp. 55–81. Editors: R. T. Acton and J. D. Lynn. Academic Press, New York.
35. Gospodarowicz, D. and Mescher, A. L. (1977): *J. Cell Physiol.*, *93*, 117.
36. Gospodarowicz, D., Ill, C., Mescher, A. L. and Moran, J. (1978): In: *Molecular Control of Proliferation and Differentiation, 35th Symposium for the Society for Developmental Biology*, pp. 33–61. Editors: J. Papaconstantinou and W. J. Rutter. Academic Press, New York.
37. Gospodarowicz, D., Weseman, J., Moran, J. S. and Lindstrom, J. (1976): *J. Cell Biol.*, *70*, 395.
38. Ross, R., Glomset, J. and Raisne, E. (1977): In: *International Cell Biology*, pp. 629–638. Editors: B. R. Ringley and K. R. Porter. Rockefeller University Press, New York.
39. Gospodarowicz, D., Moran, J. and Braun, D. (1976): *J. Cell Physiol.*, *91*, 377.
40. Gospodarowicz, D., Brown, K. D., Birdwell, C. R. and Zetter, B. R. (1978): *J. Cell Biol.*, in press.
41. Gospodarowicz, D., Moran, J., Braun, D. and Birdwell, C. R. (1976): *Proc. nat. Acad. Sci. (Wash.)*, *73*, 4120.
42. Gospodarowicz, D. (1976): In: *Progress in Clinical and Biological Research in Membranes and Neoplasia: New Approaches and Strategies*, pp. 1–19. Editor: V. T. Marchesi. A. R. Liss Inc., New York.

43. Zetter, B. R. and Gospodarowicz, D. (1977): In: *Chemistry and Biology of Thrombin*, p. 551. Editors: R. L. Lundblad, J. W. Fenton and K. G. Mann. Ann Arbor Press.
44. Gospodarowicz, D., Bialecki, H., Greenburg, G. and Zetter, B. (1978): *In Vitro, 14*, 85.
45. Gospodarowicz, D. and Zetter, B. (1977): In: *Develop. biol. Standard., V. 37*, pp. 109–130. Editors: F. T. Perkins and R. H. Regamey. S. Karger, Basle.
46. Gospodarowicz, D., Mescher, A. L. and Birdwell, C. R. (1977): *Exp. Eye Res., 25*, 75.
47. Gospodarowicz, D., Mescher, A. C., Brown, K. D. and Birdwell, C. R. (1977): *Exp. Eye Res., 25*, 631.
48. Frati, I., Danieli, S., Delogu, A. and Covelli, I. (1972): *Exp. Eye Res., 14*, 135.
49. Sun, T. T. and Green, H. (1977): *Nature (Lond.), 269*, 489.
50. Gospodarowicz, D. and Handley, H. H. (1975): *Endocrinology, 97*, 102.
51. Gospodarowicz, D., Ill, C. R., Hornsby, P. and Gill, G. N. (1976): *Endocrinology, 100*, 1080.
52. Gospodarowicz, D., Ill, C. R., Mescher A. L. and Moran, J. (1977): In: *Proceedings, 5th International Congress of Endocrinology, Hamburg, 1976, Vol. II*, p. 196. Editor: V. H. T. James. Excerpta Medica, Amsterdam–Oxford.
53. Gospodarowicz, D., Ill, C. R. and Birdwell, C. R. (1977): *Endocrinology, 100*, 206.
54. Gospodarowicz, D., Ill, C. R. and Birdwell, C. R. (1977): *Endocrinology, 100*, 219.
55. Gospodarowicz, D., Vlodavsky, I., Bialecki, H. and Brown, K. D. (1977): In: *5th Brook Lodge Meeting on Problems in Reproductive Biology*. Editor: J. Wilks. Plenum Press.
56. Rheinwald, J. C. and Green, H. (1977): *Nature (Lond.), 265*, 421.
57. Gospodarowicz, D., Rudland, P., Lindstrom, J. and Benirschke, K. (1975): *Advanc. metab. Disorders, 8*, 301.
58. Aursnes, I. (1974): *Microvasc. Res., 1*, 283.
59. Stemerman, M. B. and Spaet, T. H. (1972): *Bull. N.Y. Acad. Med., 48*, 289.
60. Bell, E. T. (1960): In: *Diabetes Mellitus*. Charles C Thomas, Springfield, Ill.
61. Boone, C. W., Takeichi, N., Paranjpe, M. and Gliden, R. (1976): *Cancer Res., 36*, 1626.
62. Buchanan, J. M., Chen, L. B. and Zetter, B. R. (1976): In: *Cancer Enzymology*, pp. 1–24. Editors: J. Schultz and F. Ahmed. Academic Press, New York.
63. Zetter, B. R., Sun, T. T., Chen, L. B. and Buchanan, J. M. (1977): *J. Cell Physiol., 92*, 233.
64. Zetter, B. R., Chen, L. B. and Buchanan, J. M. (1977): *Proc. nat. Acad. Sci. (Wash.), 74*, 596.
65. Gimbrone, M. A. (1976): *Progr. Hemostasis Thromb., 3*, 29.
66. Gospodarowicz, D., Mescher, A. L. and Birdwell, C. R. (1978): In: *Gene Expression and Regulation in Cultured Cells*. National Cancer Institute Monograph. In press.
67. Birdwell, C. R., Gospodarowicz, D. and Nicholson, G. (1978): *Proc. nat. Acad. Sci. (Wash.)*, in press.
68. Yamada, K. M., Yamada, S.S. and Pastan, I. (1976): *Proc. nat. Acad. Sci. (Wash.), 73*, 1217.
69. Ruoslahti, E. and Vaheri, A. (1975): *J. exp. Med., 141*, 497.
70. Goldstein, J. L. and Brown, M. S. (1977): *Ann. Rev. Biochem., 46*, 897.
71. Folkman, J. (1975): In: *Cancer: A Comprehensive Treatise, Vol. 3: Biology of Tumors: Cellular Biology and Growth*, pp. 355–388. Editor: F. F. Becker. Plenum Press, New York.
72. Folkman, J., Merler, E., Abernathy, C. and Williams, G. (1971): *J. exp. Med., 133*, 275.
73. Gimbrone, M. A., Leapman, S. B. and Cotran, R. (1973): *J. nat. Cancer Inst., 50*, 219.
74. Cavallo, T., Sade, R., Folkman, J. and Cotran, R. (1972): *J. Cell Biol., 54*, 408.
75. Klagsburn, M., Knighton, D. and Folkman, J. (1976): *J. Cancer Res., 36*, 110.
76. Haudenschild, C., Cotran, R., Gimbrone, M. and Folkman, J. (1975): *J. ultrastruct. Res., 50*, 22.
77. Suddith, R., Kelly, P., Hutchinson, H., Murray, E. and Haber, B. (1975): *Science, 190*, 682.
78. Fenselau, A. and Mello, R. (1976): *Cancer Res., 36*, 3269.
79. Buonassisi, V. and Venter, J. C. (1976): *Proc. nat. Acad. Sci. (Wash.), 73*, 1612.
80. Birdwell, C. R., Gospodarowicz, D. and Nicholson, G. (1977): *Nature (Lond.), 268*, 528.
81. Boone, C. W., Takeichi, N., Paranjpe, M. and Gliden, R. (1976): *Cancer Res., 36*, 1626.
82. Porter, K. R., Todaro, G. J. and Fonte, V. A. (1973): *J. Cell Biol., 59*, 633.
83. Oger, J., Arnason, B., Pantazis, N., Lehrich, J. and Young, M. (1974): *Proc. nat. Acad. Sci. (Wash.), 71*, 1554.
84. Gimbrone Jr, M. A., Cotran, R. S., Leapman, S. B. and Folkman, J. (1974): *J. nat. Cancer Inst., 52*, 413.
85. Folkman, J. and Cotran, R. (1976): *Int. Rev. exp. Path., 16*, 207.
86. Folkman, J. (1976): *Sci. Amer., 234*, 59.
87. Bassett, D. L. (1943): *Amer. J. Anat., 73*, 251.
88. Ashton, N., Ward, B. and Serpell, G. (1954): *Brit. J. Ophthal., 38*, 397.

89. Silverman, W. A. (1977): *Sci. Amer., 236,* 100.
90. Gospodarowicz, D. and Thakral, T. K. (1977): *Proc. nat. Acad. Sci. (Wash.), 75,* 847.
91. Stocker, F. W. (1959): *Amer. J. Ophthal., 47,* 772.
92. Inomata, H., Smelser, G. K. and Polack, F. M. (1970): *Amer. J. Ophthal., 70,* 48.
93. Grayson, M. and Keates, R. H. (1969): *Manual of Diseases of the Cornea.* Little, Brown and Co., New York.
94. Slick, W. C., Mannagh, J. and Yuhaz, A. (1965): *Arch. Ophthal., 73,* 229.
95. Perlman, M. and Baum, J. L. (1974): *Arch. Ophthal., 92,* 235.
96. Stocker, R. W., Eiring, A., Georgiade, R. et al. (1958): *Amer. J. Ophthal., 46,* 294.
97. Mannagh, J. and Irving, A. R. (1965): *Arch. Ophthal., 74,* 847.
98. Chi, H. H., Teng, C. C. and Katzin, H. N. (1960): *Amer. J. Ophthal., 49,* 693.

Disorders of cholesterol metabolism resulting from mutations involving the low density lipoprotein pathway*

MICHAEL S. BROWN, JOSEPH L. GOLDSTEIN and L. MAXIMILIAN BUJA

Departments of Internal Medicine and Pathology, University of Texas Health Science Center at Dallas, Dallas, Texas, U.S.A.

Three clinical disorders of cholesterol metabolism are currently recognized to result from mutations affecting the low density lipoprotein (LDL) pathway (Brown and Goldstein, 1976). The LDL pathway is the process by which extrahepatic human cells utilize a cell surface receptor to bind, take up, and catabolize plasma LDL and thereby acquire the cholesterol that they need for plasma membrane synthesis (Goldstein and Brown, 1976, 1977). Each of the clinical disorders to be discussed below involves a discrete step in the LDL pathway. In familial hypercholesterolemia, the primary genetic defect produces a decrease in the number of cell surface receptors for LDL or an alteration in their properties (Brown and Goldstein, 1974). In the Wolman disease, the primary defect causes a complete deficiency in the lysosomal acid lipase that is necessary to hydrolyze the cholesteryl esters of LDL, whereas in cholesteryl ester storage disease the activity of this same enzyme is partially deficient (Goldstein et al., 1975b; Brown et al., 1976).

SEQUENTIAL STEPS IN THE LDL PATHWAY

Studies in cultured fibroblasts first revealed that when human cells, such as fibroblasts, lymphocytes, or smooth muscle cells, are deprived of cholesterol, they synthesize a specific cell surface receptor that binds LDL, the major cholesterol-carrying lipoprotein of human plasma. Once LDL has bound to the LDL receptor in normal cells, the lipoprotein is internalized by adsorptive endocytosis and delivered to lysosomes where the protein and cholesteryl ester components of the lipoprotein are hydrolyzed. The resulting free cholesterol is then available to be used by the cell for membrane synthesis. When sufficient cholesterol has accumulated to satisfy this requirement, 3 regulatory events occur: (1) cholesterol synthesis is suppressed through a reduction in the activity of the rate-controlling enzyme, 3-hydroxy-3-methyl-glutaryl coenzyme A reductase (HMG CoA reductase); (2) excess lipoprotein-

*Supported by grants from the National Foundation–March of Dimes, the National Institutes of Health (HL 20948), and the American Heart Association, Texas Affiliate.

derived free cholesterol is re-esterified for storage as cholesteryl esters through an activation of an acyl-CoA:cholesterol acyltransferase; and (3) synthesis of the LDL receptor itself is diminished, thereby preventing further entry of LDL-cholesterol into the cell (Goldstein and Brown, 1976, 1977). The sequential steps in the LDL pathway are illustrated diagrammatically in Figure 1.

At each step in the delineation of the LDL pathway, interpretation of the data has been clarified by analysis of mutant cells derived from patients with genetic defects involving specific steps in the pathway. To date, 5 such mutations that affect the LDL pathway at the cellular level have been identified, 3 of these producing the syndrome of familial hypercholesterolemia, 1 producing the Wolman disease, and 1 producing cholesteryl ester storage disease (Goldstein and Brown, 1977; Goldstein et al., 1977).

FAMILIAL HYPERCHOLESTEROLEMIA (FH)

Of all the diseases producing hyperlipidemia in man, this disorder is the best defined clinically, genetically, and biochemically; it remains the most clear-cut example of a simply inherited defect that leads to coronary heart disease (Fredrickson et al., 1978). The disorder is characterized *chemically* by an elevated plasma concentration of LDL; *clinically* by xanthomas, arcus corneae, and premature coronary heart disease; *genetically* by autosomal dominant inheritance; and *biochemically* by a deficiency in the LDL receptor that regulates the degradation of LDL. Although the FH gene is expressed clinically as an autosomal dominant trait, the disorder is

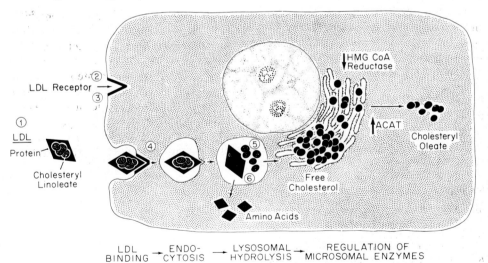

Fig. 1. Sequential steps in the LDL pathway in cultured human fibroblasts. The numbers indicate the sites at which mutations have been identified: (1) abetalipoproteinemia; (2) FH, receptor-negative; (3) FH, receptor-defective; (4) FH, internalization defect; (5) Wolman disease; and (6) cholesteryl ester storage disease. HMG CoA reductase denotes 3-hydroxy-3-methylglutaryl coenzyme A reductase, and ACAT denotes acyl-coenzyme A:cholesterol acyltransferase. (Modified from Brown and Goldstein [1976] and reproduced with permission of the publisher.)

more severe in individuals inheriting 2 doses of the gene (i.e., homozygotes) than in those inheriting 1 dose (i.e., heterozygotes).

Table 1 lists the major clinical features characteristic of patients with the heterozygous and homozygous forms of FH. About 1 in 500 persons in the general population carries 1 mutant allele at the FH locus and is thus a heterozygote for this defect, placing FH among the most common inherited diseases in man. The typical heterozygote manifests a 2.5-fold elevation in the plasma level of LDL and develops a myocardial infarction between the ages of 35 and 55. About 1 in 1 million persons in the population inherits 2 mutant alleles at the FH locus. These rare homozygotes manifest severe hypercholesterolemia with plasma LDL levels 6-fold above normal and they typically suffer myocardial infarctions before the age of 15. Although these homozygotes are relatively rare in the population, their fibroblasts were the key to understanding this disease since the homozygote cells, in contrast to the heterozygote cells, express a complete defect at the LDL receptor locus.

TABLE 1

Major clinical features characteristic of patients with the heterozygous and homozygous forms of familial hypercholesterolemia

Clinical features	Heterozygote	Homozygote
Population frequency	1 in 500	1 in 1,000,000
Plasma LDL level	↑ 2.5-fold	↑ 6-fold
Typical age for myocardial infarction	35–55 years	5–15 years

The first mutation that was shown to be present in fibroblasts from patients with homozygous FH is one that produces a complete deficiency of functional LDL receptors as determined by assays that are sufficiently sensitive to detect about 2% of the normal number (Brown and Goldstein, 1974). As a result of this receptor abnormality, these mutant cells fail to bind and take up the lipoprotein with high affinity and therefore fail to hydrolyze either its protein or cholesteryl ester components. Because they are unable to utilize LDL-cholesterol, these homozygote cells must satisfy their cholesterol requirement for growth by synthesizing large amounts of cholesterol de novo, even when high levels of LDL are present in the culture medium. Moreover, in these mutant cells LDL does not stimulate the formation of cholesteryl esters.

TABLE 2

Mutant alleles at the LDL receptor locus

R^{b^0} – – – – No binding
R^{b-} – – – – Reduced binding (1–10% of normal)
R^{b+,i^0} – – – – Normal binding, no internalization

By studying the LDL pathway in fibroblasts derived from a large number of patients with FH, we have been able to identify 2 additional mutations in the gene that specifies the LDL receptor. Table 2 lists the 3 mutant alleles at the LDL receptor locus. One of these, R^{b^0}, specifies a protein that has no binding activity as described above. The second allele, R^{b-}, specifies a protein that has reduced binding activity. The third mutant allele, R^{b+,i^o}, specifies a fascinating protein that can bind LDL normally but that cannot catalyze the internalization of the receptor-bound lipoprotein (Goldstein et al., 1975a, 1977).

Table 3 shows the distribution of these mutant alleles in fibroblast strains derived from 31 patients with the clinical diagnosis of homozygous FH. In each case the FH homozygote cells display 2 mutant alleles at the LDL receptor locus. The cells from 17 of the subjects show no binding activity and are believed to be homozygous for the R^{b^o} allele. These subjects are called receptor-negative homozygotes. The cells from 13 of the subjects show detectable but markedly reduced binding activity. Each of these subjects has one R^{b-} allele and either one R^{b^o} allele or a second R^{b-} allele. These subjects are called receptor-defective. The cells from 1 subject retain the ability to bind LDL but are unable to internalize the receptor-bound lipoprotein. Study of fibroblasts from the heterozygous parents and siblings of this subject has revealed that he is a genetic compound who carries 2 different mutant alleles at the LDL receptor locus. From his mother he has inherited the R^{b^o} allele that specifies a protein that is unable to bind LDL and is therefore biochemically silent, and from his father he has inherited the R^{b+,i^o} allele that specifies a protein that can bind LDL but not internalize it (Goldstein et al., 1977).

TABLE 3

Genetic analysis of fibroblast strains from 31 patients with the clinical diagnosis of homozygous familial hypercholesterolemia

Number of subjects	Genotype at LDL receptor locus	Biochemical phenotype
17	R^{b^o}/R^{b^o}	Receptor-negative
13	R^{b-}/R^{b^o} or R^{b-}/R^{b-}	Receptor-defective
1	$R^{b^o}/R^{b+,i^o}$	Internalization defect

We have also studied fibroblast strains from 31 FH heterozygotes. In each case, these cells exhibit 1 normal allele and 1 of the 3 mutant alleles at the LDL receptor locus. We conclude from these studies that FH, like most inborn errors of metabolism, is genetically heterogeneous in that several different mutations at a single locus can produce a similar clinical syndrome. The important point is that each of these mutations in the gene for the LDL receptor impairs the ability of cells to take up and catabolize LDL and produces severe hypercholesterolemia.

WOLMAN DISEASE

The Wolman disease is a rare inborn error of metabolism characterized by the deposition of cholesteryl esters and triglycerides in cells of the liver, spleen, adrenal glands, hematopoietic system, and small intestine. The disorder, which is transmitted as an autosomal recessive trait, becomes clinically apparent in the first few weeks of life and is invariably fatal, usually by the age of 6 months. Failure to thrive, hepatosplenomegaly, recurrent vomiting, persistent diarrhea with steatorrhea, and bilateral calcification of enlarged adrenal glands constitute the major clinical manifestations of the disorder (Sloan and Fredrickson, 1972). Since the original description of the syndrome in 1956 by Wolman and colleagues, at least 20 affected patients have been reported (Sloan and Fredrickson, 1972).

Biochemical and ultrastructural examination of excised liver tissue as well as cultured fibroblasts and freshly isolated leukocytes obtained from affected patients have shown that this disorder results from the accumulation of abnormal amounts of cholesteryl esters and triglycerides in lysosomes. The primary genetic defect appears to involve a complete absence of the activity of a lysosomal acid lipase that normally hydrolyzes cholesteryl esters and triglycerides (Patrick and Lake, 1969). In cultured human fibroblasts, this lysosomal acid lipase is responsible for hydrolyzing the cholesteryl esters of LDL that enter these cells through the LDL pathway (Fig. 1).

When fibroblasts from a patient with the Wolman disease are incubated with LDL, the lipoprotein binds to the LDL receptor and is taken up into the cell normally. Its protein component is degraded in lysosomes at a normal rate. However, because of the missing lysosomal acid lipase, the cholesteryl esters of the lipoprotein are not hydrolyzed and they accumulate within lysosomes. The reduced ability to generate free cholesterol in lysosomes leads, in turn, to a reduced ability of LDL to suppress HMG CoA reductase activity and to activate the cholesterol esterification system in the Wolman disease cells (Brown et al., 1976).

Although the heterozygous parents of affected patients have no apparent clinical abnormality, the activity of their lysosomal acid lipase, measured either in fibroblasts or in leukocytes, is decreased by 50% (Sloan and Fredrickson, 1972). Despite the decreased ability to hydrolyze cholesteryl esters, heterozygotes with the Wolman disease do not exhibit evidence of accelerated atherosclerosis. In couples who have had one affected child with the Wolman disease, the birth of a second affected child can be prevented by performing a therapeutic abortion if lysosomal acid lipase activity is absent in cultured amniotic fluid cells obtained at the 16th to 20th week of pregnancy (Patrick et al., 1976).

CHOLESTERYL ESTER STORAGE DISEASE

Like the Wolman disease, cholesteryl ester storage disease is an autosomal recessive lipid storage disorder in which the primary abnormality involves the lysosomal acid lipase enzyme (Sloan and Fredrickson, 1972). Current evidence suggests that the Wolman disease and cholesteryl ester storage disease represent allelic mutations involving the same genetic locus (Brown et al., 1976; Beaudet et al., 1977). However, in contrast to the complete absence of enzyme activity in the Wolman disease, enzyme activity is partially retained in cells of patients with cholesteryl ester storage disease (Beaudet et al., 1977).

The clinical consequences of a complete absence of lysosomal acid lipase activity (as in the Wolman disease) and the retention of 1–20% of normal acid lysosomal lipase activity (as in cholesteryl ester storage disease) are strikingly different. In contrast to patients with the Wolman disease, who invariably succumb in infancy, patients with cholesteryl ester storage disease may survive up to age 40. Of the 12 cases of cholesteryl ester storage disease that have been reported in the literature to date, the constant features have included the following: (1) delay in onset of symptoms until age 4 to 6 years; (2) lysosomal acid lipase activity varying from 1 to 20% of normal; and (3) hepatic enlargement owing to the accumulation of cholesteryl esters predominantly and triglycerides to a lesser extent (Beaudet et al., 1977). Most but not all patients also have a moderate hyperlipidemia characterized by an elevation of both plasma LDL and very low density lipoprotein (VLDL). Several of the older patients have developed portal hypertension manifest by both

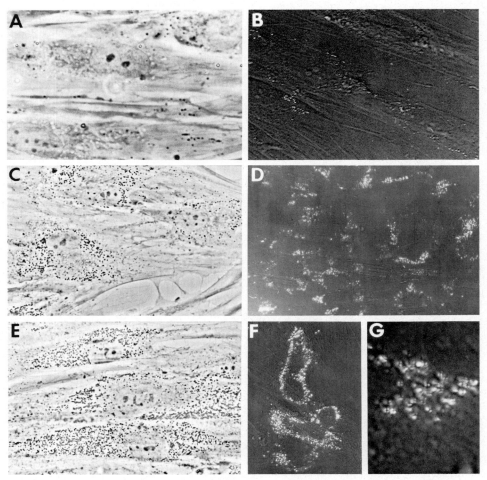

Fig. 2. Phase contrast (left column) and polarization (right column) micrographs of cultured fibroblasts from a normal subject (A,B), a patient with cholesteryl ester storage disease (C,D), and a patient with the Wolman disease (E,F,G) incubated with LDL for 24 hours. Normal fibroblasts show a few refractile inclusions (A, × 660) which exhibit weak birefringence (B, × 750). Cholesteryl ester storage disease fibroblasts contain numerous refractile inclusions (C, × 355) which have intense birefringence (D, × 355). Wolman disease fibroblasts are filled with refractile (E, × 355), birefringent (F, × 355) inclusions which frequently exhibit the formée cross pattern typical of liquid crystals of cholesteryl esters (G, × 1320). Similar formée cross patterns were observed in the cholesteryl ester storage disease fibroblasts.

splenomegaly and esophageal varices. In 2 of 3 patients in whom autopsies have been performed, severe premature atherosclerosis was evident (Sloan and Fredrickson et al., 1972; Beaudet et al., 1977).

The abnormality in the LDL pathway in cultured fibroblasts from patients with cholesteryl ester storage disease is similar to that observed in fibroblasts from patients with the Wolman disease (Goldstein et al., 1975b). If the conclusion is correct that the Wolman disease and cholesteryl ester storage disease represent allelic mutations, then genetic compounds involving these 2 abnormal alleles as well as alleles of intermediate severity are theoretical possibilities.

MORPHOLOGY OF ACCUMULATED CHOLESTERYL ESTERS IN FIBROBLASTS FROM PATIENTS WITH WOLMAN DISEASE AND CHOLESTERYL ESTER STORAGE DISEASE

The micrographs in Figure 2 depict fibroblasts from a normal subject, a patient with cholesteryl ester storage disease, and a patient with the Wolman disease. The cells were incubated with low levels of LDL for 24 hours. In each case the left panel is a phase-contrast micrograph and the right panel is a micrograph obtained with polarized light. In the normal cells a few dark-appearing inclusions are present (A) and a few of these show weak birefringence (B). In the cholesteryl ester storage disease cells the addition of LDL has led to the accumulation of moderate amounts of refractile bodies (C). When these cells are examined with polarized light, moderately large numbers of birefringent bodies are seen (D). In the cells from the patient with the Wolman disease the number of refractile bodies is markedly increased (E). When examined with polarized light these cells exhibit massive amounts of birefringent material (F). Under higher power many of these inclusions can be seen to show the typical formée crosses that represent liquid crystals of cholesteryl esters (G).

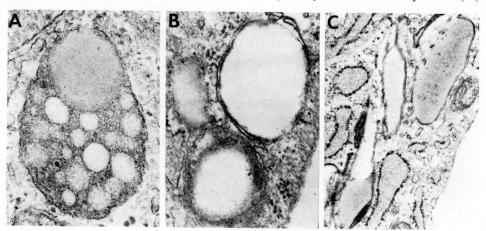

Fig. 3. Electron micrographs of typical membrane-bound, lysosomal inclusions in fibroblasts cultured from a patient with cholesteryl ester storage disease (A) and Wolman disease (B,C). The lysosomes contain discrete lipid deposits which appear as homogeneous gray or white material. A, × 56,500; B, × 37,750; C, × 20,750.

These data illustrate the pathologic consequences that occur when a cell takes up LDL normally through the LDL receptor but cannot hydrolyze the cholesteryl esters of the lipoprotein.

Figure 3 shows examples of the various forms that these lipid inclusions can exhibit by electron microscopy in the acid lipase-deficient cells. Some of these inclusions appear as multivesicular bodies (A) in which several lipid-containing vesicles are enclosed in a membrane-bound structure. Alternatively, the inclusions may contain relatively homogeneous deposits of lipid without an internal vesicular structure (B and C). Each of these types of inclusions can be seen in both the Wolman disease and cholesteryl ester storage disease cells, but not in cells from normal subjects. Histochemical stains show that each of these types of inclusions contained abundant acid phosphatase activity, confirming their identity as lysosomes. Moreover, when cells from both types of patients were grown in the absence of LDL, the number of these inclusions was reduced, as was the content of cholesteryl esters measured chemically in these cells (Brown et al., 1976). These data indicate that the accumulation of cholesteryl esters in the acid lipase-deficient cells is due to the uptake of these esters from exogenous LDL and not to their synthesis de novo within the cell.

REFERENCES

Beaudet, A., Ferry, G., Nichols Jr, B. and Rosenberg, H. (1977): *J. Pediat., 90,* 910.
Brown, M. and Goldstein, J. (1974): *Proc. nat. Acad. Sci. (Wash.), 71,* 788.
Brown, M. and Goldstein, J. (1976): *Science, 191,* 150.
Brown, M., Sobhani, M., Brunschede, G. and Goldstein, J. (1976): *J. biol. Chem., 251,* 3277.
Fredrickson, D., Goldstein, J. and Brown, M. (1978): In: *The Metabolic Basis of Inherited Disease, 4th Ed.,* Chapter 30, p. 604. Editors: J. Stanbury, J. Wyngaarden and D. Fredrickson. McGraw Hill Book Co., New York.
Goldstein, J. and Brown, M. (1976): *Curr. Top. cell. Regul., 11,* 147.
Goldstein, J. and Brown, M. (1977): *Ann. Rev. Biochem., 46,* 897.
Goldstein, J., Brown, M. and Stone, N. (1977): *Cell, 12,* 629.
Goldstein, J., Dana, S., Brunschede, G. and Brown, M. (1975a): *Proc. nat. Acad. Sci. (Wash.), 72,* 1092.
Goldstein, J., Dana, S., Faust, J., Beaudet, A. and Brown, M. (1975b): *J. biol. Chem., 250,* 8487.
Patrick, A. and Lake, B. (1969): *Nature (Lond.), 222,* 1067.
Patrick, A., Willcox, P., Stephens, R. and Kenyon, V. (1976): *J. med. Genet., 13,* 49.
Sloan, H. and Fredrickson, D. (1972): In: *The Metabolic Basis of Inherited Disease, 3rd Ed.,* Chapter 36, p. 808. Editors: J. Stanbury, J. Wyngaarden and D. Fredrickson. McGraw-Hill Book Co., New York.

Collagen: function and malfunction

S. ABE, H. K. KLEINMAN, G. R. MARTIN and B. STEINMANN

Laboratory of Developmental Biology and Anomalies, National Institute of Dental Research, National Institutes of Health, Bethesda, Md., U.S.A.

Marked changes in the connective tissues are observed in a variety of acquired and inherited diseases. Among the inherited diseases, those most likely to have altered collagen are osteogenesis imperfecta, the Ehlers-Danlos syndrome, the Marfan syndrome and certain of the chondrodystrophies (McKusick, 1972). Some of the molecular disorders with altered collagen synthesis or metabolism are listed in Table 1. Several collagens have been identified (Table 2). These proteins are chemically and genetically distinct and show different tissue distributions. Defects in each would be expected to produce unique syndromes. Each collagen type is formed by 3 chains arranged in a helix. The biosynthesis of these proteins is complex. Collagen molecules arise from biosynthetic precursors, the procollagens. Each procollagen contains 3 pro α chains. These differ from the α chains by the presence of additional peptides at both the amino and carboxyl ends of each chain. The factors determining which genes are selected for transcription are not understood. The absolute amounts of collagen produced are normally closely regulated and the rate at which collagen is synthesized varies with development, wound repair and disease. As shown in Table 1, defects at this level of biosynthesis probably occur in osteogenesis imperfecta and in certain forms of the Ehlers-Danlos syndrome (see below).

Much more information is available about the modifications the pro α chains undergo following synthesis. The formation of hydroxyproline and hydroxylysine, the glycosylation of hydroxylysine, and the crosslinking of collagen fibers by lysine-derived aldehydes are rather unique to the synthesis of collagen. (Elastin contains a low level of hydroxyproline and is crosslinked by lysine derived crosslinks.) Defects have been found at some of these steps and produce weakened connective tissues.

Cultured cells have been an important system for studying heritable diseases of collagen metabolism. Fibroblasts synthesize and secrete both types I and III procollagen, convert part of the procollagen to collagen and produce crosslinked fibers (Martin et al., 1975). They express the molecular defects in certain disorders such as the type IV and type VI forms of the Ehlers-Danlos syndrome. In addition, cultured fibroblasts produce collagenase. Altered production of collagenase has been observed in fibroblasts from patients with epidermolysis bullosa (Bauer, 1978) and rheumatoid arthritis (Dayer et al., 1977).

TABLE 1

Molecular disorders of collagen

Transcription-translation		
Gene → mRNA	Ehlers-Danlos type IV:	No type III collagen
mRNA → Pro α Chain	Osteogenesis imperfecta:	decreased type I synthesis
Hydroxylation		
Prolyl → Hydroxyprolyl	Not identified	
Lysyl → Hydroxylysyl	Ehlers-Danlos type VI:	hydroxylysine deficient collagen crosslinking defect
Glyosylation		
HO-Lysyl → Gal-O-Lysyl	Not identified	
Gal-O-Lysyl → Glc-Gal-O-Lysyl	Not identified	
Proteolysis		
Procollagen → Collagen	Ehlers-Danlos type VII:	accumulates precursor form crosslinking defect
Aldehyde formation		
Lysyl → Allysyl	Lathyrism	
HO-Lysyl → HO-Allysyl	Ehlers-Danlos type V:	crosslinking defect
	Cutis laxa (X-linked):	
Crosslinking		
Allysyl → Crosslink	Homocystinuria:	crosslinking defect

POSSIBLE TRANSCRIPTIONAL OR TRANSLATIONAL DEFECTS

Ehlers-Danlos type IV patients are quite distinct from patients with other forms of the Ehlers-Danlos syndrome (Pope et al., 1975, 1977). They have fragile but not hyperextensible skin. Their blood vessels are also unusually fragile. The defect in these patients is due to decreased levels of type III collagen. Type III collagen is widely distributed in the body (Epstein, 1974), but is a *major* component of blood vessels, skin and the stroma of certain internal organs. Fibroblasts from some type IV Ehlers-Danlos patients secrete only type I collagen. In 2 of these patients, immunological studies revealed no intracellular accumulation of type III collagen (Gay et al., 1976) suggesting that decreased synthesis rather than impaired secretion was involved. This disorder is heterogeneous. Other patients with the clinical features of this disorder have been studied (B. Steinmann, unpublished observations) whose fibroblasts synthesize some type III collagen. It is interesting that patients with decreased or deficient synthesis of type III collagen do not compensate by increasing

TABLE 2

Partial list of known collagens

	Chains	Location
Type I	$[\alpha1(I)]_2\,\alpha2$	Bone, skin, tendon, etc.
Type II	$[\alpha1(II)]_3$	Cartilage
Type III	$[\alpha1(III)]_3$	Skin, vessels, internal organs
Basement membrane (Type IV)	Procollagen-like	Sub-epithelial structure
A,B	$A_2, B(?)$	Smooth muscle

the synthesis of type I collagen. This suggests that the synthesis of type I collagen must be regulated independently from the synthesis of type III collagen.

Osteogenesis imperfecta

This disorder is clinically, genetically and biochemically heterogeneous (McKusick, 1972). Patients with certain forms may have only bone involvement while other patients have a generalized disorder with skin, teeth, cornea, etc. affected. The biochemical defects in these disorders are not known. However, 2 patients with severe forms of osteogenesis imperfecta have been identified whose skin fibroblasts synthesize a higher proportion of type III to type I collagen than normal (Penttinen et al., 1975; Müller et al., 1975). In 1 of these patients, sections of bone were found to contain depots of type III collagen in circular, hole-like structures (Müller et al., 1977). Bone was not obtained from the other patient. Since bone contains only type I collagen normally, the presence of type III collagen might weaken the tissue. In the fibroblast studies, it was suggested that a decrease in type I collagen synthesis could account for the change in proportion of type III to type I and may therefore be responsible for the general weakness of connective tissue. It should be emphasized that fibroblast cultures from most patients with osteogenesis imperfecta synthesize type I and III collagen in normal proportions (Penttinen et al., 1975).

More recently Sykes et al. (1977) reported that skin from 7 of 9 patients with mild forms of osteogenesis imperfecta and 2 of 5 patients with severe forms of the disease contained a higher proportion of type III to type I collagen than age-matched controls. They proposed that a reduction in the amount of type I collagen would account for the change and the tissue weakness in these patients.

Still other patients with osteogenesis imperfecta have bone collagen containing higher levels than normal of hydroxylysine (Trelstad et al., 1977). The level of hydroxylysine in bone collagen is variable and tends to be higher in the bones of younger animals and in hypocalcified tissue (Royce and Barnes, 1977). Such patients presumably represent a distinct form of osteogenesis imperfecta with the elevation in hydroxylysine occurring secondary to the actual lesion.

POSTTRANSLATIONAL MODIFICATIONS OF PROCOLLAGEN AND THE EHLERS-DANLOS SYNDROME (EDS)

Patients with certain recessive forms of the Ehlers-Danlos syndrome have been shown to have defects at one or another step in collagen synthesis (Table 3). It appears that these defects are related in that each leads to the impairment of the crosslinking of type I collagen. Some aspects of this disorder including increased tissue fragility, increased extensibility of skin and tendons and impaired wound healing are reminiscent of the changes observed in experimental lathyrism.

Type VI EDS   Patients with this disorder have hydroxylysine-deficient collagen (Pinnell et al., 1972). Hydroxylysines arise in collagen through the enzymatic hydroxylation of certain lysines in the pro α chains. Fibroblasts grown from patients with type VI EDS have been found to have very low levels of lysyl hydroxylase

TABLE 3

The Ehlers-Danlos syndromes

Type		Genetics	Biochemical defect
I	Severe form	Dominant	?
II	Mild form	Dominant	?
III	Benign hypermobile form	Dominant	?
IV	Ecchymotic or arterial form	Recessive	Deficiency of type III collagen
V	X-linked form	X-linked recessive	Lysyl oxidase deficiency
VI	Ocular form	Recessive	Lysyl hydroxylase deficiency
VII	Arthrochalasis multiplex congenita	Recessive	Procollagen peptidase deficiency

(Pinnell et al., 1972; Sussman et al., 1974; Steinmann et al., 1975; Krane et al., 1972). While the biological functions of hydroxylysine are not fully known, some hydroxylysine is enzymatically oxidized to aldehydes and participates in crosslinking. Crosslinks in collagen arise from both lysine and hydroxylysine residues in the molecule. However, hydroxylysine-derived crosslinks have been shown to be more stable. Type I collagen is more extractable than normal from the skin of these patients and the level of hydroxylysine-derived crosslinks is low. Normal levels of hydroxylysine were found in cartilage obtained from these patients. Cartilage contains a genetically distinct collagen and presumably a genetically distinct lysyl hydroxylase.

Type VII EDS Patients with this disorder were found to have precursor forms of collagen in their skin and a defect in the conversion of procollagen type I to collagen in culture (Lichtenstein et al., 1973). However, since these studies were done, it has been discovered that procollagen contains additional peptides at both the amino and carboxyl ends of the molecule. The conversion of procollagen to collagen requires 2 different enzymes, one removing amino and the other carboxyl terminal peptides. These enzymes have not been isolated or characterized. The defect in these patients was thought to be similar to a previously discovered disease in cattle, dermatosparaxis which is due to a defect in the conversion of procollagen to collagen (Lenaers et al., 1971). Tissue contents of collagen are normal but skin and other tissues are fragile and the collagen fibers are distorted presumably because procollagen with amino terminal peptides is incorporated into the fibers. Presumably the crosslinking of collagen in the fibers is impaired for steric reasons. In the case of the patients with type VII EDS, the nature of the precursor form accumulating should be established and more information obtained on the enzymes involved in the conversion of procollagen to collagen.

Type V EDS A possible x-linked form of the Ehlers-Danlos syndrome was described by Di Ferrante et al. (1975). Again the defects observed were related to impaired crosslinking as judged by an increased extractability of newly synthesized collagen. The level of lysyl oxidase synthesized by fibroblasts cultured from these patients was lower than normal. Lysyl oxidase carries out the sole enzymatic step in crosslinking, the oxidative deamination of lysyl and hydroxylysyl residues in collagen and elastin.

Other evidence also suggests that the gene for lysyl oxidase is located on the x-chromosome. Lowered levels of lysyl oxidase are found in mottled mice, an x-linked condition involving both coat color and the crosslinking of collagen and elastin (Rowe et al., 1974). Most recently Byers et al. (1976) reported that 2 patients with an x-linked condition resembling cutis laxa had decreased crosslinking of collagen and very low levels of lysyl oxidase in fibroblast cultures.

Type I–III EDS   The defects in the dominant forms of the EDS syndrome have not been identified. Recently, we have found that the collagen synthesized by EDS I fibroblasts in culture is more extractable than normal. This suggests that there is a crosslinking defect perhaps resulting from an amino acid substitution.

Function of the different collagens

The structural role of the various collagens is well recognized. However, if that were their only function, there would be no need for a number of genetically and chemically distinct proteins. Other functions and particularly differences in the activity of the collagens in various assays have been investigated. It is well known that collagen will induce the aggregation of platelets when added to platelet-rich plasma. In general, these studies indicate that type III collagen is the most active followed by type I. Cartilage (type II) and basement membrane collagen are much less active (Balleisen et al., 1975; Hugues et al., 1976). The binding site on the collagen molecule has not been identified but it is recognized that the fibrous form rather than the monomer is active.

Collagen promotes the fusion of myoblasts to form multinucleated muscle fibers (Hauschka and Konigsberg, 1966). Here types I–IV collagen show equal activity (Ketley et al., 1976). In this case, the collagen is active when attached to the surface of the dish but inactive if added to the medium in which the cells are grown. Presumably the collagen functions in a substrate role possibly through cell attachment.

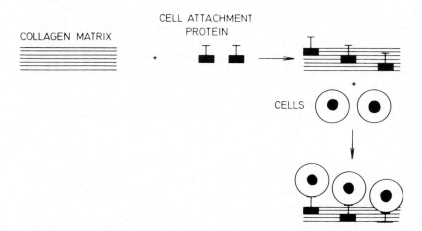

Fig. 1. Schematic description of the mechanism of binding of cells to collagen through cell attachment protein.

Types I–III collagen show differences in their susceptibility to various collagenases. Type IV and the other collagens have not been studied in this regard. The collagenase produced by an ascites tumor was found to attack type III and type I collagen similarly while type II collagen was cleaved at a much slower rate (McCroskery et al., 1975). The human leukocyte collagenase cleaves type I collagen but shows little or no activity with type III collagen (Horwitz et al., 1977). These data indicate that collagenases can distinguish between different collagens. This could be important in the remodeling of connective tissues containing more than one collagen type.

Recent studies on the manner in which cells bind to collagen indicate that specific proteins mediate the attachment. Klebe (1974) has shown that trypsinized fibroblasts bind to collagen-coated dishes through a serum-derived glycoprotein, cell attachment protein (CAP). This is shown schematically in Figure 1. Cells not treated with trypsin have CAP on their surface. The cells can produce CAP to replace that destroyed by trypsin treatment. We have shown that serum CAP binds to a specific part of the $\alpha 1(I)$ chain in the vicinity of the bond cleaved by animal collagenase. This region of the chain lacks carbohydrate, contains hydrophobic amino acids and has a low proline and hydroxyproline content. Presumably a certain sequence of amino acids in this region is recognized. Fibroblasts show little preference for different collagen types for attachment while chondrocytes bind better to types II and IV than to types I and III collagen. Presumably chondrocytes have a different CAP than that found in serum. Since CAP is a large surface-bound protein, we have assayed various other cell surface proteins for activity in cell attachment. These studies indicate that LETS-type proteins have attachment activity. Our studies indicate that the attachment proteins in different cell types may be different and show preference for one or another of the collagen types (Kleinman et al., 1976).

Studies on heritable diseases can now be extended to a variety of other disorders where suitable cell culture systems are available. It is likely that the identification of the functions of the different collagens will help to identify the pattern underlying poorly understood syndromes.

REFERENCES

Balleisen, L., Gray, S., Marx, R. and Kühn, K. (1975): *Klin. Wschr., 53*, 903.
Bauer, E. A. (1978): *Proc. nat. Acad. Sci. (Wash.), 74*, 4646.
Byers, P. H., Narayanan, A. S., Bornstein, P. and Hall, J. G. (1976): *Birth Defects, 12*, 293.
Dayer, J. M., Russell, R. G. G. and Krane, S. M. (1977): *Science, 195*, 181.
Di Ferrante, N., Leachman, R. D., Angelini, P., Donnelly, P. V., Francis, G., Almagan, A., Segni, G., Franzblau, C. and Jordan, R. E. (1975): In: *Disorders of Connective Tissue*, pp. 31–37. Editor: D. Bergsma. National Foundation, New York.
Epstein Jr, E. H. (1974): *J. biol. Chem., 249*, 3225.
Gay, S., Martin, G. R., Müller, P. K., Timpl, R. and Kühn, K. (1976): *Proc. nat. Acad. Sci. (Wash.), 73*, 4037.
Hauschka, S. D. and Konigsberg, I. R. (1966): *Proc. nat. Acad. Sci. (Wash.), 35*, 119.
Horwitz, A. L., Hance, A. J. and Crystal, R. G. (1977): *Proc. nat. Acad. Sci. (Wash.), 74*, 897.
Hugues, J. et al. (1976): *Thrombos. Res., 9*, 223.
Ketley, J., Orkin, R. W. and Martin, G. R. (1976): *Exp. Cell Res., 99*, 261.
Klebe, R. J. (1974): *Nature (Lond.), 250*, 248.
Kleinman, H. K., McGoodwin, E. B. and Klebe, R. J. (1976): *Biochem. biophys. Res. Commun., 72*, 426.
Krane, S. M., Pinnell, S. R. and Erbe, R. W. (1972): *Proc. nat. Acad. Sci. (Wash.), 69*, 2899.
Lenaers, A., Ansay, M., Nusgens, B. V. and Lapière, C. M. (1971): *Europ. J. Biochem., 23*, 533.

Lichtenstein, J. R., Martin, G. R., Kohn, L., Byers, P. and McKusick, V. A. (1973): *Science, 182,* 298.

Martin, G. R., Byers, P. H. and Piez, K. A. (1975): *Advanc. Enzymol., 42,* 167.

McCroskery, P. A., Richards, J. A. and Harris Jr, E. D. (1975): *Biochem. J., 152,* 131.

McKusick, V. A. (1972): *Heritable Disorders of Connective Tissue, 4th Ed.* C. V. Mosby Co., St Louis.

Müller, P. K., Lemmen, C., Gay, S. and Meigel, W. N. (1975): *Europ. J. Biochem., 59,* 97.

Müller, P. K., Raisch, K., Matzen, K. and Gay, S. (1977): *Europ. J. Pediat., 125,* 29.

Penttinen, R. P., Lichtenstein, J. R., Martin, G. R. and McKusick, V. A. (1975): *Proc. nat. Acad. Sci. (Wash.), 72,* 586.

Pinnell, S. R., Krane, S. M., Kenzora, J. E. and Glimcher, M. J. (1972): *New Engl. J. Med., 286,* 1013.

Pope, F. M., Martin, G. R., Lichtenstein, J. R., Penttinen, R., Gerson, B., Rowe, D. W. and McKusick, V. A. (1975): *Proc. nat. Acad. Sci. (Wash.), 72,* 1314.

Pope, F. M., Martin, G. R. and McKusick, V. A. (1977): *J. med. Genet., 14,* 200.

Rowe, D. W., McGoodwin, E. B., Martin, G. R., Sussman, M. D., Grahn, D., Faris, B. and Franzblau, C. (1974): *J. exp. Med., 139,* 180.

Royce, P. M. and Barnes, M. J. (1977): *Biochim. biophys. Acta (Amst.), 498,* 132.

Steinmann, B., Gitzelmann, R., Vogel, A., Grant, M. E., Harwood, R. and Sear, C. H. J. (1975): *Helv. paediat. Acta, 30,* 255.

Sussman, M. D., Lichtenstein, J. R., Nigra, T. P., Martin, G. R. and McKusick, V. A. (1974): *J. Bone Jt Surg., 56A,* 1228.

Sykes, B., Francis, M. J. O. and Smith, R. (1977): *New Engl. J. Med., 296,* 1200.

Trelstad, R. L., Rubin, D. and Gross, J. (1977): *Lab. Invest., 36,* 501.

Mechanisms of virus-induced birth defects*

RICHARD T. JOHNSON

Johns Hopkins University School of Medicine, Baltimore, Md., U.S.A.

Maternal infection can lead to fetal wastage and fetal malformation by a variety of mechanisms. The pathogenesis of the infection and the nature of the resultant abnormalities are dependent on the virus involved, the host species, and the gestational time of the infection. The pathways of virus dissemination will be reviewed in general, but discussion of major malformations will be limited to those involving the central nervous system.

PATHWAYS OF VIRUS SPREAD TO THE FETUS

Maternal viral infection can be acquired by respiratory spread, enteric contamination, venereal contact, or inoculation. The latter route of virus entry can occur via biting arthropods, animal bites or injections. In general, active virus replication in the mother and dissemination must occur for infections to affect the fetus. However, fetal wastage can occur without fetal infection. Severe constitutional effects on the mother may be sufficient to induce abortion, and the high abortion rate observed during smallpox epidemics has been thought to be due to this factor, since evidence of fetal infection is lacking (Dixon, 1962).

Selective placental infection can also lead to fetal loss even without severe constitutional symptoms in the mother. Although such selective localization of infection has not been documented in man, it has been demonstrated both in cytomegalovirus infections of mice (Johnson, 1969) and equine abortion virus infections in hamsters (Burek et al., 1975). In these cases the placenta presents new cell types which are selectively vulnerable to viral replication, and abortion can occur without evidence of fetal infection. For example, equine abortion virus in female hamsters does not infect normal uterine cells, but the syncytial trophoblasts of the placenta are selectively involved leading to widespread necrosis and resultant abortion.

For the development of specific malformations infection of the fetus must occur, and at least 4 pathways of potential spread of virus to the fetus must be considered. Vertical and transovarian infection have been demonstrated in laboratory animals but not in man. Vertical transmission has been most extensively studied with murine

*Studies supported by grants from the United Cerebral Palsy Research and Educational Foundation (R-230-77) and U. S. Public Health Service (NS 10920).

leukemia viruses, so-called endogenous viruses, which are transmitted as provirus apparently integrated with the parental genes (Rowe, 1972). Transovarian infection can occur with exogenous non-cytopathic viruses such as lymphocytic chorio-meningitis virus in mice. Following fetal or neonatal infection virtually all the cells of the mouse are infected for life. This includes infection of the germinal epithelium of the ovary and the ovum establishing the potential for transovarian transmission (Mims, 1966) (Table 1).

TABLE 1

Pathogenesis of viral infections affecting fetal development

Systemic effect on mother
Placental infection
Fetal infection
   Vertical
   Transovarian
   Ascending
   Transplacental

    Ascending infection along the birth canal is often considered but is yet unproven as a route of intrauterine virus infection. In man neonatal herpes virus infections with the type 2 or venereal strains of herpes simplex has been postulated to spread via this pathway; but most evidence suggests that neonatal infection occurs during parturition with passage through the contaminated cervix and vagina (Nahmias et al., 1970).

    In general, most fetal infections occur by transplacental passage of virus. This, of course, requires the presence of a viremia in the mother of sufficient magnitude and duration to allow penetration across the placental membranes. In the human hemochorial placenta the outer embryonic fetal membrane, the chorion, lies in intimate contact with the modified mucosal coat of the uterus, the desidua. Maternal blood flows through an outer coat of trophoblasts arising from the fetal chorion into open intervillous spaces. The fetal villi extending into these spaces contain the fetal blood vessels surrounded by trophoblasts of the fetal chorion. Thus, fetal blood is separated from maternal blood by a layer of trophoblasts derived from the fetus, a basement membrane and the endothelial cells of the fetal vessels. These are the membranes that must be infected or transversed by virus in order to gain access to the fetal circulation. Alternatively, growth or penetration of virus within the chorionic plate can give rise to infection of the amnionic membranes and allow shedding of virus into the amnionic cavity exposing the skin, respiratory and gastrointestinal tracts of the fetus.

    The differences in placental structure at various stages of gestation and the differ-ences between different animals may be important determinants in fetal infection. For example, the rodent placenta contains 3 layers of trophoblasts, 2 of which are syncytial in character, rather than the single layer in man. Such differences may explain why viruses such as human cytomegalovirus crosses the placenta, whereas murine cytomegalovirus does not, or why equine abortion virus infects the fetal foal but fails to cross the hamster placenta.

In addition, placental infection may cause structural or functional damage altering the barrier function of the placenta and allowing virus penetration to the fetus. Indeed, cellular damage has been found in the human placenta in both congenital rubella and cytomegalovirus infections (Töndury and Smith, 1966; Benirschke et al., 1974).

MECHANISMS OF VIRUS-INDUCED MALFORMATIONS

Entry of virus into the amnionic fluid or the fetal circulation is of no significance, unless there are fetal cells susceptible to virus infection. Furthermore, this infection may have different effects on susceptible cells. The mechanisms that may alter central nervous system development are summarized in Table 2.

TABLE 2

Mechanisms of viral-induced CNS disease of fetus

Acute or chronic generalized encephalitis
Chromosomal alterations
Mitotic inhibition
Selective infection of specific cells
   Alterations in organogenesis
   Selective destruction of mitotic or undifferentiated cell populations
   Obstruction of CSF pathways and hydrocephalus

Acute and chronic encephalitis are the recognized forms of viral cytopathology seen in fetal rubella, cytomegalovirus and herpes simplex virus infections in man. In each case there is evidence of cell destruction, an inflammatory reaction and resultant necrotic areas with mineralization. When widespread, microcephaly may be evident. In both rubella and cytomegalovirus infections the infection is persistent, and a chronic inflammatory encephalitis persists in the neonatal period. These pathological changes have become accepted as the hallmarks of antecedent or ongoing viral infection.

Viruses are also capable of producing cytogenetic abnormalities, and in cell culture a variety of chromosomal breakages, pulverizations and alterations or chromosome distribution or number have been produced (Nichols, 1970). Although the potential of viruses to lead to chromosomal abnormalities is well recognized, convincing evidence has not been presented for virus-induced chromosomal damage as a mechanism of teratogenesis in animals. The early reports correlating a temporal and geographic clustering of Down syndrome with infectious hepatitis have not been substantiated by subsequent studies (Siegel, 1973).

Non-cytopathic infections can lead to inhibition or slowing of mitotic activity without obvious cell destruction. This phenomena may explain some features of the congenital rubella syndrome in which the children appear to be small for gestational age, have reduced number of cells in organs (Naeye and Blanc, 1965), and may have asymmetrical hypoplasia such as unilateral microphthalmia. Focal clones of cells appear to be infected in their tissues (Woods et al., 1966), and cells grown from rubella virus-infected fetuses have been shown to have depressed mitotic activity (Rawls and Melnick, 1966).

Selective infection of specific cell populations can potentially lead to symmetrical, non-inflammatory malformations. A variety of such malformations have been observed in animals, and most lack the inflammation, mineralization and necrosis which pathologically might suggest a viral etiology. Thus, these malformations resemble malformations of man thought to result from toxic, genetic or vascular abnormalities (Johnson, 1972).

Interference with organogenesis of the central nervous system has been demonstrated only with viruses in embryonated eggs. The first was reported by Hamburger and Habel (1947). Influenza A virus was inoculated in eggs at 48 hours of incubation, and over the subsequent 24–48 hours collapse of the primitive brain, abnormalities of tube flexion and failure of closure of the neural tube were demonstrated (Robertson et al., 1960). Similar effects can also be induced with Newcastle disease virus (Robertson et al., 1955). In both cases the neural tube shows no histological abnormalities, and mitotic activity along the luminal surface is normal. However, immunofluorescence studies to localize virus replication at a cellular level have shown that influenza and Newcastle disease viruses infected different cell populations. Newcastle disease virus does infect cells within the neural tube (Williamson et al., 1965), whereas influenza virus infection has not been identified in neuroectoderm, the surrounding mesenchymal tissue, or the notochord. The influenza infection appears limited to the chorionic and amnionic membranes, the non-neural ectoderm and focal areas of the primitive myocardium and gut (Johnson et al., 1971). Thus, in 1 case infection of the neural tube itself and in the other infection of non-contiguous extraneural tissues appear to result in the same defect in organogenesis. The genesis of this malformation appears less dependent on the involvement of specific cell populations than on the developmental time of the infection.

Anomalies resulting from destruction of immature cell populations are highly dependent on which cells are infected. Some viruses such as the parvoviruses, which are small single-stranded DNA viruses, are restricted to replication in cells undergoing cellular DNA synthesis. Therefore, a parvovirus such as feline panleukopenia virus causes gastroenteritis and leukopenia in the mature cat. On the other hand, late fetal or neonatal infection causes selective destruction of the germinal cells of the cerebellum prior to their post-natal migration to form the granular cell layer. This infection results in a small cerebellum with abnormalities of foliation, total or subtotal absence of the granular cell layer and abnormal synaptic organization. The resultant disease, spontaneous ataxia of kittens, is the commonest neurological disease of the domestic cat and was previously thought to be a genetic disorder (Kilham and Margolis, 1966). Although mitotic activity appears prerequisite for infection, it is not the sole determinant of susceptibility. Studies of other parvoviruses have shown that within the brain as well as in extraneural tissues not all cells undergoing DNA synthesis are susceptible to infection (Lipton and Johnson, 1972).

Other viruses may selectively infect immature cells not because of their limitation to cells undergoing cellular DNA synthesis, but because immature cells may have undifferentiated membranes allowing for viral attachment or pluripotential metabolic functions including the potential to replicate virus. For example, bluetongue virus does not infect cells of the mature sheep or rodent brain. On the other hand, it selectively infects germinal cells of the ependymal plate in fetal lambs or neonatal mice, even though the undifferentiated germinal cells of the cerebellum are unaffected (Osburn et al., 1971a, b; Narayan and Johnson, 1972). Infection of the subependymal zone can lead to major anomalies of the forebrain. Direct intramuscular inoculation of the ovine fetus with the vaccine strain of bluetongue virus

TABLE 3

Experimental malformations induced by viruses

Malformation	Virus	Host species
Defects in neural tube	Myxoviruses	
	Influenza	Chick embryo
	Newcastle disease	Chick embryo
Encephalocele	Togavirus	
	St. Louis encephalitis	Mouse
Cerebellar hypoplasia	Parvoviruses	
	Rat virus	Hamster, rat, cat, ferret
	Feline panleukopenia	Cat, ferret
	Minute virus of mice	Mouse
	Arenaviruses	
	Lymphocytic choriomeningitis	Rat
	Tamiami	Mouse
	Unclassified	
	Bovine viral diarrhea	Cow, sheep
	Hog cholera	Pigs
Hypomyelinization	Unclassified	
	Hog cholera	Pigs
	Border disease	Sheep
Hydranencephaly	Orbivirus	
	Bluetongue	Sheep
	Togavirus	
	Akabane	Cow
Porencephaly	Orbivirus	
	Bluetongue	Sheep, mouse, hamster
	Togavirus	
	Venezuelan equine encephalitis	Monkey
Hydrocephalus	Myxoviruses	
	Mumps	Hamster
	Parainfluenza, Type 1 and 2	Hamster, mouse
	Influenza	Hamster, mouse, monkey
	Measles (mutant)	Hamster
	Newcastle disease	Mouse
	Reovirus	
	Type 1	Mouse, hamster, rat, ferret
	Type 3 (mutant)	Mouse
	Togaviruses	
	Japanese encephalitis	Pig
	Ross River	Mouse
	St. Louis encephalitis	Mouse

Modified from Johnson, 1978.

leads to consistent malformation. Fetuses inoculated at the end of the first trimester develop hydranencephaly, those inoculated at mid-gestation develop porencephaly, and those inoculated in the third trimester have only microscopic microglial nodules. Sequential virological and histological studies have shown infection of the early fetal subventricular zone causes widespread destruction of the entire forebrain. By mid-gestation most of the cortical mantle has differentiated in the ovine fetus, and infection at this time involves primarily glial precursor cells leading to cystic lesions largely within the white matter. In either case, at the time of the acute infection, there is widespread necrosis and inflammation, but this has resolved by the time of birth leaving only glial walled cavities with no histopathological footprints to suggest the earlier acute infection (Osburn et al., 1971a).

Cerebrospinal fluid pathways can be obstructed subsequent to infection of both meningeal or ependymal cells, and a variety of viruses selectively infect these cells in fetal or neonatal animals (Johnson, 1975). For example, mumps virus causes a clinically inapparent infection in neonatal hamsters limited largely to the ependymal cells. After the clearance of infection and the resolution of the inflammatory response, the aqueduct becomes stenosed or totally occluded and hydrocephalus develops (Johnson et al., 1967). Thus, although acute cell destruction and inflammation accompany the clinically inapparent infection, studies at the time of clinical disease show no residual signs of the infectious process and no persistence of virus or viral antigens. The pathology appears similar to that seen in agenesis of the aqueduct of Sylvius in man. The area of the aqueduct is replaced by relatively normal brain stem tissue rather than glial tissues, the remaining ependymal cells form rosettes or aqueductules, and normal brain stem appears to traverse areas between these islands of residual ependymal cells (Johnson and Johnson, 1968).

This malformation, due to selective infection of ependymal cells, appears to have a human counterpart. After the description of mumps virus-induced hydrocephalus in hamsters, a number of children were reported with hydrocephalus following mumps virus infections (Johnson, 1975). Evidence that mumps virus selectively infects ependymal cells in man has also been obtained by electron microscopical examination of spinal fluid sediment in patients with mumps meningitis. Numerous ependymal cells are found, and these cells contain cytoplasm inclusions composed of tubules corresponding in size and localization to the nucleocapsids of mumps virus (Herndon et al., 1974). It is unknown, however, whether mumps or other viruses cross the human placenta and cause ependymal cell destruction in the human fetus.

SUMMARY

The magnitude of the problem of birth defects due to viral infections is unknown. At the present time we recognize only rubella and cytomegaloviruses as major causes of fetal infection of the central nervous system. Association of these viruses with neonatal neurological diseases was relatively easy because of the characteristic clinical signs of disease and the presence of the histopathological features which we have come to associate with fetal viral infection. On the other hand, we recognize that acute fetal infection in animals may occur in which virological and histopathological evidence of infection are no longer evident at the time of birth or first manifestation of clinical signs. In man such malformations would be exceedingly difficult to associate with prior maternal infection. Yet in animals there is evidence that viruses can cause defects in neural tube closure, encephalocele, cerebellar hypoplasia, hypomyelinization, hydranencephaly, porencephaly, and hydrocephalus (Table 3).

In the National Institutes of Health's perinatal study 3% of newborns were found to have greater than 22 mg% of IgM in cord blood, and half of these infants exhibited major clinical abnormalities in the first year of life. However, in only 20% of those children could the increased IgM be accounted for by antibodies to cytomegalovirus, rubella, herpes simplex virus, toxoplasmosis, or syphilis, the 5 infectious agents considered to be major infectious teratogens. The remaining 80% with elevated IgM remain unexplained (Sever, 1973). Furthermore, transient infections cleared early in gestation, such as those which we have associated with some malformations of the brain in animals, might not show elevated IgM at time of birth. Therefore, even the above figures may give only a small indication of the potential magnitude of the problem.

REFERENCES

Benirschke, K., Mendoza, G. R. and Bazeley, P. L. (1974): *Virchows Arch. path. Anat., 16,* 121.
Burek, J. D., Roos, R. P. and Narayan, O. (1975): *Lab. Invest., 33,* 400.
Dixon, C. W. (1962): *Smallpox.* Churchill, London.
Hamburger, V. and Habel, K. (1947): *Proc. Soc. exp. Biol. (N.Y.), 66,* 608.
Herndon, R. M., Johnson, R. T., Davis, L. E. and Descalzi, L. R. (1974): *Arch. Neurol. (Chic.), 30,* 475.
Johnson, K. P. (1969): *J. infect. Dis., 120,* 445.
Johnson, R. T. (1972): *New Engl. J. Med., 287,* 599.
Johnson, R. T. (1975): *Develop. Med. Child Neurol., 17,* 807.
Johnson, R. T. (1978): In: *Handbook of Clinical Neurology, Vol. 33.* Editors: P. S. Vinken and G. W. Bruyn. North-Holland Publishing Co., Amsterdam.
Johnson R. T. and Johnson, K. P. (1968): *J. Neuropath. exp. Neurol., 27,* 591.
Johnson, R. T., Johnson, K. P. and Edmonds, C. J. (1967): *Science, 157,* 1066.
Johnson, K. P., Klasnja, R. and Johnson, R. T. (1971): *J. Neuropath. exp. Neurol., 30,* 68.
Kilham, L. and Margolis, G. (1966): *Amer. J. Path., 48,* 991.
Lipton, H. L. and Johnson, R. T. (1972): *Lab. Invest., 27,* 508.
Mims, C. A. (1966): *J. Path. Bact., 91,* 395.
Naeye, R. L. and Blanc, W. (1965): *J. Amer. med. Ass., 194,* 1277.
Nahmias, A. J., Alford, C. A. and Korones, S. B. (1970): *Advanc. Pediat., 17,* 185.
Narayan, O. and Johnson, R. T. (1972): *Amer. J. Path., 68,* 1.
Nichols, W. W. (1970): *Ann. Rev. Microbiol., 24,* 479.
Osburn, B. I., Johnson, R. T., Silverstein, A. M., Prendergast, R. A., Jochim, M. M. and Levy, S. E. (1971a): *Lab. Invest., 25,* 206.
Osburn, B. I., Silverstein, A. M., Prendergast, R. A., Johnson, R. T. and Parshall, C. J. (1971b): *Lab. Invest., 25,* 197.
Rawls, W. E. and Melnick, J. L. (1966): *J. exp. Med., 123,* 795.
Robertson, G. G., Williamson, A. P. and Blattner, R. J. (1955): *J. exp. Zool., 129,* 5.
Robertson, G. G., Williamson, A. P. and Blattner, R. J. (1960): *Yale J. Biol. Med., 32,* 449.
Rowe, W. P. (1972): *J. exp. Med., 136,* 1272.
Sever, J. L. (1973): In: *Pathobiology of Development,* p. 97. Editors: Perrin and Finegold. Williams and Wilkins, Baltimore.
Siegel, M. (1973): *J. Amer. med. Ass., 226,* 1521.
Töndury, G. and Smith, D. W. (1966): *J. Pediat., 68,* 867.
Williamson, A. P., Blattner, R. J. and Robertson, G. G. (1965): *Develop. Biol., 12,* 498.
Woods, W. A., Johnson, R. T., Hostetler, D. D., Lepow, M. L. and Robbins, F. C. (1966): *J. Immunol., 96,* 253.

PREVENTION AND DIAGNOSIS

Chairman: Mary Ellen Avery, Boston, Mass.

The environment and prenatal origins of human disease

ROBERT W. MILLER

Clinical Epidemiology Branch, National Cancer Institute, Bethesda, Md., U.S.A.

Patterns of discovery of environmental effects on the embryo

Environmental agents that cause birth defects have usually first been recognized by alert practitioners (Miller, 1978). The history of the teratologic effects of X-rays is typical. In the 1920's individual cases were reported of infants with small head circumference and mental retardation attributed to maternal exposure to radio-therapy early in pregnancy. In 1928–29 Goldstein and Murphy, Philadelphia obstetricians, created a case series from the literature, and added a series of their own, assembled by the simple procedure of a mail survey inquiring about cases at other obstetric centers. After the relationship between exposure and teratogenic effects was observed by retrospective study in man, similar effects were induced experimentally in rats in 1938. When the atomic explosions occurred in Japan, a prospective study was made, that defined the dose-response, gestational interval of susceptibility, and the range of effects (Fig. 1) (Miller and Mulvihill, 1976).

Agents known to be teratogenic or fetopathic but not (yet) known to be carcinogenic in man are shown in Table 1. Five other chemicals are known to be both teratogenic and carcinogenic (Table 2), but the dissimilarities of the organs affected by a given agent in the 2 processes implies that dissimilar biologic mechanisms are involved – except perhaps for DES which causes minor anomalies and, far less frequently, cancer of the cervix or vagina in young women (Herbst et al., 1975, 1977). Other possible transplacental carcinogens include any chemical that can cross the placenta and is known to cause cancer in man; e.g., benzene, melphalan, immuno-suppressants after renal transplantation, vinyl chloride, or diphenylhydantoin (DPH) (Hoover and Fraumeni, 1975). DPH is thought to induce lymphoma, and is teratogenic (the fetal hydantoin syndrome) (Hanson and Smith, 1975). One might expect children with the syndrome to be at increased risk of *lymphoma*, so it came as a surprise when 2 cases with *neuroblastoma* were reported in quick succession in the United States (Pendergrass and Hanson, 1976; Sherman and Roizen, 1976).

Predicting teratogenesis

Animal screening tests are uncertain predictors of the human response. Aspirin and cortisone are teratogenic in rats but not in man. Thalidomide produces limb-reduction

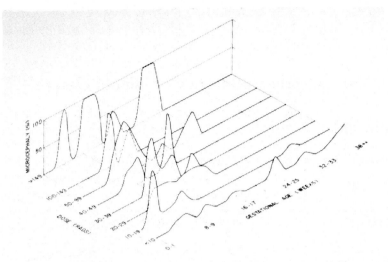

Fig. 1. Small head circumference after intrauterine exposure to the atomic bomb in Hiroshima. Percentage of cases according to gestational age and estimated radiation dose in air to the mother (from Miller and Mulvihill, 1976).

deformities in man, but not in the usual experimental animals (Schardein, 1976). Laboratory screening tests seem to be well on their way to becoming effective predictors of carcinogenesis (or mutagenesis) (Sugimura et al., 1976; McCann and Ames, 1976). The same is not true for teratogenesis, because of the diversity of mechanisms involved.

Monitoring for new human teratogens

Registries for congenital malformations or cancer have been more useful in testing hypotheses than in generating them (Miller and Flynt, 1976). Confirmation of the transplacental carcinogenicity of DES, for example, was quickly provided by the

TABLE 1

Agents known to be teratogenic or fetopathic but not carcinogenic in man *

Chemicals	Viruses
Aminopterin	Rubella
Antithyroid drugs	Cytomegalovirus
Busulfan	Herpes virus hominis 1 and 2
Mercury, organic	Varicella
Methotrexate	Venezuelan equine encephalitis
PCBs	
Tetracycline	
Thalidomide	
Warfarin	

*From Miller (1977a).

TABLE 2

Agents that are both carcinogenic and teratogenic*

Agent	Cancer sites	Organs affected
Alcohol	Mouth, larynx, esophagus	Brain, face
Diphenylhydantoin	Lymph glands	Brain, face, nails (hypoplasia)
Ionizing radiation	Various	Brain, stature
Androgens	Liver	Masculinization of the external genitalia of females
Diethylstilbestrol	Cervix or vagina	Cervix and vagina

*From Miller (1977a).

New York State Tumor Registry (Greenwald et al., 1971). Monitoring systems for sudden regional increases in rates for specific malformations now exist in at least 12 countries or areas (Miller, 1977).

Teratogenic pollutants

Occurrences that initially appear to be remote local problems have soon thereafter become international problems. An epidemic of chloracne, and to a lesser extent adverse fetal effects, occurred in Kyushu, Japan, from PCBs, a heat-transfer agent that leaked into cooking oil during its manufacture. Soon after, contamination of chicken feed in the United States occurred in the same fashion, but no human disease was reported. Since then, as is now well known, PCBs have become a widespread problem through contamination of fish in river waters of the U.S. and elsewhere (reviewed by Miller, 1977b).

In 1955, exposure to methylmercury-contaminated fish from Minamata Bay caused an epidemic of neurological disabilities in children and adults, but it was not realized until 7 years later that a concomitant epidemic of congenital cerebral palsy had occurred as a result of maternal exposure during pregnancy. Dr. M. Harada of Kumamoto University has been particularly active in studying intrauterine chemical effects in Kyushu, Japan, and he published a composite photograph of 10 Minamata children with congenital cerebral palsy waiting to be examined in 1962 (Harada, 1976).

The lesson of Minamata disease was not too well known or learned, for the disease occurred later in at least 5 other locales, from the ingestion of meat or baked products in which methylmercury-coated grain was used (Koos and Longo, 1976; Center for Disease Control (U.S. Publ. Hlth Service), unpublished data). The grain, so coated and stained with a warning dye, was meant for planting.

Stored specimens as measures of environmental changes

In 1971 Dr. Harada hit upon the ingenious idea of studying the methylmercury content of dried umbilical cords, traditionally kept for decades as a souvenir of birth in Japan. He studied the children in 2 families, born between 1927 and 1966, and discovered from the results that an earlier episode of Minamata disease had gone undetected (Nishigaki and Harada, 1975). Dr. Harada's study revealed the value in using easily preserved specimens as biologic measures of changes in the environment which may indicate past exposures that affect the health of the newborn (Miller, 1976).

Other possible specimens for such preservation include a spot of blood (the Guthrie test for PKU), which has recently been used to study the lead levels of newborn infants in Glasgow, Scotland (Moore et al., 1977), and the hair of the newborn, which can be studied millimeter by millimeter for certain chemicals deposited at various times from the 19th week of gestation until term.

Interaction of genetics and the environment

It is important to know not only what causes disease, but who is most or least susceptible and why. Alert clinicians have contributed substantially to this aspect of etiology.

Clinical observations led to recognition of the gamma-ray analog of xeroderma pigmentosum (reviewed by Miller, 1977c). Ataxia telangiectasia (AT) is a rare genetic disorder first described in 1941 by the French physician, Madame Louis-Bar. By 1965 several clinicians had reported the development of lymphoma in these patients, presumably due to their congenital immunodeficiency. In 1967 a child with AT and lymphoma was reported to have had a severe acute reaction to conventional radiotherapy for the lymphoma. The following year a second case was reported. In 1974, another such patient was observed in Birmingham, England, and studies made of skin fibroblasts in culture. Cell survival was diminished in proportion to the radiation dose and, in another laboratory at about the same time, it was found that defective repair of DNA was apparently responsible. Thus, this chain of events, in conjunction with those concerning xeroderma pigmentosum, is leading to a new understanding of the fundamental biology of sensitivity to environmental agents as it relates to aging and neoplasia. Use of such supersensitive cells in culture should help in screening environmental agents for their capacity to induce mutagenesis, and possibly carcinogenesis in man.

Some ethnic groups are peculiarly resistant to certain forms of cancer (reviewed by Miller, 1977c). Among Blacks, for example, rates for Ewing's sarcoma are low, and in the Chinese and Japanese, chronic lymphocytic leukemia is almost nonexistent. Subgroups of other populations may, for genetic reasons, have diminished susceptibility to such carcinogens as cigarette smoke.

Recommendations to enhance etiology at the bedside

Enlarge the number of alert practitioners   Persons who select medicine as a career and are selected for admission to medical schools tend to think of one patient at a time, and concentrate on diagnosis and therapy. They tend not to think very deeply about peculiarities in the occurrence of disease that might reveal new information about its origins.

A latent aptitude to think etiologically might be detected by giving screening examinations to medical students, or better yet to college or high-school students. In Australia, national science talent quests have been made among high-school students, with those scoring the best given assistance in developing their ability. A similar approach in the United States might greatly add to the very thin ranks of etiologists/epidemiologists.

Channel unusual observations for evaluation Physicians should know how to refer unusual clinical observations for evaluation by experts at national, university or other research centers. For example, congenital malformations thought to be due to an environmental exposure might be referred to the Committee on Environmental Hazards of the American Academy of Pediatrics or to the Birth Defects Branch, Bureau of Epidemiology, Center for Disease Control.

Formally train a few epidemiologists There is a need for deep training of enough classical epidemiologists to fill positions in Schools of Public Health, Federal Agencies and a few universities. Classical epidemiologists specialize in statistical and methodological detail essential to good scientific design. In the main, these physicians are teachers, critics and investigators of complex epidemiologic studies.

Develop clinical etiologists There is a wide need, with virtually no established positions, for medical specialists familiar with epidemiology. One might argue that each university should have one such person to make the most of new observations of etiologic interest on the wards and in the clinics. These physicians, trained in traditional medical specialties, would draw on their expert knowledge to ask questions that can be investigated through simple epidemiologic methods. The medical specialist with an interest in etiology and enough knowledge of epidemiology to avoid its pitfalls, can set an example for medical students by inquiring into the origins of disease. His attention to etiology would complement the usual attention given in medical schools to diagnosis, mechanism and therapy.

Although physicians should have a special advantage in detecting features of etiologic interest in their patients, occasionally non-medical observers have a remarkable talent for doing so.

Broaden thinking about new environmental hazards Small groups of scientists from different disciplines need to think creatively about environmental agents recently identified as hazardous. Without an appropriate specialist in attendance, there has been a tendency, for example, to overlook the special susceptibility or exposures of the fetus or child (Miller, 1974). It would be well to include at such meetings one free-thinking participant, who is not a member of the establishment, and will challenge traditional ideas or patterns of thought.

Establish an annual award for clinical astuteness in etiology Perhaps the Australians have excelled in identifying human teratogens because they have followed an example set by Gregg in 1941. Without special laboratory instruments, he made a monumental contribution to scientific knowledge by noting a peculiar clinical occurrence, asking the right questions and recognizing a response in common, which led to the cause.

In other countries a similar example might be set by establishing an annual award for the person, not necessarily a physician, whose medical astuteness has led to the recognition of a new factor in the causation of disease. A symposium might be held at which the steps are described, from clinical discovery, through confirmation and laboratory elucidation, to the benefits for patients and the public health. Description of the chain of events might point the way for others to bring observations to scientific attention.

REFERENCES

Greenwald, P., Barlow, J. J., Nasca, P. C. and Burnett, W. S. (1971): *New Engl. J. Med., 285,* 390.
Hanson, J. W. and Smith, D. W. (1975): *J. Pediat., 87,* 285.
Harada, M. (1976): *Bull. Inst. constitut. Med. (Kumamoto Univ.), 25 (Suppl.),* 1.
Herbst, A. L., Cole, P., Colton, T., Robboy, S. J. and Scully, R. E. (1977): *Amer. J. Obstet. Gynec., 128,* 43.
Herbst, A. L., Poskanzer, D. C., Robboy, S. J., Friedlander, L. and Scully, R. E. (1975): *New Engl. J. Med., 292,* 234.
Hoover, R. and Fraumeni Jr, J. F. (1975): In: *Persons at High Risk of Cancer: An Approach to Cancer Etiology and Control,* p. 185. Editor: J. F. Fraumeni, Jr. Academic Press, New York.
Koos, B. J. and Longo, L. D. (1976): *Amer. J. Obstet. Gynec., 126,* 390.
McCann, J. and Ames, B. N. (1976): *Proc. nat. Acad. Sci. (Wash.), 73,* 950.
Miller, J. R. (1977): *Congenital Anomalies, 17,* 1.
Miller, R. W. (Ed.) (1974): *Pediatrics, 53 (Suppl.),* 777.
Miller, R. W. (1976): *Lancet, 1,* 315.
Miller, R. W. (1977a): *J. nat. Cancer Inst., 58,* 471.
Miller, R. W. (1977b): *J. Pediat., 90,* 510.
Miller, R. W. (1977c): In: *Genetics of Human Cancer,* p. 1. Editors: J. J. Mulvihill, R. W. Miller and J. F. Fraumeni, Jr. Raven Press, New York.
Miller, R. W. (1978): In: *Chemical Mutagens,* V. Editors: A. Hollaender and F. J. de Serres. Plenum Press, New York. In press.
Miller, R. W. and Flynt Jr, J. W. (1976): In: *Prevention of Embryonic, Fetal, and Perinatal Disease, Vol. 3,* p. 287. Editors: R. L. Brent and M. I. Harris. Fogarty International Center Series on Preventive Medicine, DHEW Publication No. (NIH) 76-853, United States Government Printing Office, Washington, D.C.
Miller, R. W. and Mulvihill, J. J. (1976): *Teratology, 14,* 355.
Moore, M. R., Meredith, P. A. and Goldberg, A. (1977): *Lancet, 1,* 717.
Nishigaki, S. and Harada, M. (1975): *Nature (Lond.), 258,* 324.
Pendergrass, T. W. and Hanson, J. W. (1976): *Lancet, 2,* 150.
Schardein, J. L. (1976): *Drugs as Teratogens.* CRC Press, Inc., Cleveland, Ohio.
Sherman, S. and Roizen, N. (1976): *Lancet, 2,* 517.
Sugimura, T., Yahagi, M., Nagao, M., Takeuchi, M., Kawachi, T., Hara, K., Yamasaki, E., Matsushima, T., Hashimoto, Y. and Okada, M. (1976): In: *Screening Tests in Chemical Carcinogenesis, Vol. 12,* p. 81. Editors: R. Montesano, H. Bartsch and L. Tomatis. IARC Scientific Publications, Lyon.

The growth retarded infant

303

JOSEPH B. WARSHAW

Yale University School of Medicine, Division of Perinatal Medicine, Department of Pediatrics and Obstetrics and Gynecology, New Haven, Conn., U.S.A.

A normal pregnancy carries with it the implication of normal intrauterine development of the fetus and an absence of factors which may restrict growth or affect the length of gestation. While the normal program of embryonic and fetal development is dictated by the genetic potential of the fetus, a multitude of environmental factors may supervene and thwart the course of normal development. A frequent final expression of adverse genetic and environmental influences is low birthweight. Low birthweight generally refers to an infant of less than 2500 g birthweight. Within the category of low birthweight are infants small for gestational age and those who are born before expected term. Infants born 2 or 3 months prior to term because of premature labor may suffer a variety of postnatal difficulties such as hypoxic injury, nutritional restriction, infection and ventricular hemorrhage, all of which can result in subsequent impairment. However, if the low birthweight premature infant manages to avoid these and other hazards to normal development by effective intervention and newborn intensive care, normal development can be attained. It is important to differentiate infants with low birthweight from those who are small for gestational age because of extrinsic and intrinsic constraints on fetal growth. It is the latter group which will be considered primarily.

Recognition of the growth retarded fetus

The terms 'small for gestational age' or 'small for date' are reserved for those infants whose weight is at or below the third percentile for gestational age. The key to prevention of low birthweight and development of rational approaches to therapy is recognition during pregnancy. Abnormal fetal growth can often be detected through careful clinical examination including monitoring of maternal weight gain and increase in uterine size and through the application of such modern methods of obstetric surveillance as ultrasound and tests of fetal-placental function. Ultrasound has been particularly useful. Using ultrasound criteria, Campbell (1974) has confirmed 2 patterns of abnormal fetal growth. The more common pattern is normal growth until some time during the third trimester when growth shows abrupt slowing. This alteration of normal growth is related to disruption of the maternal supply line such as would be caused by maternal hypertension or toxemia. Disruption of the maternal supply lines does not commonly cause growth retardation prior to the 26th to the 28th week of gestation. Apparently, only after that time does the fetal mass represent a sufficiently large 'sink' so that transfer of nutrients to the fetus becomes restrictive for normal growth.

Another group of small for date fetuses are defined by ultrasound (Campbell, 1974) as early as the second trimester. In this group there is no tendency for slowing in later gestation, and there is little association with toxemia or intrapartum asphyxia. When born, these infants are symmetrically small and appear to be small for date because of decreased potential for growth such as would occur in chromosome abnormalities or with congenital infection. Newer ultrasound techniques, including quantitation of fetal bladder volume and urinary output, may also be useful in assessing growth (Campbell et al., 1973). Fetal urine production is decreased in the growth retarded infant (Wladimiroff and Campbell, 1974). More recently, Hobbins and his associates (Gohari et al., 1976) have utilized total intrauterine volume as an indicator of fetal growth retardation.

Chemical monitoring of the high risk pregnancy has also been invaluable in monitoring fetal well being. Maternal urinary estriols tend to be low in intrauterine growth retardation (Kushinsky and Chi, 1973). Placental lactogen can also provide an index of placental size during gestation; in conditions with impaired uterine blood flow resulting in small placentas, the placental lactogen level tends to be low (Spellacy and Cohn, 1973).

The growth retarded newborn

Growth standards used to chart the progress of small for date and premature infants warrant careful scrutiny. Drillien (1974) has commented that the growth standards used in the United States are based on lower socio-economic class populations in Denver and that the 10th percentile in Denver approximates the 3rd percentile for general populations at sea level in North America. The original data base utilized by Dancis to compile the premature infant weight gain grid in 1948 used a base of 100 infants between 1000 and 2500 grams birthweight in whom nutrition was designed to reach 120 calories per kg by the 10th day of life (Dancis et al., 1948). When these grids are applied to prematures with birthweights of less than 1500 grams, infants will be below the 10th percentile of the Denver curves by 1 month of age.

Although there are these difficulties in applying standards to the initial assessment and subsequent growth of both premature and small for date low birthweight infants the first step in evaluation of low birthweight is to measure accurately the standard growth parameters of weight, length, and head circumference and to evaluate the overall appearance of the infant, including neurologic status. It is important to distinguish the immature infant from the infant small for gestational age. The small for gestational age newborn reflects the 2 patterns of fetal growth noted above (Thomson, 1970). There may be a major compromise of weight, some decrease in length and a head circumference that is spared or affected only mildly. The second pattern is a uniform compromise of all growth parameters at birth usually associated with postnatal failure to grow despite adequate provision of calories and proteins. This latter pattern of symmetrical small size is more frequent in infants

with decreased growth potential but may be seen with profound intrauterine malnutrition.

While there are degrees of overlap between small for gestational age infants and
those born prematurely, the small for gestational age infant exhibits a number of
distinctive features.

These infants often have a wasted malnourished appearance, yet the infants look
alert and frequently appear older than their weights would indicate; they frequently
have decreased caloric reserves particularly glycogen. The incidence of perinatal
asphyxia and its complication are higher in these infants than in normal newborns
(Scott and Usher, 1966; Low and Galbreith, 1974; Laga and Cassady, 1971; Low
et al., 1972). Many of the problems encountered reflect complications of asphyxia
during labor and delivery. These include meconium aspiration and its attendant
postnatal complications of pneumonia, pneumothorax and persistent fetal circulation. Growth retarded infants may be symptomatically polycythemic and exhibit
symptoms of hyperviscosity such as lethargy, irritability, seizures and decreased renal
function. Polycythemia exhibited by the growth retarded infant may be a response
to intrauterine hypoxia, or as suggested by Oh and Omori (1975) result from placental
to fetal transfusion during periods of hypoxic insult. The growth retarded infant is
also prone to problems with thermoregulation because of decreased subcutaneous
fat and relatively large surface area for body weight.

Metabolic features of the growth retarded newborn

During the second half of gestation, the human fetus increases in weight from
approximately 45 to 3500 grams. Protein and fat accumulate in the fetus at different
rates. Protein accumulation occurs at a very high incremental rate during early
pregnancy, and plateaus after the 26th to the 27th week as the rate of growth slows.
On the other hand, the accumulation of fat does not increase until after the middle
of gestation when there is an almost exponential increase in the deposition of fat in
body tissues (Southgate and Hey, 1976). Energy stored as fat shows a remarkable
increase in the last weeks of gestation when over 100 Kcal per day are deposited in
the fetus. During the last 2 months of gestation subcutaneous fat increases from
20 grams to 350 grams and deep body fat from 10 grams to approximately 80 grams
to give the full term infant approximately 13–16% of body mass as fat. Infants with
intrauterine growth retardation exhibit deficiencies of both subcutaneous and deep
fat, presumably because of insufficient calories to meet the energy cost of fat
deposition and storage. Failure of fat stores to develop may limit the postnatal oxidation of fuels alternative to glucose such as long chain fatty acids and ketone bodies
(Warshaw, 1972).

An absence of glycogen from liver and other tissues (Shelley and Neligan, 1966)
in the growth retarded newborn limits glucose availability in the immediate newborn
period. Infants small for gestational age may also have a functional delay in the
development of gluconeogenesis. These infants do not show a normal glycemic
response to alanine infusion despite elevated levels of serum glucagon (Williams
et al., 1975). Infants with a depleted muscle mass may also lack sufficient protein
reserves to support gluconeogenesis. In view of these multiple factors, it is not

surprising that small for gestational infants may exhibit severe hypoglycemia and are at serious nutritional risk because of inadequate caloric reserves.

Biochemical aspects of intrauterine growth retardation

Numerous studies have documented abnormalities of cell kinetics in infants with various categories of intrauterine growth retardation. In large part these studies are based on the now classic work of Enesco and LeBlond (1962). Since the DNA content of mammalian cells is constant, an estimation of cell number in a given tissue specimen can be obtained by dividing the amount of DNA in the sample by the constant amount of DNA per cell. Similarly, the protein to DNA ratio can be utilized as an index of cell size. In these estimations, 3 overlapping stages of cell growth have been defined: (1) cell division with rapid increases in DNA and relative constancy of cell size, (2) slower cell division and an increase in cell size, (3) an increase in cell size without an increase in cell number. A number of investigators have utilized these measures to document cell growth under various conditions of maternal, fetal and newborn nutritional deprivation (Winick and Rosso, 1969; Hill et al., 1971; Dickenson et al., 1971). These studies have demonstrated that early malnutrition can result in a permanent decrease in cell number in brain and other organs. Winick (1970) showed that rats subjected to either prenatal malnutrition alone or to postnatal malnutrition alone showed a 15 to 20% reduction in brain cell number. However, if rats were malnourished both prenatally and postnatally the animals demonstrated a 60% reduction in total brain cell number at the time of weaning. There is considerable evidence that after such major nutritional insult the brain may not show complete catch-up growth during the period of nutritional rehabilitation. Work by others has documented changes in brain cell growth, myelination and protein synthesis following nutritional deprivation during the period of the brain growth spurt which in humans begins in mid-pregnancy and continues for 3 or 4 years postnatally (Dobbing and Sands, 1973). Widdowson et al. (1972) showed that human tissues obtained between 14 and 25 weeks of intrauterine life showed hyperplastic growth whereas in tissue obtained during the last 10 weeks of gestation, there was a rapid growth in cell size and a slowing of cell division. Organs of small for date infants showed fewer cells than normal controls.

More recently, in an interesting follow-up to the Dutch Famine study, Ravelli et al. (1976) reported that survivors of that catastrophe who were subjected to nutritional restriction during the last trimester of uterine life had a decreased incidence of obesity in later life presumably because of a permanent effect on adipocyte number induced during the period of nutritional restriction.

Winick (1976) and his colleagues have extended their observations of nutritional influences on cell kinetics to investigations of enzymes important for nucleic acid metabolism. Both DNA polymerase and alkaline RNAse have been used as indices of nutritional status in rats exposed to maternal protein restriction. The results indicate that malnutrition results in decreased DNA polymerase activity and increased alkaline RNAse activity in placenta. Of considerable interest is the observation that alkaline RNAse activity of serum obtained from a malnourished central American population was also increased.

Maternal leukocyte metabolism has been used as an index of fetal growth. Urrusti et al. (1972) showed a significant correlation between maternal leukocyte RNA polymerase activity and the birthweight of infants in a malnourished Mexican population. The changes in white cell metabolism may reflect nutritional constraints on a rapidly dividing maternal tissue similar to what occurs in the fetus. These data also suggest that maternal factors may influence both maternal and fetal cell development. The significance of these observations are not clear, but they do provide possible indices with which to gauge effects of nutrition on growth.

FACTORS AFFECTING FETAL GROWTH

Normal development of the fetus depends on the genetic potential for growth, adequacy of the maternal supply line and the absence of negative influences on growth potential. Since the genetic potential for fetal growth in normal populations is relatively fixed, the adequacy of placental function and transport of nutrients from the maternal to the fetal circulation is a major determinant of growth. This subject has been extensively reviewed (Longo, 1972; Dancis and Schneider, 1975). Factors controlling normal and abnormal growth are outlined in Table 1 and will be discussed in more detail below.

TABLE 1

Influences on fetal growth

I. *Genetic*
    Population differences
    Maternal size
    Litter size
    Y chromosome
    Chromosomal defects

II. *Environmental*
    Maternal nutrition
    Uteroplacental insufficiency,
      maternal medical disease, altitude, litter size
    Congenital infection
    Drugs: cigarettes, alcohol, heroin
    Hormones and growth factors

III. *Synergisms*

Genetic influences on growth

Fetal growth is markedly constant in different species and high correlation is found between maternal size and newborn birthweight. Ounstead (1971) has emphasized that tall adequately nourished mothers have larger babies than mothers on the shorter side of the spectrum. Genetic influences on growth may also be expressed on a population basis. In a survey of birthweights of different geographic and ethnic groups Meredith (1970) showed that American Indians of the Cheyenne Tribe had mean birthweights of 3700 grams as contrasted with offspring of the Lumi Tribe in New Guinea with mean birthweights of 2400 grams. The high birthweight of the American Indian infants had a favorable effect on neonatal mortality. In a group surveyed by Norris and Shipley (1971), it was found that neonatal mortality was the same as for American whites, even though postnatal Indian mortality was 3 to 4 times that of the rest of the US population.

An unexplained genetic influence on birthweight is the effect of the Y chromosome. Males weigh approximately 200 grams more than females at term. Ounsted (1970) has suggested that the difference in birthweight between males and females is due to the larger male placenta caused by the antigenic dissimilarity between the mother and the male fetus. In mixed multiple pregnancies, the presence of a male fetus enhances the rate of fetal growth of the female twin. However, an indirect effect of testosterone on placental growth is also a possibility.

Growth retardation is frequently found in infants with congenital malformations, and the association of chromosome disorders with decreased growth potential is well appreciated. McKeown et al. (1976) for example, have shown that at all gestational ages, infants with Down's syndrome had lower weights than normal single births suggesting an association of the abnormal karyotype with decreased potential for fetal growth.

Environmental influences on fetal growth

A final common pathway for a variety of environmental influences on fetal growth is low birthweight. There may be considerable interaction between genetic and environmental influences on growth as for example, the lower birthweights observed in multiple pregnancies. Litter size is influenced genetically and products of multiple pregnancy may have nutritional constraints on growth during the latter part of pregnancy. McKeown et al. (1976) have shown that an increase in the number of fetuses in a given human pregnancy reduces the rate of growth. They have suggested that the human uterus normally functions at or below its capacity to support maximal growth so that any increase in litter size may constrain growth. If such is the case, maternal medical factors or environmental influences may easily exert a restrictive influence on growth during late pregnancy when nutrient supply becomes even more critical. In species such as the sheep which frequently produce twins, the uterus has sufficient reserve so that twin pregnancies are associated with little or no growth retardation.

Ounsted and Ounsted (1966) have suggested that the rate of intrauterine growth in a growth retarded fetus may be limited by a predetermined maternal regulator. Data supporting this hypothesis is that in any given sibship, newborn weights tend to be relatively constant. Further evidence for such a regulator is the absence of placental abnormalities in low birthweight newborn infants included in this survey (Ounsted, 1966). The placentas were significantly smaller than normal by weight but showed no clear morphologic abnormality suggesting that maternal regulation rather than nutritional or environmental influences were responsible for growth retardation in this population examined. The influence of such a maternal regulator may be multigenerational. Mothers with growth retarded infants have a significantly lower mean birthweight themselves than do mothers of normally grown infants.

Further support for a multigenerational influence on growth regulation is work reported by Stewart (1973) showing that more than one generation is required to rehabilitate a nutritionally deprived rat colony. These studies emphasize the long-term implications of nutritional deprivation in a high risk population. Such regulation may be an adaptive mechanism that has survival benefit to the species when food supply becomes restrictive.

Fetal environment and nutrition

Among the most important influences on fetal growth are restrictions on substrate flow to the fetus caused either by inadequate maternal nutrition or by restriction of nutrient flow to the placenta and fetus. In general the more a mother gains during a pregnancy, the larger will be the baby (Alexander and Downes, 1953). While the optimal amount of maternal weight gain during pregnancy has not been determined, the Committee on Maternal Nutrition of the National Academy of Science in the U.S.A. has recommended a weight gain of at least 25 pounds in previously well-nourished women (Proceedings of Workshop on Nutritional Supplementation on the Outcome of Pregnancy, 1973). Further data supporting a direct relationship between maternal nutrition and growth of the fetus is the striking decrease in birth-weight observed during the Dutch Famine of 1944–45. The overall drop in birthweight in a previously well-nourished population was about 200 grams (Smith, 1947). Winick (1976) has commented that this 200 gram decrease corresponds to the average birthweight differences found between rich and poor countries in the developed countries of the world. Children born during the siege of Leningrad showed an even more marked reduction in birthweight, about 400 grams. Other data showing a maternal nutritional effect is the increased birthweight observed in Japan over the past 3 decades (Gruenwald et al., 1967).

Roberts and Thomson (1976) have reported on the increase in birthweight with increasing parity in 44,000 newborns in Hong Kong. A progressive increase in birthweight with increasing parity is well recognized and may relate to development of a more favorable uterine bed with each pregnancy. Highest birthweights in the Hong Kong population were seen in the winter months, again possibly related to changes in maternal nutrition during the hotter months of the year.

Altitude is an additional environmental factor affecting birthweight. Infants born in the Peruvian Andes at 5000 meters altitude weighed 2.95 kg as compared with controls born at sea level who weighed 3.49 kg. Although maternal size and nutrition were less favorable in the high altitude group, placental weights were 60 g greater than at sea level; the combination of low birthweight and large placenta suggests a restrictive effect of altitude on fetal growth (Kruger and Arias-Stella, 1970). Similar data at high altitude have been collected in Lake County, Colo., USA (Howard et al., 1957).

Intrauterine infection can also cause low birthweight and impairment of cell and organ growth (Naeye and Blanc, 1965). This subject has been reviewed extensively and will not be considered here.

Since the fetus is ultimately dependent on substrates delivered via the utero-placental circulation, decreases in uterine blood flow or in the transport properties of the placenta will restrict nutrient flow to the fetus and limit and restrict growth.

Considerable information has been gained through the use of models for intrauterine growth retardation in which there is restriction of substrate flow to the fetus. Wigglesworth (1964) has created such a model by ligating the distal end of the uterine artery in one of the uterine horns of the pregnant rat. The fetuses close to the point of ligation showed growth restriction with decreases in weight, protein, DNA and RNA whereas those closest to an intact circulation showed normal growth. Hill (1974) and his colleagues have created a model of placental insufficiency by removing a segment of the placenta in pregnant monkies. A marked reduction in organ weight, as well as reduced muscle mass and fat content was observed in newborns at term. While there were decreases in wet weight, DNA, RNA and protein in cerebellum, the cerebrum showed only minimal changes, again reflecting a relative sparing of brain growth as found in other species. In a model developed by Alexander (1964), surgical reduction in the number of carnucles of the sheep uterus resulted in a reduction of placental weight and fetal size at term. Growth retardation has also been reported following unilateral ovariectomy in the rat which results in an increased fetal number in the remaining uterine horn with resultant crowding and nutrient restriction. In most of these models there is relative sparing of brain growth with marked reductions in the ratio of liver to brain weight.

The sparing of brain growth may relate to a redistribution of fetal blood flow to the brain during hypoxic or nutritional insult to the fetus (Assali and Brinkman, 1973). In low birthweight, the placenta itself may reflect abnormalities of utero-placental blood flow and maternal nutritional state. Aherne and Dunnill (1966) found placental blood volumes of 350 ml in small for gestational age infants as compared with 480 ml in placentas of normal fullterm pregnancies. Laga et al. (1972) showed marked reductions in trophoblastic mass and decreases in villous surface area in placentas from a poorly nourished Guatamalan population, further suggesting that severe malnutrition may influence placental transport properties.

Drug effects on growth

Examples of drug effects on the fetus are the association of low birthweight with cigarette smoking (Rush and Kass, 1972), heroin use, (Zelson et al., 1971) and in infants of alcoholic mothers. Although there were early reports that infants of alcoholic mothers exhibited mental retardation (MacNicoll, 1905), it is only recently that the constellation of features known as the fetal alcohol syndrome has been widely recognized (Jones et al., 1973). These infants show intrauterine growth retardation, a rather striking developmental delay and characteristic craniofacial and other abnormalities. While cigarette smoking in pregnancy has been associated with low birthweight, a recent report by Davies et al. (1976) has suggested that a large part of the growth deficiency observed among cigarette smoking mothers is related to decreased food intake in the smoking population rather than uteroplacental insufficiency.

Hormonal regulation of growth

During the initial period of pregnancy, growth and development occurs largely in the absence of secretions of endocrine glands. By about the 100th day of development, the fetus will begin to produce hormones such as insulin and thyroxin which influence metabolic and phenotypic differentiation. The peptide hormones produced by the placenta are present from the time of implantation; however, clear evidence of direct effects of these hormones on fetal growth is lacking. Human placental lactogen may have an indirect effect on fetal growth through its stimulation of maternal lipolysis (Grumbach et al., 1968). The increase in maternal free fatty acids may spare maternal glucose utilization and make glucose more available for uteroplacental transport in support of fetal growth and metabolism. Kim and Felig (1971) showed an increase in maternal concentrations of placental lactogen in response to short-term starvation in mid-pregnancy, suggesting a feedback system when maternal caloric intake is restricted.

Insulin has been of considerable interest to those concerned with fetal growth. The presence of somatic hypertrophy in poorly regulated infants of diabetic mothers has long suggested a direct effect of insulin on fetal growth. Infants of diabetic mothers do not appear to be overgrown prior to the 28th week of gestation. As is the case for other hormones, insulin may affect fetal growth only after certain critical developmental periods have been achieved (Cardell, 1953). There are considerable data supporting a direct effect of insulin on late fetal growth. Ashworth et al. (1973) demonstrated a linear relationship between fetal weight and in vitro insulin secretion by human fetal pancreases obtained at 15–24 weeks' gestation. Picon (1967) showed that injection of insulin into rat fetuses produces overgrowth and obesity similar to that seen in human newborns of diabetic mothers. Again these effects were only observed at the end of gestation in the rat. Clark et al. (1968) demonstrated that insulin injected into rat fetuses before 17 days of gestation failed to increase incorporation of ^{14}C-glucose into lipids, carbohydrates and proteins whereas a significant effect was observed with insulin injection after that time. The development of insulin responsiveness possibly relates to the appearance of surface receptors for insulin on cell membranes (Blazquez et al., 1976). Further evidence for a direct effect of insulin on growth are reports of decreased fetal growth in congenitally diabetic infants (Sherwood et al., 1974; Liggens, 1974). Effects of insulin on fetal growth may relate more to stimulation of protein synthesis than of glucose transport itself. Grasso et al. (1968) showed that although amino acids result in a brisk discharge of insulin from the premature pancreas, glucose is a poor stimulator of insulin secretion.

Similar to insulin, thyroxin does not seem to be required for expression of early morphogenic potential. The hormone is, however, critical for normal development, particularly that of the central nervous system during late gestation. Deficiency of thyroxin is associated with hypoplasia of neural elements (Eayrs, 1955; Geel and Timiras, 1967) and with decreased brain myelination (Walravens and Chase, 1969). The decreased cell number in hypothyroidism appears to be related to a slower rate of cell proliferation. More recently, Erenberg et al. (1974) have investigated growth and development of the thyroidectomized ovine fetus. The results show that thyroid hormone deficiency during the last trimester of gestation in the sheep fetus impairs lung growth, delays bone and skin maturation, inhibits myelination of the central nervous system and limits cell growth in a variety of other tissues. The demonstrated effect on lung growth may have relevance to human disease in view of the report of Cuestas et al. (1976) showing a higher incidence of hypothyroidism in infants developing the respiratory distress syndrome of the newborn. Thyroxin thus appears to have effects on multiple systems and important influences on lung and brain development. Its presence is important for the timing of normal cell maturation and development of certain metabolic functions.

Growth factors

Potentially important but largely unexplored influences on fetal growth are those possibly mediated by a number of recently described growth factors. These factors include the somatomedins, epidermal growth factor, nerve growth factor and fibroblastic growth factor. A common property of these proteins is their ability to bind with high specific activity to plasma membranes of target cells.

Salmon and Daughaday (1957) first reported that growth hormone stimulated the in vitro incorporation of labeled sulfate by cartilage by inducing a secondary substance measurable in serum. This substance first called sulfation factor was later characterized as somatomedin. It has been demonstrated that perfusion of rat liver in vivo with growth hormone is accompanied by production of a somatomedin-like factor in the medium (McConaghey, 1972). Somatomedin activity can also be obtained from other tissues such as muscle and kidney. The factor stimulates growth of a number of different cell types. Recently, Gluckman and Brinsmead (1976) demonstrated that somatomedin levels rose with gestational age and showed a positive correlation with birthweight, length and head circumference. Infants in their series with renal agenesis had normal levels of somatomedin suggesting that the kidney is not an important source of somatomedin in the fetus.

Fibroblast growth factor, a polypeptide isolated from bovine pituitary gland by Gospodarowicz (1974), has also been shown to enhance proliferation of a variety of cell lines even when cells exhibit density-dependent inhibition of growth. This may also play a role as a neurotrophic factor in amphibian limb regeneration and may also have a role in cell and organ growth in human development.

The biological and chemical properties of epidermal growth factor have been extensively examined by Cohen and his colleagues (Taylor et al., 1972). This factor, isolated from extracts of the submaxillary gland of the male mouse, induces precocious opening of the eyelids and premature eruption of teeth when injected into newborn mice (Cohen, 1962). Administration of high concentrations of epidermal growth factor resulted in decreased growth of newborn mice suggesting that the maturational enhancement seen after its administration is associated with restricted growth.

Nerve growth factor first described by Levi-Montalcini and Hamburger (1953) is important for the development and maintainance of sensory and sympathetic neurons. The hormone binds to the target cell plasma membranes and has biological properties similar to insulin with which it shares structural similarities (Hogue-Angeletti et al., 1975).

These factors may exert important synergistic influences on growth and may be important in the causation of abnormal growth. Investigation of somatomedin and other growth factors in development may well provide important clues to the regulation of growth in the low birthweight infant and the adaptive mechanisms leading to small size.

This survey has covered clinical, epidemiologic, environmental, genetic and biological aspects of low birthweight. Only through multidisciplinary approaches ranging from studies of population influences to biological investigations of regulation of cell growth will continued progress be made in eliminating this most serious and important developmental defect of low birthweight.

REFERENCES

Aherne, W. and Dunnill, M. S. (1966): *Brit. med. Bull., 22,* 5.
Alexander, G. (1964): *J. Reprod. Fertil., 7,* 289.
Alexander, S. A. and Downes, J. T. III (1953): *Amer. J. Obstet. Gynec., 66,* 1161.
Ashworth, M. A., Leach, F. N. and Milner, R. D. G. (1973): *Arch. Dis. Childh., 48,* 151.
Assali, N. S. and Brinkman, C. R. III (1973): *Amer. J. Obstet. Gynec., 117,* 643.
Blazquez, E., Rubalcava, B., Montesano, R., Lelio, O. and Unger, R. H. (1976): *Endocrinology, 98,* 1014.
Campbell, S. (1974): *Clin. Obstet. Gynaec., 1,* 41.
Campbell, S., Wladimiroff, J. W. and Dewhurst, C. J. (1973): *J. Obstet. Gynaec. Brit. Cwlth, 80,* 680.
Cardell, B. S. (1953): *J. Obstet. Gynaec. Brit. Cwlth, 60,* 834.
Clark Jr, C. M., Cahill, G. F. and Soeldner, J. S. (1968): *Diabetes, 17,* 362.
Cohen, S. (1962): *J. biol. Chem., 237,* 1555.
Cohen, S., Carpenter, G. and Lembach, K. J. (1975): *Advanc. metab. Disorders, 8,* 265.
Cuestas, R. A., Lindall, A. and Engel, R. R. (1976): *New Engl. J. Med., 295,* 6.
Dancis, J., O'Connell, J. and Holt Jr, L. (1948): *J. Pediat., 33,* 570.
Dancis, J. and Schneider, H., (1975): In: *The Placenta and its Maternal Supply Line,* p. 95. Editor: P. Gruenwald. University Park Press, Baltimore.
Davies, D. P., Gray, O. P., Ellwood, P. C. and Abernethy, M. (1976): *Lancet, 1,* 385.
Dickenson, J. W. T., Merat, A. and Widdowson, E. M. (1971): *Biol. Neonate, 19,* 354.
Dobbing, J. and Sands, J. (1973): *Arch. Dis. Childh., 48,* 757.
Drillien, C. M. (1974): *Clin. Perinatol., 1,* 197.
Eayrs, J. T. (1955): *Acta anat. (Basel), 25,* 160.
Enesco, M. and LeBlond, C. P. (1962): *J. Embryol. exp. Morphol., 10,* 530.
Ehrenberg, A., Omori, K., Menkes, J. H., Oh, W. and Fisher, D. A. (1974): *Pediat. Res., 8,* 783.
Geel, S. E. and Timiras, P. S. (1967): *Brain Res., 4,* 135.
Gluckman, P. D. and Brinsmead, M. W. (1976): *J. clin. Endocr., 43,* 1378.
Gohari, P., Berkowitz, R. L. and Hobbins, J. C. (1976): *Amer. J. Obstet. Gynec., 127,* 255.
Gospodarowicz, D. (1974): *Nature (Lond.), 294,* 123.
Grasso, S., Saproprito, N., Messina, A. and Restano, G. (1968): *Lancet, 2,* 735.
Grumbach, M. M., Kaplan, S. L., Sciarra, J. J. et al: (1968): *Ann. N.Y. Acad. Sci., 148,* 501.
Gruenwald, P., Funakawa, H., Mitani, S., Nishimura, T. and Takeuchi, S. (1967): *Lancet, 1,* 1026.
Hall, K. and Olin, P. (1972): *Acta endocr., 69,* 417.
Hill, D. E. (1974): In: *Size at Birth,* p. 99. Editors: K. Elliott and J. Knight. Elsevier, Amsterdam.
Hill, D. E., Myers, R. E., Holt, A. B., Scott, R. E. and Cheek, D. B. (1971): *Biol. Neonate, 19,* 68.
Hogue-Angeletti, R. A., Bradshaw, R. A. and Frazier, W. A. (1975): *Advanc. metab. Disorders, 8,* 285.
Howard, R. L., Lichty, J. A. and Bruns, P. D. (1957): *Amer. J. Dis. Childh., 93,* 670.
Jones, K. L., Smith, D. W., Ulleland, C. N. and Streissguth, P. A. (1973): *Lancet, 1,* 1267.
Kim, Y. J. and Felig, P. (1971): *J. clin. Endocr., 32,* 864.
Kruger, H. and Arias-Stella, J. (1970): *Amer. J. Obstet. Gynec., 106,* 586.
Kushinksy, S. and Chi, D. (1973): *Obstet. and Gynec., 41,* 343.
Laga, E. M., Driscoll, S. G. and Munroe, H. N. (1972): *Pediatrics, 50,* 33.
Laga, G. and Cassady, G. (1971): *Amer. J. Obstet. Gynec., 109,* 615.
Levi-Montalcini, R. and Hamburger, V. (1953): *J. exp. Zool., 123,* 233.
Liggins, G. C. (1974): In: *Size at Birth,* p. 165. Editors: K. Elliott and J. Knight. Elsevier, Amsterdam.
Longo, L. D. (1972): In: *Disorders of Placental Function, Vol. 1,* p. 2. Editor: N. S. Sahling. Academic Press, New York.
Low, J. A., Boston, R. W. and Pancham, S. R. (1972): *Amer. J. Obstet. Gynec., 113,* 351.
Low, J. A. and Galbraith, R. S. (1974): *Obstet. and Gynec., 44,* 122.
MacNicoll, T. A. (1905): *Quart. J. Inebriety, 27,* 113.

McConaghey, P. (1972): *J. Endocr.*, *52*, 1.

McKeown, T., Marshall, T. and Record, R. G. (1976): *J. Reprod. Fertil.*, *47*, 167.

Meridith, P. V. (1970): *Human Biol.*, *42*, 217.

Naeye, R. L. and Blanc, W. (1965): *J. Amer. med. Ass.*, *194*, 1277.

Norris, F. D. and Shipley, P. W. (1971): *HSMHA Hlth Rep.*, *86*, 810.

Oh, W. and Omori, K. (1975): *Amer. J. Obstet. Gynec.*, *122*, 316.

Ounsted, C. (1970): *Lancet*, *2*, 857.

Ounsted, M. (1971): In: *Recent Advances in Paediatrics*, p. 2. Editors: D. Gairdner and D. Hull. Churchill, London.

Ounsted, M. and Ounsted, C. (1966): *Nature (Lond.)*, *212*, 995.

Picon, L. (1967): *Endocrinology*, *81*, 1419.

Proceedings, Workshop on Nutritional Supplementation on the Outcome of Pregnancy (1973): National Academy of Science, Washington, D.C.

Ravelli, G. P., Stein, Z. A. and Susser, M. V. (1976): *New Engl. J. Med.*, *295*, 353.

Roberts, D. F. and Thomson, A. M. (1976): In: *The Biology of Human Fetal Growth*, p. 267. Editors: D. F. Roberts and A. M. Thomson. Halsted Press, New York.

Rush, D. and Kass, E. H. (1972): *Amer. J. Epidemiol.*, *96*, 183.

Salmon Jr, W. D. and Daughaday, W. H. (1957): *J. Lab. clin. Med.*, *49*, 825.

Scott, K. E. and Usher, R. (1966): *Amer. J. Obstet. Gynec.*, *94*, 951.

Shelley, H. J. and Neligan, G. A. (1966): *Brit. med. Bull.*, *22*, 34.

Sherwood, W. G., Chance, G. W. and Hill, D. E. (1974): *Pediat. Res.*, *8*, 360.

Smith, C. A. (1947): *Pediatrics*, *530*, 229.

Southgate, D. A. T. and Hey, E. N. (1976): In: *The Biology of Human Fetal Growth*, p. 195. Editors: D. F. Roberts and A. M. Thomson. Halsted Press, New York.

Spellacy, W. N. and Cohn, J. E. (1973): *Obstet. and Gynec.*, *42*, 330.

Stewart, R. J. C. (1973): *Nutr. Rep. Int.*, *7*, 487.

Taylor, J. M., Mitchell, W. M. and Cohen, S. (1972): *J. biol. Chem.*, *247*, 5928.

Thomson, A. M. (1970): *Amer. J. Dis. Child.*, *120*, 398.

Urrusti, J., Yoshida, P., Velasco, L., Frenk, S., Rosado, A., Sosa, A., Morales, M., Yoshida, T. and Metcoff, J. (1972): *Pediatrics*, *50*, 4.

Van De Brande, J. L., Van Buul, S., Heinrich, U., Van Roon, F., Zurcher, T. and Van Steirtegem, A. C. (1974): *Advanc. metab. Disorders*, *8*, 171.

Walravens, P. and Chase, H. P. (1969): *J. Neurochem.*, *16*, 1477.

Westermark, B. and Wasteson, A. (1975): *Advanc. metab. Disorders*, *890*, 19.

Warshaw, J. B. (1972): *Develop. Biol.*, *28*, 537.

Widdowson, E. M., Crabb, D. E. and Milner, R. D. G. (1972): *Arch. Dis. Child.*, *47*, 665.

Wigglesworth, J. S. (1964): *J. Path. Bact.*, *81*, 1.

Williams, P. R., Fisher Jr, R. H., Sperling, M. A. and Oh, W. (1975): *New Engl. J. Med.*, *292*, 612.

Winick, M. E. (1970): *Fed. Proc.*, *29*, 1510.

Winick, M. A. (1976): In: *Prevention of Embryonic Fetal and Perinatal Disease*, p. 97. Editors: R. L. Brent and M. I. Harris. Fogarty International Center Series on Preventive Medicine, Vol. 3. DHEW Publication Number (NIH) 76-853.

Winick, M. and Rosso, P. (1969): *Pediat. Res.*, *3*, 181.

Wladimiroff, J. W. and Campbell, S. (1974): *Lancet*, *1*, 151.

Zelson, C., Estrellita, R. and Wasserman, E. (1971): *Pediatrics*. *48*, 178.

The high risk pregnancy
with particular reference to birth defects

R. A. H. KINCH

Department of Obstetrics and Gynaecology, McGill University and Montreal General Hospital, Montreal, Canada

A major concern of modern obstetrics is the concept of the 'high risk pregnancy' which evolved from the identification of those factors which were associated with increased fetal morbidity and mortality. This was a natural evolution from historical paramount concern with the prevention of maternal mortality which has almost reached an irreducible minimum. It appears that 15–20% of the obstetrical population give rise to 70–80% of perinatal morbidity and mortality. Consequently the concept of the 'high risk pregnancy' was devised as a rescue operation for those fetuses in an actual or potentially morbid or even lethal situation. This has led to regionalization of delivery of these high risk pregnant women in well-equipped obstetrical units with intramural neonatal intensive care units.

In a symposium on birth defects, this strict definition of high risk pregnancy clearly does not apply. However, it is the aim of this conference to attempt to prevent the 25% of this perinatal loss wich is due to congenital malformations. Up until now this group has been written off as non-preventable.

For this reason technological advances for rescuing the high risk fetus, such as fetal monitoring, do not come into the scope of this discussion. However, 2 techniques specifically devoted to detection of birth defects early enough to allow for safe therapeutic termination of pregnancy must be mentioned. The first is the use of ultrasound monitoring for neural tube defects. The optimum time for scanning is between the 15th and 17th week. Campbell (1977) maintains that all cases of dorsal lumbar spina bifida can be detected. There is difficulty in defining spina bifida in the lumbosacral region. The advantage of this method is that it can detect the closed spina bifida by a non-invasive technique.

The second technique is fetoscopy. Patrick et al. (1974, 1976) have described our technique and point out that the method allows direct observation of the fetus and placenta, giving opportunity to observe obvious congenital defects, to take blood from the placental vessels and carry out skin biopsy of the fetus. Ultimately it might be possible to inject blood or medications into the fetus. Blood sampling is successful in 60–80% of cases, depending on the location of the placenta. Fetal skin biopsy, however, according to Benzie and Doran (1975), does not culture as successfully as a biopsy of fetal amnion. With this instrument fetal complications appear to be low, the main problem is fetal or placental hemorrhage and premature labour. At this moment it is still in the experimental stage and may be superseded by fetal biopsy under ultrasound direction.

As a clinician trying to follow the ways of sophisticated basic scientists who move with practiced ease amongst the complexity of molecular biology, who do not only see a cell as a world but also are familiar with its intricate workings, with the analysis, function and mechanism of construction and repair of genes and chromosomes, I listen fascinated with the technology of this microcosmic world and speculate about how this knowledge can be applied by a clinician to the care of those high risk non-pregnant or pregnant patients predisposed to birth defects. The resounding message is that the cell, the chromosome, and the gene are all very tender and, in the early phases following conception and particularly during morphogenesis, can be easily damaged.

Dr. Barton Childs in his superb keynote address spoke of studying the attitudes of patients and doctors to various problems in this field. The most important attitudinal change is to turn the 'rescueing' physician into a 'preventing' physician and instead of saving the patients after the catastrophe has occurred, preventing the catastrophe from occurring. This is a very trite remark but to change physicians' attitudes in any area is still difficult. Rescue is exciting; prevention is boring.

The preventive approach to the high risk pregnancy has been greatly improved in the last decade. However, as yet, the same service is not given to the high risk sperm and the high risk ovum and the process of fertilization is almost totally unsupervised and often an unplanned event. Even now, 44% of babies delivered are unplanned and 15% are unwanted.

How should the clinician and his patient be influenced? The answer is in the content of this Conference. Mass screening for genetic defects is well developed in many centers and often in a more advanced stage than clinical genetic counselling. In many cases, genetic counselling is carried out after the tragic event of a baby with a birth defect so this is very often applied as therapy for both parents and doctor. More stress should be given to preconceptual genetic counselling, individually or in groups, particularly in such common situations as the young, newly married diabetic patient.

Both the patient and physician are aware of the dangers of rubella infection during pregnancy. Although there are certain hazards to rubella vaccination, this should be carried out more consistently. A simple precaution is to take blood in early pregnancy and keep it in reserve for determining rubella titers should the patient have an accidental exposure during the vulnerable phase of pregnancy. This should be as routine as Rh typing and of course can be done at the same time. Although diagnostic X-rays may not produce sufficient dosage to risk birth defects in the embryo and fetus, it is a simple precaution to make sure that diagnostic radiological procedures involving relatively heavy dosage of irradiation should be carried out prior to ovulation.

The physician should be very acutely aware of when he is possibly endangering the environment of the early embryo. Three obvious examples will suffice. In this Conference, Janerich has emphasized the sensible advice that patients should wait 3–4 months following discontinuation of oral contraceptive medication before attempting to get pregnant. This advice is still often not heeded either by physician or patient.

Boué and Boué (1975) point out that there is an increased incidence of abortion associated with chromosomal anomalies following stimulation of ovulation using human menopausal gonadotrophin, human chorionic gonadotrophin and Climiphene citrate. This increased incidence lasts for 2 cycles and to quote, 'the indications of induction of ovulation should be considered carefully especially in the cases of women with previous abortions. A prospective study of 473 women has shown that such therapy may increase the risk of having a conceptus with chromosomal anomalies'.

Finally, the persistence of physicians who use a progesterone or progestational steroid withdrawal test for pregnancy diagnosis must be discouraged. Levy et al. (1973) and Janerich point out that following the use of progestational steroids as a pregnancy test, the pregnancy may be at risk for an increased incidence of cardiac anomalies.

Patients' work habits must be studied. Miller *(This Volume)* points out the danger of noxious fumes, pollutants, etc. Smith (1974), and Yeager (1973) have emphasized the increased risk of abortion and of congenital anomalies, and stillbirths experienced by female anesthetists.

To be an effective counsellor, the obstetrician must have all this information and use it.

The thalidomide disaster of 1961, although producing the tragic consequences of phocomelia for many young children and their families, undoubtedly saved many more from drug-induced birth defects. This well-publicized tragedy, at least in North America, has resulted in 2 beneficial effects. Firstly, it is almost impossible to persuade any woman to take any drug for nausea and vomiting in early pregnancy or in fact for anything in early pregnancy. Secondly, it completely stopped the procedure of sending unsolicited free samples of drugs to physicians. This latter practice encouraged physicians to hand out samples of recently heavily detailed drugs. This attitude of the patients towards drugs in early pregnancy should certainly be reinforced by the obstetrician.

It takes a jolt like the thalidomide tragedy to convince most people in our contemporary society of the need for closer drug supervision in pregnancy. To quote Allan Barnes (1968), 'they, as well as their physicians, seem to regard life as a drug-deficient disease to be cured or even endured only with the aid of innumerable medications'. It can therefore be seen that in contemporary society the fetus is always at risk. People do not recognize when they are exposing themselves and their fetus to possible chemical injury. The proposed cure is to move the obstetrician from the place of rescue to a place of prevention; that he should be the fetal pediatrician and educate the child-bearing public to a sensible attitude to drug taking and pre-pregnancy planning.

Complete safety from untoward drug effects can only be obtained by therapeutic nihilism in the child-bearing age for women between the ages of 14 and 45. To ensure safety to all is to deny therapy to any; therefore every drug must be medically indicated and the therapeutic value must be weighed against possible adverse effects before and after birth. Patients under treatment for chronic diseases, i.e. epilepsy, must be carefully scrutinized for the teratogenic effects of the drugs they are taking.

However, even with this sensible advice, one must remember that most pregnancies are still unplanned. Pregnancies happen to women taking drugs more often than drugs are taken by women who are pregnant. Patients rarely see their doctors until they are 3 months pregnant when organogenesis is complete and the damage has been done. It is an interesting fact that patients desirous of abortion nearly always manage to reach an obstetrician before 6 weeks of pregnancy. At present we are engaged in studying this motivation and perhaps future birth defects conferences should have a section on the 'Madison Avenue' approach to physician and patient education. Physicians are still reticent to use the television medium for education of patient and doctor but maybe the day for one to one educational or genetic consultation is nearly over and intelligent use of the media could perhaps be more emphasized. However, in certain cases such as smoking and alcohol, the ear thus bombarded does not listen and we come again to Dr. Childs important question: 'why?'.

The future must see better methods of drug testing, a registry of congenital malformations, improved reporting of possible drug effects to enable rapid detection of epidemics of congenital anomalies and increased knowledge of fetal pharmacology, all of which should guard the future from the mistakes of the past.

REFERENCES

Barnes, A. C. (1968): In: *Intrauterine Development*. Editor: A. C. Barnes. Lea and Febiger, Philadelphia.
Benzie, R. J. and Doran, T. A. (1975): *Amer. J. Obstet. Gynec., 121*, 460.
Boué, J. G. and Boué, A. (1975): In: *Physiology and Genetics of Reproduction*. Editors: E. M. C. Coutinho and F. Fuchs. Plenum Press, New York.
Campbell, S. (1977): *Clin. Obstet. Gynec., 20*, 351.
Levy, E. P., Cohen, A. and Fraser, F. Clarke (1973): *Lancet, 7803/1*, 611.
Patrick, J. E. (1976): *Clin. Obstet. Gynec., 19*, 909.
Patrick, J. E., Perry, T. B. and Kinch, R. A. H. (1974): *Amer. J. Obstet. Gynec., 119/4*, 539.
Smith, B. E. (1974): *Clin. Obstet. Gynec., 17*, 145.
Yeager, J. W. (1973): *J. occup. Med., 15*, 724.

Alphafetoprotein and the prenatal diagnosis of neural tube defects*

D. J. H. BROCK

Department of Human Genetics, University of Edinburgh, Western General Hospital, Edinburgh, United Kingdom

The neural tube defects, of which anencephaly and spina bifida cystica are the most common, are a group of congenital malformations showing a remarkable geographical variation. The highest incidence is found in the British Isles where the overall rate is about 4 per 1000 births. Intermediate rates are found in other parts of Europe and North America and low rates are experienced in Africa, Asia and South America. Nonetheless, in most populations the neural tube defects are among the more common of the serious birth malformations. Despite intense investigation their causation remains obscure, though both genetic and environmental factors have been suggested (Carter, 1976). Approaches to the prevention of spina bifida and anencephaly have been consistently foiled by the inability to locate any of the major factors responsible, and it has been necessary to confront the problem by a manifestly second-best solution, namely the early prenatal recognition and selective abortion of affected fetuses.

Before the advent of serum alphafetoprotein screening, recognition of pregnancies with an increased risk of bearing a child with a neural tube defect depended upon empirical studies. A number of categories of family history suggesting increased risk have now been identified (Table 1). These are largely based on British data where

TABLE 1

Empirical risk of neural tube defect (NTD) in various family situations

Family history	Risk (%)	Reference
One child with NTD	5	Carter et al., 1968
Two children with NTD	10	Carter and Roberts, 1967
Three children with NTD	21	Smith, 1973
Parent with NTD	4.5	Carter, 1976
One child with multiple vertebral anomalies	5	Wynne-Davies, 1975
One child with spina dysraphism	4	Carter et al., 1976

*The work reported here was supported by a grant from the Medical Research Council.

birth incidences are high and should be modified for countries where incidences are lower. Indeed preliminary data from the United States of America suggest that the recurrence risk for a mother who has had one affected child with a neural tube defect is nearer to 1 % than the 5 % shown in Table 1 (Holmes et al., 1976; Milunsky and Alpert, 1976).

AMNIOTIC FLUID STUDIES

Alphafetoprotein

The value of measuring amniotic fluid alphafetoprotein (AFP) concentrations in the early prenatal diagnosis of both anencephaly and open spina bifida was discovered about 5 years ago (Brock and Sutcliffe, 1972, 1973; Brock and Scrimgeour, 1972). The first prospective diagnoses were reported soon thereafter (Lorber et al., 1973; Seller et al., 1973; Allan et al., 1973). The technique rapidly passed into routine clinical usage and is now an important part of the armentarium of laboratories offering prenatal diagnostic services.

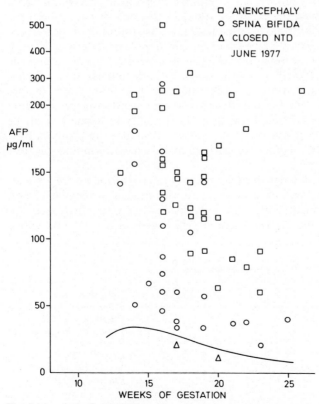

Fig. 1. Amniotic fluid AFP concentrations in neural tube defects. Prospective diagnoses in author's laboratory to June 1977.

AFP concentrations in amniotic fluids from pregnancies where the fetus has a neural tube defect are usually very high indeed (Fig. 1). Anencephalic values tend to be higher than those in spina bifida (Brock et al., 1975a), in accordance with the theory that the protein leaks from the lesion into the surrounding fluid (Brock, 1976a). If 'rocket' electrophoresis is the assay method used, neural tube defects often reveal themselves as open peaks, making precise quantitation largely redundant (Fig. 2). However, less clear-cut, but nonetheless abnormal values may sometimes be observed with small, open spina bifidas (Laurence et al., 1975; Henry and Robinson, 1977).

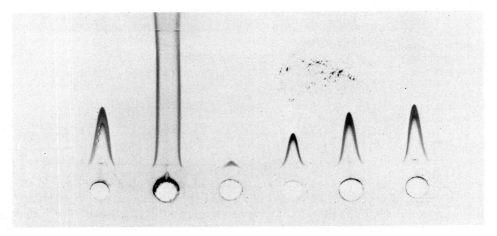

Fig. 2. Rocket immunoelectrophoresis of amniotic fluid AFP. Open-topped rocket indicates a neural tube defect.

Amniotic fluid AFP will not allow the detection of all types of neural tube defect. This was first pointed out by Laurence et al. (1973) who reported a large, slack occipital encephalocele with a normal amniotic fluid AFP value at 16 weeks. There is now a general belief that a closed neural tube defect will not be detectable through assay of AFP in amniotic fluid. It is not yet clear what proportion of the total number of cases of neural tube defects are represented by the closed lesions. It is generally reckoned at between 5 and 10% (Laurence, 1974), though studies on maternal serum AFP suggest that it may be substantially larger. It is also not yet clear how serious these failures will be. Many will be represented by the comparatively harmless meningocele spina bifidas, but as Laurence (1974) has pointed out, encephaloceles and small, skin-covered myelocele spina bifidas are serious disorders, and may cause great distress to mothers who were expecting to be protected against the birth of a child with a neural tube defect.

Measurements of amniotic fluid AFP have been criticised on the grounds of their relative non-specificity, it being suggested that the association of other fetal conditions with raised values compromises the usefulness of this diagnostic tool. A close inspection of the reported facts do not entirely support this criticism. It must be remembered that the objective of AFP analysis is to make diagnoses early enough in pregnancy to permit termination should the fetus be shown to be abnormal.

TABLE 2

Fetal abnormalities where elevated amniotic fluid AFP concentrations may be found[a]

Probable
    Anencephaly
    Spina bifida (open)
    Intrauterine death
    Congenital nephrosis
    Exomphalos (omphalocele)
    Sacrococcygeal teratoma

Possible
    Turner's syndrome
    Duodenal atresia
    Esophageal atresia
    Polycystic kidneys
    Hydrocephalus
    Fallot's tetralogy
    Pilonidal sinus
    Annular pancreas
    Congenital skin defects

---

[a]Detailed references in Brock (1977).

Thus the observation that amniotic fluid AFP is raised in Fallot's tetralogy in the third trimester of pregnancy (Seppala, 1975) has little bearing on the specificity of AFP assay until such conditions can be shown to be associated with an elevated value at or around the 16th week of pregnancy. A more valid comment relates to the variability of AFP elevations in many fetal conditions. Exomphalos (omphalocele) is a case in point. Both normal and raised AFP concentrations have been observed early in pregnancy and there is as yet no data on the correlation of the AFP value and the possible surgical repair of such lesions (Brock and Sutcliffe, 1973; Kunz and Schmid, 1976; Clarke et al., 1977). The conditions listed in Table 2 are thus arranged into those where AFP elevation is probable and those where it is possible.

A common source of apparent false positive amniotic fluid AFP values are those deriving from fluids contaminated with fetal blood. AFP levels in fetal serum parallel those in amniotic fluid quite closely, but with concentrations between 100- and 200-fold higher (Brock, 1974). This means that the admixture of a comparatively small amount of fetal blood with the amniotic fluid can increase the AFP value to a point where it mimics the values found in neural tube defects. Once this problem is recognised there is little difficulty in avoiding it. Current practice in many laboratories is to set aside an aliquot of whole amniotic fluid from any sample where there is visible blood contamination. Should the AFP value be elevated, the cell button is then examined for the presence of fetal red cells either by Kleihauer's test, or by electrophoresis which will show the characteristic band of hemoglobin F or by the use of commercially available antisera which are directed specifically against hemoglobin F. Contaminated samples with moderately raised AFP values which contain a major proportion of fetal blood may be rejected and a fresh amniocentesis called for. Alternatively an attempt may be made to calculate the expected contribution of AFP from fetal blood, by estimating the number of fetal erythrocytes in

TABLE 3

Effect of fetal blood contamination on amniotic fluid AFP

Gestation (weeks)	Mean fetal serum AFP (mg/ml)	Amniotic AFP, mean + 3 SD (μg/ml)	Addition due to 1% contamination (μg/ml)
14	2.7	18 + 14	14
15	2.5	17 + 16	13
16	2.3	14 + 14	12
17	2.1	12 + 16	11
18	1.9	10 + 12	10
19	1.7	10 + 16	9
20	1.5	6 + 10	8

1% contamination = 1×10^7 fetal RBC/ml AF.

the fluid and the mean level of AFP in fetal serum at the appropriate stage in gestation (Table 3).

When allowance has been made for fetal blood-contaminated samples it is still difficult to estimate the proportion of genuine false positives. As has been pointed out by Wald and Cuckle (1976) much depends on the accepted upper limit of the normal range. The limited data in Table 4 suggest that between 3 and 4 standard deviations above the mean for the gestational period is the critical point. The precise figure is of considerable importance in view of the fact that it is now widely recommended that all amniotic fluid samples should be subjected to AFP analysis, whatever the reason for amniocentesis. Since the most common indications for amniocentesis remain advanced maternal age or a previous history of chromosome abnormality, neural tube defects will be encountered infrequently in these samples. It is therefore of the greatest importance that the false positive rate in AFP assay be kept as low as possible lest more normal pregnancies than those in which the fetus has a neural tube defect be identified as abnormal.

TABLE 4

Cumulative false positive and false negative results in amniotic fluid AFP at various cut-off points

Cut-off in S.D. above mean	False positives	False negatives	
		Anencephaly	Open spina bifida
< 3	1500	0	0
3	4	0	1
4	0	0	4
5	0	0	5
6	0	0	5
7	0	0	6
8	0	0	8
9	0	0	12
10	0	0	17
Totals	1504	36	29

Amniotic fluid cell morphology

When amniotic fluid cells are plated out for in vitro culture, they adhere slowly and are usually left undisturbed for a period of days. Sutherland et al. (1973) observed that amniotic fluids from pregnancies in which the fetus had a neural tube defect contained a comparatively high proportion of cells which became firmly fixed to a glass or plastic surface in as little as 12 hours. They showed that the cells had the properties of macrophages and that they were fetal in origin. Sutherland et al. (1975) devised a simple counting procedure for the estimation of the cells and used it in the early identification of both anencephaly and spina bifida (Nelson et al., 1974). However, there were a number of false positives (large numbers of rapidly adhering cells in pregnancies which subsequently turned out to be normal), and this lack of specificity prevented quantitative macrophage estimation from being used as a primary method for the diagnosis of neural tube defects.

Recently Gosden and Brock (1977) have refined and extended the exploitation of the morphology of amniotic fluid cells in early prenatal diagnosis of congenital defects. The amended procedure described rapidly adherent (RA) cells as a proportion of the *viable* cells rather than of the *total* cells. In 12 amniotic fluids from anencephalic fetuses the proportion of RA cells ranged from 10% to 100% and in 8 fluids from fetuses with spina bifida the proportions ranged from 9% to 52%, while in 92 normal amniotic fluids the proportion of RA cells did not exceed 6%.

More importantly the morphological characteristics of RA cells were shown to be an important indicator of the nature of the fetal defect. Seven different types of cells were identified and tentatively named. In amniotic fluids from neural tube defects there were substantial proportions of long bipolar cells, cells with multiple filamentous processes, large vacuolated cells with inclusions and giant cells with multiple nuclei (Table 5). Though high proportions of RA cells were also observed when the placenta had been traversed, the morphology of these was quite distinct from those seen in neural tube defects and also different from those seen in a case of exomphalos (Gosden and Brock, 1977). This suggested the possibility that other types of fetal defect might be associated with special cells with distinctive morphology.

Further studies on RA cell morphology (Gosden et al., 1977) have shown that a majority of the distinctive types seen in amniotic fluids from neural tube defects originate from brain and spinal cord. This emphasises the importance of regarding any amniotic fluid containing long bipolar cells, cells with multiple processes, large vacuolated cells or giant cells with multiple nuclei as indicating a probable neural

TABLE 5

Range of RA cell types found in anencephaly and spina bifida

Condition	RA cell types			
	Long bipolar (%)	Multiple processes (%)	Vacuolated (%)	Multiple nuclei (%)
Anencephaly (12)	0–50	0–34	14–48	8–58
Spina bifida (8)	2–13	4–13	9–69	9–55

tube defect even when the amniotic fluid AFP is not greatly elevated. Brock and Gosden (1977) have described their experience in prenatal diagnosis in 2 cases where amniotic fluid AFP was marginally elevated. Though the AFP concentrations were virtually identical one fluid contained distinctive RA cells while the other was essentially free of anything but epithelioid-like cells. The former case lead to an infant with spina bifida while the latter was normal. RA cell morphology will also obviously be of some importance in diagnosing neural tube defects in amniotic fluids which are substantially contaminated with maternal and fetal blood.

Other parameters

Several other parameters have been suggested as being useful adjuncts to AFP in early prenatal diagnosis of neural tube defects. These include β-trace protein (Macri et al., 1974; Brock and Olsson, 1976), α_2-macroglobulin, IgM (Brock, 1975), fibrin and fibrinogen degradation products (Purdie et al., 1975), fibrinogen degradation fragment E (Gordon et al., 1976) and β-lipoprotein (Brock, 1976b). None of these has been shown to have adequate specificity and all suffer from the disadvantage that maternal blood contamination of the fluid distorts their values (Brock, 1977).

Screening for neural tube defects

Though the categories of mothers at increased risk of bearing children with neural tube defects are now well established (Table 1), complete ascertainment of these families would have a comparatively small impact on the overall incidence of the abnormalities. More than 90% of infants with anencephaly and spina bifida are born to mothers who have no previous history to suggest increased risk. Unless early amniocentesis were to become routine in all pregnancies (which given its uncertain risk to the fetus and the load that such a policy would throw on obstetrical services, seems unlikely) screening through amniotic fluid AFP assay is impossible. Likewise monitoring all pregnancies through a non-invasive technique like ultrasonography is not feasible. For the present, screening for spina bifida and anencephaly must depend on rapid chemical tests made in the maternal body fluids.

The possibility of *maternal serum* AFP measurements being used in screening for neural tube defects was predicted by Brock and Sutcliffe (1972). The first report of raised maternal serum AFP levels in pregnancies in which the fetuses had anencephaly was made by Hino et al. (1972), though only in the third trimester. A similar finding was made by Leek et al. (1973), again late in pregnancy. Of more relevance to prenatal diagnosis was the observation by Brock et al. (1973) of increased maternal serum AFP at 16 weeks and again at 21 weeks in a pregnancy, which after amniocentesis and confirmatory amniotic fluid AFP determination, was terminated to yield a fetus with anencephaly. Within a few months a number of papers appeared directed towards the assessment of this new diagnostic procedure (Harris et al., 1974; Seller et al., 1974; Brock et al., 1974, 1975b; Wald et al., 1974). All were guarded in their conclusions, but the general consensus was that measurement of maternal serum AFP would allow the early detection of some but by no means all cases of neural tube defects. It was clear that serum measurements were to be seen as a preliminary screen, and that wherever high values were found follow-up should include ultrasonar scan, amniocentesis and confirmatory amniotic fluid AFP determination. A workshop was convened in London to compare results and to discuss refinements to assay techniques (Editorial, 1974). It was decided to institute a collaborative study which by pooling of results might define the prospects and limitations of the AFP screening technique.

The Report of the UK Collaborative Study on Alphafetoprotein in Relation to Neural Tube Defects (1977) has been recently published. It is based on data from 19 participating laboratories and comprises serum AFP determination from 18,684 singleton pregnancies, 163 twin pregnancies without fetal neural tube defect, 146 pregnancies with anencephalic outcome, 142 with spina bifida outcome and 13 where the fetus had an encephalocele. Since absolute AFP values ranged widely from center to center, each laboratory reported its median AFP values and all values above the 90th percentile for normal singleton pregnancies within 3 week gestational periods. AFP values from neural tube defect and twin pregnancies could therefore be related to each laboratory's median value for that period of pregnancy, and results from all the laboratories pooled without the necessity of bringing them into absolute numerical agreement. Data was collected in 6 separate reporting periods, so that it was possible to monitor the results over time. A quality control survey was carried out at the same time which allowed an estimate of the proportion of variation in serum AFP levels which could be attributed to assay imprecision.

In this way it was possible to express each serum AFP value from a neural tube defect pregnancy as a multiple of the median value for the particular gestational period and also to determine its relationship to given percentiles of the normal range. In Table 6 the dectection efficiency (the proportion of cases lying on or above given percentiles) is shown for both anencephaly and open spina bifida. Detection efficiencies rise with increasing gestation though the data are not sufficiently extensive to indicate whether there is a statistically significant difference between the 16- to

TABLE 6

Numbers and proportions of singleton pregnancies with neural tube defects where maternal serum AFP levels were equal to or greater than various percentiles of the normal range[a]

Gestation (weeks)	Number of NTD pregnancies	Percentiles of the normal range		
		95th	97th	99th
ANENCEPHALY				
10–12	20	4 (20%)	3 (15%)	3 (15%)
13–15	47	34 (72%)	28 (60%)	23 (49%)
16–18	51	45 (88%)	44 (86%)	43 (84%)
19–21	19	19 (100%)	19 (100%)	18 (95%)
22–24	9	7 (78%)	7 (78%)	7 (78%)
SPINA BIFIDA (OPEN)				
10–12	22	4 (18%)	4 (18%)	1 (5%)
13–15	35	16 (45%)	13 (37%)	10 (29%)
16–18	33	29 (88%)	25 (76%)	23 (70%)
19–21	13	7 (54%)	7 (54%)	6 (46%)
22–24	5	5 (100%)	5 (100%)	5 (100%)

[a]Adapted from the UK Collaborative Study (1977).

TABLE 7

Twin pregnancies at 16–18 weeks' gestation with serum AFP values at or above defined percentiles of the normal range[a]

Number	Percentiles of the normal singleton range				
	95th	96th	97th	98th	99th
47	16 (34%)	14 (30%)	11 (23%)	11 (23%)	8 (17%)

[a]From the UK Collaborative Study (1977)

18-week group and later periods. Since the confirmatory diagnostic test of amniotic fluid AFP measurement does not appear to increase in efficiency with advancing gestational age, there is probably nothing to be gained by delaying the serum test beyond the 18th week of pregnancy. At this point the detection efficiency for both anencephaly and open spina bifida at the 95th percentile of the normal range is 88%. As shown in Table 7 some 34% of twin pregnancies will have serum AFP values above the 95th percentile at 16 to 18 weeks of gestation. The Collaborative Report also details the advantages for laboratories with comparatively small sets of data in using multiples of the median value in place of percentiles of the normal range in determining the cut-off level (Table 8). It points out that the proportion of affected

TABLE 8

Percentage of pregnancies with maternal serum AFP levels at 16–18 weeks' gestation equal to or greater than specified multiples of the normal median[a]

Pregnancy	Multiples of the median				
	2.0 (%)	2.5 (%)	3.0 (%)	3.5 (%)	4.0 (%)
Anencephaly	90.0	88.0	84.0	82.0	76.0
Open spina bifida	91.0	79.0	70.0	64.0	45.0
Normal singleton	7.2	3.3	1.4	0.6	0.3

[a]From U.K. Collaborative Study (1977).

pregnancies with serum AFP levels exceeding a given multiple of the median is unlikely to vary significantly from one laboratory to another or over time, though the proportion of 'false positives' will depend on the precision with which serum AFP and gestation are measured. Using different multiples of the normal median as cut-off points it is possible to calculate the chances of a pregnancy being affected in different areas of neural tube defect incidence (Table 9).

The UK Collaborative Study has thus defined over a large body of data the optimal stage of pregnancy for serum AFP screening and the likely detection efficiencies for anencephaly and spina bifida. It has not, however, been able to define the problems encountered when serum AFP screening is introduced into the clinical arena. A number of ongoing prospective intervention trials in different parts of the world should point out the difficulties more clearly. Common to all of them will be the

TABLE 9

Odds of a woman with serum AFP at or above various multiples of the normal median having a fetus with a neural tube defect (multiple pregnancy excluded by ultrasonography)[a]

Multiple of median	Local incidence of neural tube defects per 1000				
	2	4	6	8	10
2	1:41	1:21	1:14	1:10	1:8
2.5	1:21	1:10	1:7	1:5	1:4
3	1:10	1:5	1:3	1:2	1:2
3.5	1:4	1:2	2:3	1:1	1:1
4	1:3	1:1	1:1	3:2	2:1

[a]From UK Collaborative Study (1977).

incomplete nature of the test which may generate among expectant mothers the anticipation that they are being protected from the birth of a child with a neural tube defect which screening cannot completely justify. There are, however, obvious hopes that the efficiency of the test will rise with more practice, and it is a notable fact that the various prospective intervention trials being conducted in the United Kingdom seem to be recording higher detection efficiencies than had been anticipated. Even if detection efficiency is maintained at levels lower than indicated by the Collaborative Study it will be hard to deny the introduction of a simple test which can have such an enormous impact on the incidence of a group of congenital malformations which bring so much suffering to the families affected.

REFERENCES

Allan, L. D., Ferguson-Smith, M. A., Donald, I., Sweet, E. M. and Gibson, A. A. M. (1973): *Lancet*, *2*, 522.

Brock, D. J. H. (1974): *Clin. chim. Acta*, *57*, 315.

Brock, D. J. H. (1975): *Clin. Genet.*, *8*, 297.

Brock, D. J. H. (1976a): *Lancet*, *2*, 345.

Brock, D. J. H. (1976b): *Hum. Hered.*, *26*, 401.

Brock, D. J. H. (1977): In: *Progress in Medical Genetics, New Series, Vol. 2*, pp. 1–37.

Brock, D. J. H., Bolton, A E. and Monaghan, J. M. (1973): *Lancet*, *2*, 923.

Brock, D. J. H., Bolton, A. E. and Scrimgeour, J. B. (1974): *Lancet*, *1*, 767.

Brock, D. J. H. and Gosden, C. M. (1977): *Brit. med. J.*, *2*, 934.

Brock, D. J. H. and Olsson, J. E. (1976): *Clin. Genet.*, *9*, 385.

Brock, D. J. H. and Scrimgeour, J. B. (1972): *Lancet*, *2*, 1252.

Brock, D. J. H., Scrimgeour, J. B., Bolton, A. E., Wald, N. J., Peto, R. and Barker, S. (1975b): *Lancet*, *2*, 195.

Brock, D. J. H., Scrimgeour, J. B. and Nelson, M. M. (1975a): *Clin. Genet.*, *7*, 163.

Brock, D. J. H. and Sutcliffe, R. G. (1972): *Lancet*, *2*, 197.

Brock, D. J. H. and Sutcliffe, R. G. (1973): *Trans. biochem. Soc.*, *1*, 149.

Carter, C. O. (1976): *Brit. med. Bull.*, *32*, 21.

Carter, C. O., David, P. A. and Laurence, K. M. (1968): *J. med. Genet.*, *5*, 81.

Carter, C. O., Evans, K. A. and Till, K. (1976): *J. med. Genet.*, *13*, 343.

Carter, C. O. and Roberts, J. A. F. (1967): *Lancet*, *1*, 306.

Clarke, P. C., Gordon, Y. B., Kitau, M. J., Chard, T. and McNeal, A. D. (1977): *Brit. J. Obstet. Gynaec.*, *84*, 285.

Editorial (1974): *Lancet*, *1*, 907.

Gordon, Y. B., Ratky, S. M., Leighton, P. C., Kitau, M. J. and Chard, T. (1976): *Brit. J. Obstet. Gynaec.*, *83*, 771.

Gosden, C. M. and Brock, D. J. H. (1977): *Lancet*, *1*, 919.

Gosden, C. M., Brock, D. J. H. and Eason, P. (1977): *Clin. Genet.*, *12*, 193.

Harris, R., Jennison, R. F., Barson, A. J., Laurence, K. M., Ruoslahti, E. and Seppala, M. (1974): *Lancet*, *1*, 429.

Hino, M., Koki, Y. and Nishi, S. (1972): *Igaku no Ayumi (Progr. in Med.)*, *82*, 512.

Henry, G. P. and Robinson, A. (1977): *Amer. J. Obstet. Gynec.*, *127*, 204.

Holmes, L. B., Driscoll, S. G. and Atkins, L. (1976): *New Engl. J. Med.*, *294*, 365.

Kunz, J. and Schmid, J. (1976): *Lancet*, *1*, 47.

Laurence, K. M. (1974): *Lancet*, *2*, 939.

Laurence, K. M., Turnbull, A. C., Harris, R., Jennison, R. G., Ruoslahti, E. and Seppala, M. (1973): *Lancet*, *2*, 860.

Laurence, K. M., Walker, S. M., Lloyd, M. and Griffiths, B. L. (1975): *Lancet*, *2*, 81.

Leek, A. E., Ruoss, C. F., Kitau, M. J. and Chard, T. (1973): *Lancet*, *2*, 385.

Lorber, J., Stewart, C. R. and Milford Ward, A. (1973): *Lancet*, *1*, 1187.

Macri, J. N., Weiss, R. R. and Joshi, M. S. (1974): *Lancet*, *1*, 1109.

Milunsky, A. and Alpert, E. (1976): *Obstet. and Gynec.*, *48*, 1.

Nelson, M. M., Ruttiman, M. T. and Brock, D. J. H. (1974): *Lancet*, *1*, 504.

Purdie, D. W., Howie, P. W., Edgar, W., Forbes, C. D. and Prentice, C. R. M. (1975): *Lancet*, *1*, 1013

Report of U.K. Collaborative Study on Alpha-Fetoprotein in Relation to Neural Tube Defects (1977): *Lancet*, *1*, 1323.

Seller, M. J., Campbell, S., Coltart, T. M. and Singer, J. D. (1973): *Lancet*, *2*, 73.

Seller, M. J., Singer, J. D., Coltart, T. M. and Campbell, S. (1974): *Lancet*, *1*, 482.

Seppala, M. (1975): *Ann. N.Y. Acad. Sci.*, *259*, 59.

Smith, C. (1973): In: *Antenatal Diagnosis of Genetic Disease*. Editor: A. E. H. Emery. Churchill-Livingstone, London.

Sutherland, G. R., Brock, D. J. H. and Scrimgeour, J. B. (1973): *Lancet*, *2*, 1098.

Sutherland, G. R., Brock, D. J. H. and Scrimgeour, J. B. (1975): *J. med. Genet.*, *12*, 135.

Wald, N. J., Brock, D. J. H. and Bonnar, J. (1974): *Lancet*, *1*, 765.

Wald, N. J. and Cuckle, H. (1976): *Lancet*, *1*, 1292.

Wynne-Davies, R. (1975): *J. med. Genet.*, *12*, 280.

Prenatal diagnosis of genetic defects –
where it is and where it is going

MITCHELL S. GOLBUS

Department of Obstetrics, Gynecology and Reproductive Sciences, University of California Medical Center, San Francisco, Calif., U.S.A.

CURRENT INDICATIONS AND WORLD STATISTICS

The 4 years since this conference last met have witnessed significant advances in genetic counseling, and many of the most noteworthy have occurred in the area of prenatal diagnosis. Prenatal diagnosis has evolved during that time span from a procedure offered experimentally in a limited number of centers to one of proven safety offered on a service basis to thousands of families annually in dozens of centers. For the most part, prenatal diagnosis relies upon the cytogenetic or biochemical analysis of cultured amniotic fluid cells. These techniques are familiar to most of this audience and will not be further elaborated on at this time.

The most common indication for prenatal diagnosis is a fetus at risk for a chromosomal abnormality. The relationship of the incidence of trisomic offspring to increased maternal age is well established (Penrose, 1933). There is no rigid definition of 'advanced' maternal age, but most centers are using either 35 or 37 years as their criterion. Almost 6000 pregnancies have been tested for this indication. Of the fetuses studied because of advanced maternal age 2.4% were found to be aneuploid. It now appears that the risk of finding an aneuploid fetus rises from approximately 1% for the 35-year-old woman to approximately 10% for the 45-year-old woman (Polani et al., 1976).

The second largest group of patients tested are women who have borne a previous trisomic child and are at a 1 to 2% recurrence risk, irrespective of age (Mikkelson and Stene, 1970). It is considered appropriate to provide prenatal diagnosis in subsequent pregnancies. Of the almost 2000 such pregnancies studied, 1.2% were aneuploid.

Although affecting a much smaller segment of the population, the greatest risk of producing a chromosomally abnormal fetus exists for those individuals who are carriers of a balanced translocation. The magnitude of the risk is different for each specific translocation. However, for all known examples the risk is greater if the female rather than the male is the translocation carrier (Hamerton, 1968). Taking this heterogeneous group as a whole, 30 of the 299 fetuses studied were aneuploid.

An interesting lesson is present in Table 1 on the line depicting miscellaneous chromosomal indications for prenatal diagnosis. Although the miscellaneous indications were not detailed by all authors, most of these gestations were studied because of a history of children with the Down syndrome elsewhere in the family, a previous child with a non-trisomic chromosomal abnormality or a previous child with multiple congenital anomalies. With these 'softer' indications the frequency of chromosomally abnormal fetuses was 2%.

TABLE 1

Cumulative experience of prenatal detection centers

Indication	Pregnancies studied	'Affected' fetuses found	Per cent 'abnormal' fetuses
Chromosomal			
Maternal age > 35 years	3,516	85	2.4
> 40 years	1,043	45	4.3
35–39 years	1,284	22	1.7
Previous trisomy 21	1,970	24	1.2
Translocation carriers	299	30	10.0
Miscellaneous	1,316	28	2.1
X-linked diseases	438	202[a]	46.2 (males)
Biochemical defects	565	132	23.4
Total	10,431	568	5.5%

[a]Includes one trisomy-21 fetus.

Another type of chromosomal indication for prenatal diagnosis has been to determine the sex of the fetus of a woman known or suspected to be a carrier of a deleterious X-linked gene. Currently, affected and unaffected males can be distinguished from one another for only 4 X-linked disorders. These are Fabry disease, Menkes disease, the Lesch-Nyhan syndrome, and the Hunter syndrome. Since it now appears that there may be an autosomal recessive form of the Hunter syndrome, it is mandatory that appropriate enzymatic studies be performed on amniotic fluid and cultured amniotic fluid cells of any pregnancy being studied for this indication, regardless of fetal sex (Neufeld et al., 1977). It is now widely accepted that for fetal sexing a complete karyotype must be done. The worldwide experience has been that close to the expected 50% of fetuses monitored for X-linked diseases were male (Table 1).

The prenatal diagnosis of a biochemical defect is generally carried out by assay of enzyme activities in cultured amniotic fluid cells. At the present time approximately 40 disorders have actually been diagnosed prenatally and another 35 are capable of diagnosis (Golbus, 1976). 565 pregnancies have been monitored for an inborn error of metabolism of which 132 were affected. Tay-Sachs disease, Pompe disease, and the mucopolysaccharidoses have been the commonest indications for prenatal biochemical studies thus far. The programs of mass screening for heterozygote detection now being developed and executed will increase the demand for prenatal diagnosis of certain biochemical defects. One limiting factor in the diagnosis of hereditary enzyme defects has been the 4–8 weeks required to grow sufficient amniotic fluid cells for enzyme analysis. More sensitive techniques, developed by Galjaard and collaborators (1974) and by Hösli (1974), are based on the measurement of enzyme activities in small numbers of cells, on the order of 10's to 1000's, using quantitative microspectrophotometry or microfluorometry. These more rapid assays are now available for all of the clinically important lysosomal enzymes.

FETAL VISUALIZATION

Most multifactorially inherited congenital malformations and many Mendelian disorders occur without demonstrable chromosomal or biochemical abnormalities. The prenatal diagnosis of such disorders has been attempted by both indirect and direct fetal visualization. The indirect techniques have been sonography and radiography. With the introduction of gray-scale and real-time sonography, a number of congenital anomalies have already been prenatally diagnosed. These include anencephaly (Campbell et al., 1972), myelomeningocele (Campbell et al., 1975), omphalocele, and polycystic kidneys (Bartley et al., 1977). Serial measurements of ventricular size to evaluate hydrocephalus or microcephaly may be of value in diagnosing some instances of these abnormalities in the first half of pregnancy.

Direct radiography appears to be limited in its potential for prenatal diagnosis. It has been used to demonstrate fetal radii and, therefore, determine that a fetus was not affected by the thrombocytopenia-absent radii syndrome (Omenn et al., 1973) and to diagnose Saldino-Noonan dwarfism (Richardson et al., 1977). However, X-rays of 3 achondroplastic fetuses and of a fetus with infantile osteopetrosis, all at 20 weeks' gestation, did not result in diagnoses of existing abnormalities (Golbus and Hall, 1974; J. Hall, personal communication).

Contrast radiography with a water-soluble radio-opaque dye has been used to demonstrate an absence of fetal swallowing in the presence of esophageal or duodenal atresia (White and Stewart, 1973). This technique also can be used to outline the fetal silhouette to detect an abnormal mass or short limbed dwarfism (Golbus et al., 1977). The use of both direct and contrast radiography will probably be superseded by the development of better sonographic techniques.

Direct fetal visualization is performed using a small bore fiberoptic endoscope. Practicality dictated that a fetoscopic method be developed which can be performed as an out-patient procedure under local anesthesia. This has been made possible by the production of a 1.7-mm diameter endoscope by Dyonics Inc. containing a solid lens surrounded by fiber bundles transmitting the light. The introducing cannula has an outer diameter of 2.2 mm and accepts a sharp trocar for transabdominal insertion into the amniotic sac. Initial use of the fetoscope in 287 volunteers undergoing elective second trimester abortions with saline or prostaglandin $F_{2\alpha}$ resulted in successful entry into the amniotic sac in 275 instances (Benzie and Doran, 1975; Hobbins and Mahoney, 1976; Golbus, unpublished data). Although isolated parts of the fetal anatomy are sporadically identified, visualization of the entire fetus is rarely accomplished. Nevertheless, 4 pregnancies at risk for either the Ellis-van Creveld syndrome or for the autosomal dominant split-hand syndrome have been examined fetoscopically (J. C. Hobbins, personal communication). On the basis of visualization of polydactyly, 1 fetus was diagnosed as having the Ellis-van Creveld syndrome and this was verified when the pregnancy was terminated.

FETAL TISSUE SAMPLING

However, the major use of fetoscopy has been as one of the three techniques devised, thus far, for sampling fetal tissue other than amniotic fluid constituents. Many genetic defects are not reflected in amniotic fluid constituents but are demonstrable using other fetal tissues or cells. The most readily accessible and easily sampled tissue after birth is blood, and the most serious attempts to sample fetal tissues have also concerned fetal blood. It already has been shown that examination of as little as 10 μl of fetal blood in the second trimester of pregnancy permits the prenatal diagnosis of aberrant hemoglobin chains, as in sickle cell anemia, or of abnormal rates of hemoglobin synthesis, as in the β-thalassemias (Alter et al., 1976; Kan et al., 1977).

Using fetoscopy, it has been possible to obtain sufficient fetal red blood cells for hemoglobin synthesis studies from approximately 90% of the patients (Hobbins and Mahoney, 1976). Of 40 pregnancies subjected to such endoscopic sampling with the intention of being allowed to proceed to term, 5 terminated in spontaneous abortions (Hobbins and Fairweather, personal communication).

Our Center has primarily used a second technique, that of sonographically directed placental aspiration through a 20-gauge needle to obtain fetal erythrocytes (Golbus et al., 1976). The technique involves placing the needle bevel against the fetal surface of the placental plate and then inserting it 2 to 4 mm further for blood aspiration. In the case of an anterior placenta, the placenta is traversed by the 20-gauge needle until amniotic fluid is obtained. The needle is withdrawn to the placental plate and then withdrawn 2 to 4 mm further into the fetal surface of the placenta.

Both of these methods for obtaining fetal cells produce a mixture of fetal and maternal blood. Since fetal red cell volume is greater than that of adult cells, the presence of fetal erythrocytes is determined by analysis of cell volume by a Coulter particle size analyzer (Kazazian et al., 1972). The presence of maternal cells is not an insurmountable problem since the overall globin synthetic rate of the fetal cells is more than 500 times greater than that of maternal cells (Nathan et al., 1975). Thus, even though β-chain synthesis is approximately 50% of the total in maternal cells and only 5% of the total in fetal cells, the maternal cells do not make a great contribution to the β-chain radioactivity of the sample.

In 41 pregnancies at risk we have been successful in 87% of anterior placentas, obtaining positive samples with a mean value of 65% fetal cells, and in 94% of posterior placentas, obtaining positive samples with a mean of 66% fetal cells. In the 4 cases where there was a failure to obtain fetal cells either we or the patients or both felt that a second attempt was inappropriate. Six of the 35 fetuses successfully tested when the indication was β-thalassemia were found to be homozygous affected (Kan et al., 1977). After termination each of these prenatal diagnoses has been confirmed. Both of the successfully sampled fetuses at risk for sickle cell anemia were also homozygous affected and these diagnoses, likewise, were confirmed after pregnancy termination.

The third technique that has been employed to obtain fetal blood cells is the fluorescence activated cell sorter. This machine sorts droplets containing single cells according to the cell size and the amount of fluorescent dye bound to the cell (Herzenberg et al., 1976). It has been utilized to separate out the fetal cells that have crossed the placental barrier and are present in the maternal circulation. If we consider fetal red cells for the diagnosis of hemoglobinopathies, the technique has not been applicable. Even though the machine can scan and sort 5000 cells per second it would take it over a month to sort out sufficient fetal red cells from an estimated 1 in 1000 mixture in maternal blood. If we consider fetal white blood cells for karyotyping, then the problems are (1) that the white cells obtained do not respond well to PHA stimulation and another mitogen will have to be found, and (2) that white blood cells from previous pregnancies have been found circulating in maternal blood up to a year after that gestation (Schroeder et al., 1974). Whether or not these difficulties can be overcome and this methodology applied to prenatal diagnosis remains to be seen.

We should consider the fetoscope further because it will be used for directed sampling of fetal tissues for other prenatal diagnoses. The next application of this technique will be for X-linked Duchenne muscular dystrophy. Up until the present time, only fetal sexing could be carried out for the pregnant woman who was a carrier of this gene. If the fetus was a male, it would still have an equal chance of being affected or normal. However, Duchenne muscular dystrophy is known to result postnatally in very high activities of serum creatine phosphokinase, presumably because of leakage of the enzyme from diseased muscle (Zundel and Tyler, 1965). If plasma CPK is similarly elevated in an affected fetus in the second trimester of pregnancy, then assay of this enzyme may be useful for the prenatal diagnosis of Duchenne muscular dystrophy. Correction of the aspirate sample CPK activity for the maternal and amniotic fluid contributions, if any, allow calculations of the fetal CPK activity.

We, and others, are in the process of defining the normal ranges of CPK activity in fetal plasma obtained either in utero or following a prostaglandin $F_{2\alpha}$ induced therapeutic abortion, in amniotic fluid, and in newborn male serum. The first pregnancy of a possible carrier of the Duchenne muscular dystrophy gene was monitored in collaboration with Drs. Hobbins and Mahoney of Yale University and Dr. Caskey of Baylor School of Medicine (Mahoney et al., 1977). After amniocentesis demonstrated the counselee to be carrying a male, the family requested that an attempt at a more specific prenatal diagnosis be made. The fetal plasma CPK activity was within normal limits and the pregnancy was continued. At birth, the child had a serum CPK of 248, which is also within normal limits, and this fell to 69 by the 14th day of life. A second pregnancy at risk has been tested at Yale University at the time of therapeutic abortion and found to have an in utero CPK of over 700 mIU/ml. Fetal muscle has been read as microscopically abnormal. The third pregnancy at risk tested was at the University of California, San Francisco, also at the time of therapeutic abortion, and the in utero CPK was 80 mIU/ml. The fetal muscle was read as normal. Clearly, one difficulty is the lack of a diagnostic marker to 'prove' a fetus was or was not affected. Further evaluation of this technique in a small number of at risk pregnancies should be informative of whether the prenatal diagnosis of Duchenne muscular dystrophy can be reliably made by studying fetal plasma CPK.

The ability to obtain fetal blood potentially makes possible the prenatal diagnosis of many other inherited abnormalities. Fetal erythrocytes may be used to demonstrate the numerous red cell enzyme defects that lead to hemolytic anemias, or to demonstrate enzyme deficiencies that are not demonstrable in amniotic fluid cells.

An example of the latter is arginase where deficiency causes hyperargininemia associated with progressive neurologic deterioration (Spector et al., 1977). Fetal polymorphonuclear leukocytes could be used to prenatally diagnose the Chediak-Higashi syndrome or chronic granulomatosus disease. Fetal lymphocytes might be used for the in utero diagnosis of combined immunodeficiency states. Platelet size may be useful to diagnose Wiscott-Aldrich syndrome in utero. Also, a number of genetically important serum proteins are synthesized early in development (Gitlin and Biasucci, 1969). Examples include C1 esterase inhibitor which is defective or missing in hereditary angioneurotic edema, ceruloplasmin which is decreased in Wilson's disease, α-1-antitrypsin which is defective or absent in familial neonatal hepatitis, fibrinogen which is absent in afibrinogenemia, and Factor VIII which is defective in hemophilia A. I feel that medical genetics will soon make more frequent use of fetal blood than of amniotic fluid fibroblasts for the prenatal diagnosis of single gene defects.

OTHER APPROACHES

Despite the large number of enzyme defects and other hereditary and congenital abnormalities which can be identified directly or indirectly in amniotic fluid cells, amniotic fluid and fetal blood, or which can be visualized by one of several physical techniques, there are still a great number of genetic disorders which cannot be so diagnosed. These approaches are not of value either because the biochemical defects are not detectable in the available materials, because the underlying defects have not been identified, or because there are no easily visible structural defects. Efforts are therefore being made to develop other approaches to prenatal diagnosis, and prototypes for 2 of these 'new' approaches now exist.

A fundamental tenet of genetics is that the genome of all cells from an individual is identical. Therefore, if a hereditary defect can be identified at the level of the gene or DNA sequences involved, DNA from any tissue should be suitable for analysis. The validity of this approach has now been established in the prenatal diagnosis of α-thalassemia. This disorder is produced by an absence of hemoglobin α-chain synthesis which, in turn, is the result of a deletion of all 4 α genes from the genome (Ottolenghi et al., 1974). The technique involved is based on using reverse transcriptase to produce a radioactively labeled copy of DNA complementary to a specific messenger RNA. The rapidity with which this complementary or cDNA for the α-globin structural gene binds to DNA from a cell sample is proportional to the number of copies of the structural gene in the cell samples' genome. Although α chains are not normally made by amniotic fluid cells, the genes which govern their synthesis are present. Therefore, it has been possible, using these molecular hybridization techniques, to detect α-thalassemia-1 (2 genes deleted), hemoglobin H disease (3 genes deleted) and α-thalassemia (4 genes deleted) by analysis of DNA derived from cultured amniotic fluid cells (Kan et al., 1976). This approach should be applicable to any genetic disorder in which the defect results from the deletion of a gene for which the specific messenger RNA can be obtained or synthesized. Although these requirements have not been met for any non-hemoglobin related conditions, the recent explosion in molecular research suggests that they ultimately will be.

Another way to make use of the presence of unexpressed genes in amniotic fluid cells is to develop methods for inducing the expression of these genes. That this is feasible has been demonstrated in somatic cell hybridization experiments in which fibroblasts or leukocytes were observed to initiate the synthesis of albumin, a liver cell protein, after fusion with hepatoma cells (Peterson and Weiss, 1972; Darlington et al., 1974). Successful development of methods for the activation of unexpressed genes would be particularly useful for the prenatal diagnosis of conditions such as urea cycle defects, certain mucopolysaccharidoses, muscle abnormalities, and phenylketonuria which cannot be approached by our present techniques.

An entirely different approach to the diagnosis of conditions for which available materials or molecular techniques are not suitable is the utilization of linked genetic markers. With the application of somatic cell hybridization techniques to the mapping of the human genome, genes for readily detectable biochemical or immunologic markers which are closely linked to genes for inherited disorders are being discovered. In favorable situations, when the carrier of a deleterious gene is also heterozygous for such a closely linked marker and when the mate is of an appropriate genotype, it may be possible to follow the transmission of the gene to a fetus indirectly by actually following the transmission of the marker. The proximity of the disorder locus and the marker locus is of great importance since meiotic crossing over is proportional to the distances between loci and can lead to false negative and false positive results.

This approach has already been applied to the prenatal diagnosis of myotonic dystrophy (Schrott et al., 1973; Insley et al., 1976). The gene for this disorder is closely linked to the secretor locus which controls the secretion of ABH blood group substance (Renwick et al., 1971). Since amniotic fluid reflects the secretor status of the fetus, this linkage can be used for the prenatal diagnosis of myotonic dystrophy. The distance between these linked genes gives an 8 % probability that any specific gamete will be recombinant (Renwick et al., 1971). This risk of a misleading prenatal diagnosis must be understood and accepted by the couple being counseled. Other potentially useful linkages for prenatal diagnoses include glucose-6-phosphate dehydrogenase and hemophilia A (particularly in blacks, who have a high frequency of G6PD variants) (Boyer and Graham, 1965), HLA and the various complement loci, and HLA and dominantly inherited spinocerebellar ataxia (Jackson et al., 1977). This last linkage, which is reasonably tight, opens the prospect of being able to make the prenatal diagnosis of a condition which does not ordinarily become manifest until adult life.

CONCLUSION

In conclusion, I believe that prenatal diagnosis holds great promise for exciting advances. The number of disorders diagnosable in utero will increase steadily and amniocentesis will become routine for women at increased risk of producing defective offspring. The family which is unwilling to risk reproduction because of a genetic risk will be able to have children without fearing the birth of a child with a specific serious genetic disorder.

REFERENCES

Alter, B. P., Modell, C. B., Fairweather, D., Hobbins, J. C., Mahoney, M. J., Frigoletto, F. D., Sherman, A. S. and Nathan, D. G. (1976): *New Engl. J. Med.*, *295*, 1437.

Bartley, J. A., Golbus, M. S., Filly, R. A. and Hall, B. D. (1977): *Clin. Genet.*, *11*, 5.

Benzie, R. J. and Doran, T. A. (1975): *Amer. J. Obstet. Gynec.*, *121*, 460.

Boyer, S. H. and Graham, J. B. (1965): *Amer. J. hum., Genet.*, *17*, 320.

Campbell, S., Johnstone, F. D., Holt, E. M. and May, P. (1972): *Lancet, 2*, 1226.

Campbell, S., Pryse-Davies, J., Coltart, T. M., Seller, M. J. and Singer, J. D. (1975): *Lancet, 1*, 1065.

Darlington, G. J., Bernhard, H. P. and Ruddle, F. H. (1974): *Science*, *185*, 859.

Galjaard, H., Hoogeveen, A., Keijzer, W., DeWit-Verbeek, E. and Vlek-Noot, C. (1974): *Histochem. J.*, *6*, 491.

Gitlin, D. and Biasucci, A. (1969): *J. clin. Invest.*, *48*, 1433.

Golbus, M. S. (1976): *Obstet. and Gynec.*, *48*, 497.

Golbus, M. S. and Hall, B. D. (1974): *Lancet, 1*, 629.

Golbus, M. S., Hall, B. D., Filly, R. A. and Poskanzer, L. B. (1977): *J. Pediat.*, *91*, 464.

Golbus, M. S., Kan, Y. W. and Naglich-Craig, M. (1976): *Amer. J. Obstet. Gynec.*, *124*, 653.

Hamerton, J. L. (1968): *Cytogenetics*, *7*, 260.

Herzenberg, L. A., Sweet, R. G. and Herzenberg, L. A. (1976): *Sci. Am.*, *234*, 108.

Hobbins, J. C. and Mahoney, M. J. (1976): *Clin. Obstet. Gynec.*, *19*, 341.

Hösli, P. (1974): In: *Birth Defects*, p. 226. Editors: A. G. Motulsky and W. Lenz. Excerpta Medica, Amsterdam.

Insley, J., Bird, G. W. G., Harper, P. S. and Pearse, G. W. (1976): *Lancet, 1*, 806.

Jackson, J. F., Currier, R. D., Terasaki, P. I. and Morton, N. E. (1977): *New Engl. J. Med.*, *296*, 1138.

Kan, Y. W., Golbus, M. S. and Dozy, A. M. (1976): *New Engl. J. Med.*, *295*, 1165.

Kan, Y. W., Golbus, M. S., Trecartin, R. F., Filly, R. A., Valenti, C., Furbetta, M. and Cao, A. (1977): *Lancet, 1*, 269.

Kazazian, H. H., Kaback, M. M., Woodhead, A. P., Leonard, C. O. and Nersesian, W. S. (1972): *Advanc. exp. Med. Biol.*, *28*, 337.

Mahoney, M. J., Hazeltine, F. P., Hobbins, J. C., Banker, B. Q., Caskey, C. T. and Golbus, M. S. (1977): *New Engl. J. Med.*, *297*, 968.

Mikkelson, M. and Stene, J. (1970): *Hum. Hered.*, *20*, 457.

Nathan, D. G., Alter, B. P. and Frigoletto, F. (1975): *Semin. Hematol.*, *12*, 305.

Neufeld, E. F., Liebaers, I., Epstein, C. J., Yatziv, S., Milunsky, A. and Migeon, B. (1977): *Amer. J. hum. Genet.*, *29*, 455.

Omenn, G. S., Figley, M. M., Graham, C. B. and Heinrichs, W. L. (1973): *New Engl. J. Med.*, *288*, 777.

Ottolenghi, S., Lanyon, W. G., Paul, J., Williamson, R., Weatherall, D. J., Clegg, J. B., Pritchard, J., Poutrakull, S. and Boon, W. H. (1974): *Nature (Lond.)*, *251*, 389.

Penrose, L. S. (1933): *J. Genet.*, *27*, 219.

Peterson, J. W. and Weiss, M. C. (1972): *Proc. nat. Acad. Sci. (Wash.)*, *69*, 571.

Polani, P. E., Alberman, E., Berry, A. C., Blunt, S. and Singer, J. D. (1976): *Lancet, 2*, 516.

Renwick, J. H., Bundey, S. E., Ferguson-Smith, M. A. and Izatt, M. M. (1971): *J. med. Genet.*, *8*, 407.

Richardson, M. M., Beaudet, A. L., Wagner, M. L., Malini, S., Rosenberg, H. S. and Lucci Jr, J. A. (1977): *J. Pediat.*, *91*, 467.

Schroeder, J., Tiilikainen, A. and Chapelle, A. de la (1974): *Transplantation, 17*, 346.

Schrott, H. G., Karp, L. and Omenn, G. S. (1973): *Clin. Genet.*, *4*, 38.

Spector, E. B., Cederbaum, S. D. and Bernard, B. (1977): *Pediat. Res.*, *11*, 464 (abst.).

White, P. R. and Stewart, J. H. (1973): *Brit. J. Radiol.*, *46*, 706.

Zundel, W. S. and Tyler, F. H. (1965): *New Engl. J. Med.*, *273*, 537 and 596.

Genetic screening. An outlook en route

CHARLES R. SCRIVER[1] and CLAUDE LABERGE[2]

[1]*Departments of Pediatrics and Biology, McGill University, Montreal, and Montreal Children's Hospital; and* [2]*Centre Hospitalier, Université Laval, Ste-Foy, Quebec. Canada*

It is not the custom of the International Conference on Birth Defects to have more than one author for plenary session papers; in this case the medium is part of the message. Although we and our colleagues* work at different universities, in different cultures, we have achieved a program of genetic screening which transcends traditional 'boundaries' and encompasses many activities. This program – The Quebec Network of Genetic Medicine – has been described in detail elsewhere (Clow et al., 1973; Laberge et al., 1975; Nat. Acad. Sci., 1975a; Scriver et al., 1977). It is the source of experience which encouraged us to select 2 rather low-key themes for emphasis at this time. These themes are: teaching of human genetic principles to physicians and citizens; and the organization of genetic screening programs. We believe the real importance of these themes will be revealed in the future if and when the principles of genetic screening are applied to common multifactorial disease.

GENETIC SCREENING: RATIONAL AND EXPERIENCE

Genetics is the science of biological variation. Interpretation of variation, as to cause and effect, and in terms of health, or equilibrium, and of disease or disequilibrium is the medical geneticist's most important task. Genetic screening can discern variation in populations and individuals (Levy, 1973).

Screening in the medical context is an investigation that is *not* initiated by a patient's specific problem or request for advice. Screening is a 'presumptive identification of unrecognized disease or defect by the application of tests, examinations or other procedures which can be applied rapidly'. Screening tests sort out apparently well persons who probably have a disease from those who probably do not (Wilson and Jungner, 1968). Large-scale (mass) screening can encompass whole populations

---

*Claude Laberge (Laval Univ.) is Chairman, and Charles Scriver (McGill Univ.) is Vice-Chairman of the Quebec Network of Genetic Medicine. The other members of the Committee are: Jean Dussault, André Grenier (Laval Univ.); Carol Clow, Harvey Guyda (McGill Univ.); Louis Dallaire, Jacques Letarte, Serge Melançon (Univ. de Montréal); Bernard Lemieux, Denis Shapcott (Sherbrooke Univ.); Pierre Bergeron (Government member); Lina Roy (secretary).

in open-ended fashion or it can be selectively directed at high-risk sub-populations. Screening can encompass case finding which is a directive form of investigation to detect disease and initiate treatment; such activity is in contrast to epidemiological surveys. Diagnosis is a specific activity by which the cause for a finding is identified.

Genetic screening is a search in a population for persons with genotypes associated with incipient and established disease or which may lead to disease in their descendants. Accordingly, the major objectives of genetic screening are (Nat. Acad. Sci., 1975a):

1. To detect genetic disease and to minimize its effect by medical intervention.
2. To identify carriers who possess genes of potential harm to offspring, so as to provide information about reproductive decisions.
3. To enumerate the prevalence of certain genes in populations and to determine their biological significance (Harris and Hopkinson, 1972).

Genetic screening to meet the first objective has usually been concerned with the identification of extreme forms of variation. More often than not, it has been directed at homozygotes (or genetic compounds) who possess rare alleles which are expressed in the universal environment. This form of screening detects the incipient stage of disease expression, and upon confirmation of diagnosis a treatment process is initiated to neutralize the effect of the mutant gene. The prototype is screening for hyperphenylalaninemia, in the newborn period. The pitfalls, lessons and benefits of 'PKU screening' learned from practice on many millions of newborn infants in many nations has been described elsewhere in considerable detail (viz. Levy, 1973; Nat. Acad. Sci., 1975a; Scriver, 1977).

There has been much less experience with genetic screening for medical intervention in the older age population. The individual, in possession of a 'silent' genetic variant can be at high specific risk for a common multifactorial disease under certain conditions (Motulsky, 1974; Scriver, 1976; Childs, *This Volume*). Such persons might benefit from a change in lifestyle or from a specific prophylaxis, if the presence of risk were known and if the conditions under which that risk is converted to disease were also known. The extension of genetic screening to children, adolescents and adults for purposes of mass medical intervention is likely to occur in the near future. In our opinion, this practice will evince major problems in the absence of certain changes which we mention below.

Genetic screening to provide reproductive options has been applied to the prevention of the Down syndrome and other chromosomal anomalies in the offspring of older age women. The techniques of amniocentesis and prenatal diagnosis (Nadler, 1968; Milunsky et al., 1970) have served well this form of screening. The most important result to arise from antenatal screening of the at-risk pregnancy is the conversion of statistical probability regarding an outcome to a binary case (affected; non-affected). The process of decision making by the affected couple regarding reproductive options is considerably different in the latter situation from that which prevails in the absence of prenatal diagnosis (Abby Hand, unpublished observations, and personal communication). Mass screening for purposes of heterozygote detection has been attempted for the prevention of sickle cell anemia and Tay-Sachs disease. In this case, a relatively simple laboratory procedure can be applied to a blood sample for the detection of heterozygotes who are at risk with respect to their offspring. Moreover, such screening can be focussed upon specific populations (or communities and demes) where the prevalence of the genetic variant in question is high.

Yet the worthy objective of helping couples at risk to avert harm to their offspring has run into difficulty, particularly in sickle cell trait screening programs but even in some Tay-Sachs carrier screening programs. The persons at potential risk often do not participate numerously; when they do, the self knowledge gained from the screening experience is often not a welcome event. And doctors usually do not advocate such programs; sometimes they even oppose them. The reasons for these problems of advocacy and participation are complex. They relate to matters of knowledge and attitudes and they deserve careful consideration (Nat. Acad. Sci., 1975b; Kaback et al., 1974; Beck et al., 1974; Mentzer et al., 1970; Culliton, 1972). On the other hand, screening the newborn for a rare genetic disease usually evokes a satisfactory physician acceptance (Nat. Acad. Sci., 1975b). The process resembles both a medical and a public health procedure. An apparent 'cause' for an illness is identified and a so-called 'treatment' can be prescribed. Moreover, the physician probably has little familiarity with the rare disease brought to his attention by the screening program and he welcomes the process which takes care of it. Citizens can also hold a similar view of newborn screening for medical intervention (Clow et al., 1969). They welcome a simple procedure that can be applied to their offspring to prevent a potential handicap. There is a lesson to be learned and a message to be heard in the contrasting attitudes of physicians and citizens toward genetic screening for 'rare' disease in the newborn or the prevention of Down syndrome related to advanced maternal age, and toward screening for heterozygosity which places the client or his offspring at risk for a disease.

Screening for enumeration and research has revealed, for example, that about 10 % of hyperlipidemic myocardial infarction can be traced to the expression of one mutant allele carried by about 0.2 % of the North America population (Goldstein et al., 1973). The allele is responsible for the condition known as familial hypercholesterolemia. The cellular mechanisms which lead to the hypercholesterolemia have been studied intensively (M. Brown, *This Volume*). The risk to health for a carrier of the allele is now quite well understood and methods to offset the process of premature atherosclerosis in such a person are under investigation. But as yet there is no simple mass screening method for reliable identification of the familial hypercholesterolemia heterozygote. Assuming that a method for detection will soon be available, and that its application will be desirable, we come face to face with two of the major issues in genetic screening today. One involves knowledge and attitudes among advocates and clients; the other involves the structure, efficiency and effectiveness of screening programs.

Education, knowledge and attitudes

Childs has identified deficits in the education and perception of physicians with respect to medical genetics (Nat. Acad. Sci., 1975b; Childs, 1974, and *This Volume*) (Table 1). The genetic view of health and disease, that is, the appreciation of genetic origins of equilibrium between the organism and the environment, is largely missing from our modern medical curriculum. The serious deficiency in physician advocacy of genetic screening for heterozygotes (Table 1) reflects the lacunae in knowledge

TABLE 1

Genetic screening: physician and citizen views

Context	Physician	Citizen
1. Approve genetic screening in principle	95.6 %[a]	83.1 %[b]
2. Participated in genetic screening	4 % (as advocate)[a]	(i) 8.1 % as adult client[c] (ii) 75 % as student client[d]
3. Average hours of instruction/education in genetics	< 15 (in medical curriculum)[e]	< 15 (in secondary schools)[b]

Sources: [a]Nat. Acad. Sci. (1975a); [b]Clow et al. (1977); [c]Beck et al. (1974); [d]Clow and Scriver (1977); [e]Scriver (unpublished data).

which physicians can have with respect to some aspects of genetic disease. A parallel deficit exists also in the contemporary education of citizens. High-school students are anxious to learn more human genetics (Clow et al., 1977). They also favor genetic screening (Clow and Scriver, 1977). Yet they have only imperfect information about their own genes. They are confused about the nature of genes and chromosomes; they have almost no appreciation about their own prevalent heterozygosity. They do not perceive that they could be 'at risk' for a specific disease because of their particular genotype. The serious deficiency in participation in screening programs among the parents of these high-school students (Beck et al., 1974; Clow and Scriver, 1977) presumably reflects deficits in knowledge which they possess with respect to their own genetic identity. Accordingly, it is unlikely that physicians will be better advocates or that citizens will be more active participants in any screening programs of the future with a focus on common disease and subtle genetic variation until they are better informed about the genetic basis of human nature. Attainment of the goals of genetic screening is apparently tied to education of health workers and their clients.

Genetic screening services: structure and process

Genetic screening programs require a suitable structure to serve the process. This unglamorous aspect of screening has been slow to elicit attention and interest. Yet it is clear that failures in structure have been largely responsible for failures to achieve objectives in many genetic screening programs (Clow et al., 1973; Nat. Acad. Sci., 1975a; Scriver et al., 1977). The aggregate objective of genetic screening services is to reduce the burden and cost of genetic disease to society. A repeating series of structures (Fig. 1) concerned with screening, patient retrieval, diagnosis and management is required to maintain the various processes which serve several sub-objectives in an integrated program.

Screening   The structure must achieve and maintain high specificity and sensitivity in the testing process. If the screening is multiphasic, the structure must allow tests to be added or deleted as required in the progress of the program. Modifications in a multiphasic structure should incur only marginal costs. The process of screening

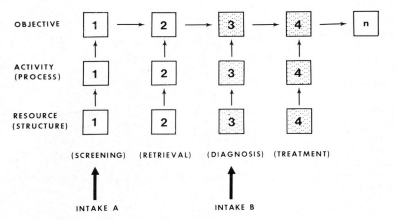

Fig. 1. Organization diagram for genetics services whose objective is to reduce the burden of 'genetic' disease through screening. Each sub-objective requires the appropriate process and resource (structure). Intake A (and unstippled 'objectives') indicate activities relating to (mass) screening; intake B and stippled objectives can also serve activities relating to *medical referral* of patients (another form of screening). Treatment includes counseling and follow-up.

should be centralized rather than fragmented into many independent structures (laboratories) in order to maintain maximum sensitivity, specificity and flexibility (Nat. Acad. Sci., 1975a).

Patient retrieval   Inefficient patient retrieval defeats the objectives of screening. Efficiency increases when there is direct communication between patient and the genetic structure (Scriver et al., 1977). Efficiency is also related to the structure of the medical care system in which the program operates (Starfield and Holtzman, 1975).

Diagnosis   The cause of a 'positive' screening test requires a precise diagnosis before prophylaxis and counseling can be prescribed. For example, 'hyperphenylalaninemia' which is the signal generated in the screening process reflects several conditions at the diagnostic level, each with its own prognosis and requirements for treatment and counseling. Centralization of expertise in the clinical and technical facets of diagnosis enhances the attainment of the aggregate objective of screening programs. Accordingly the organization of regional clinical centers is a logical development.

Treatment, counseling and follow-up   How self knowledge, achieved by genetic screening is accepted and utilized requires careful evaluation. This is true also, of course, for patients whose intake into a program is through specific referrals for diagnosis and counseling (Fig. 1). If treatment is required, close supervision of the process and regular monitoring of the treatment response will influence outcome. A mechanism in the program which allows the patients to be treated at home or on an ambulatory basis can improve the quality of treatment and reduce its cost (Clow et al., 1971). Supervision of treatment for rare genetic disease is particularly efficient when it is initiated from centers with regional influence (Comm. for Improvement of Hered. Dis. Management, 1976).

We had the opportunity recently to demonstrate the importance of structure in a genetics service program in traditional and dramatic terms. Our experience with screening for congenital hypothyroidism might convince skeptics that organization does matter. We have now screened more than a quarter million newborn infants in Quebec for congenital hypothyroidism. As a result, cretinism, a 'classic' birth defect, shows evidence of a rapid decline in frequency in our population. Efficient screening for congenital hypothyroidism would not have been possible without an organized program. The powerful example of thyroid hormone screening deserves a brief case analysis here to illustrate our theme. Specific and detailed recommendations for such screening have now been published (Amer. Acad. Ped., 1976) and deserve careful examination if the mistakes of PKU screening (Nat. Acad. Sci., 1971a; Scriver, 1977) are not to be repeated.

The thyroid hormone screening experiment

We stated earlier that the third objective of genetic screening is enumeration and research. Research and development of a mass screening test for congenital hypothyroidism was initiated as a pilot study in the Quebec Network of Genetic Medicine in 1973. Pilot studies are mandatory in the Network, prior to implementation of mass screening procedures. This policy conforms to the principles enumerated by the National Academy of Science in its report on genetic screening (Nat. Acad. Sci., 1975a). The Quebec pilot study revealed the effectiveness of a new microradioimmune assay for thyroid hormone (T_4) when it is applied to dried blood spots. We found the prevalence of congenital hypothyroidism to be about 1 per 7,000 live births in the pilot study (Dussault et al., 1975), a figure confirmed at 1 per 5,900 births in the later programs (Amer. Acad. Ped., 1977).

The specificity (exclusion of false positive tests) and sensitivity (exclusion of false negative tests) of thyroid hormone screening was of great concern in the pilot study. An elaborate system of statistical analysis to define maximum specificity and sensitivity, provision of a second back-up test (TSH determination on the same blood spot) and a protocol for repeat testing were each established. The T_4/TSH testing program was set up in one central laboratory for the whole province (95,000 births per year) to maximise specificity and sensitivity and to increase recall efficiency for follow-up tests (Dussault et al., 1976).

Direct contact with the patients after identification of a presumptive positive test, and referral to one of the regional genetic centers has reduced the follow-up time. The cumulative diagnostic investigation in this program reveals that about 60% of patients investigated for positive tests (low blood T_4 level) have athyrotic congenital hypothyroidism; about 10% have aberrations of thyroid hormone biosynthesis other than athyrotic T_4 deficiency; about 30% have hereditary deficiency of thyroxine-binding globulin. A few positive tests reflect miscellaneous diagnoses such as the congenital nephrotic syndrome.

When diagnosis is established, treatment is begun under the supervision of the patient's own physician in consultation with the regional center. The mean length of time elapsed between birth and initiation of treatment on 45 patients with congenital hypothyroidism is 29 days in our program.

Evaluation of the program after 3 years of formal activity following the pilot study, indicates that specificity of the test is 0.989 and sensitivity is 0.97. The medical care system of Quebec is likely to bring any patient who has been missed by screening to attention. One of the patients missed by T_4 screening had not been screened; in this case the drop in specificity reflects a flaw in the program and not in the test. At the time of diagnosis half of the patients showed no clinical signs of congenital hypothyroidism. Follow-up of treated patients at 1 year of age by a single observer in the program is yielding preliminary evidence for normal growth and development in both physical and mental dimensions. Untreated patients with low thyroxine-binding globulin activity are serving as controls in the screening program. Our program is now enrolled in a larger, long-term collaborative evaluation study with other programs under the sponsorship of the American Thyroid Association.

This brief résumé reveals several points of interest to the discussion. A structured program can have the flexibility to integrate new activities. The global budget, which is a feature of our program, has allowed us to drop one screening activity with low yield in our population (galactosemia screening) and replace it with thyroid screening. The infrastructure of the existing program supports, at marginal cost, all aspects of the new high-yield component except a portion of the cost for the immune assay testing system; the latter is an additional (marginal) cost. The testing program is centralized in one laboratory, yet it serves 95,000 births per year throughout a large geographic region. The screening has satisfactory specificity and sensitivity. Retrieval of patients is efficient and diagnosis is not delayed. Treatment is prescribed appropriately. Follow-up and evaluation of treatment is part of the formal program. This total activity which is directed at a non-genetic birth defect has been readily incorporated into a genetic screening program because the existing structure made it possible to do so. Of course structure alone is not enough. It is people working together with good will who achieve such objectives.

COMMENT

We anticipate that many readers will regard with little interest or sense of relevance the separate yet interacting issues of public and professional attitudes toward genetic screening, genetic instruction/education of public and profession, and structure and process in screening programs. Yet such issues are of concern to everyone in health care systems. Gene-dependent illness is a large segment of the disease burden in most developed countries today. Moreover, there is an increasing concern among the public about issues in medical genetics, as revealed by articles on related topics in the popular press. And some official organizations have already committed themselves to the surveillance and maintenance of health care standards in the area of medical genetic problems. Therefore a person who is now unconcerned with these issues must soon be; public policy will demand it. As individuals, we can participate in the development of informed public attitudes, in the knowledge about human and medical genetics and in the maintenance of efficient genetics service programs. Our performance as individuals will eventually influence performance of the collective system.

ACKNOWLEDGEMENTS

We are grateful to successive Ministers of Social Affairs in the Government of Quebec who have supported genetic services and the Quebec Network of Genetic Medicine.

REFERENCES

American Academy of Pediatrics. The Task Force on Genetic Screening (1976): *Pediatrics, 58,* 757.
Beck. E., Blaichman, S., Scriver, C. R. and Clow. C. L. (1974): *New Engl. J. Med., 291,* 1166.
Childs. B. (1974): *Amer. J. hum. Genet., 26.* 120.
Clow, C. L., Fraser, F. C., Laberge, C. and Scriver, C. R. (1973): In: *Progress in Medical Genetics, Vol. 9,* 159. Editors: A. C. Steinberg and A. G. Bearn. Grune and Stratton, New York.
Clow, C., Reade, T. and Scriver, C. R. (1971): *New Engl. J. Med., 284,* 1292.
Clow, C. L., Schok, M., Scriver, C. R. and Scriver, D. E. (1977): *Amer. J. hum. Genet., 29,* 32A.
Clow, C. L. and Scriver, C. R. (1977): *Pediatrics, 59,* 86.
Clow, C. L., Scriver, C. R. and Davies, E. (1969): *Amer. J. Dis. Child., 117,* 48.
Committee for Improvement of Hereditary Disease Management (1976): *C.M.A.J., 115,* 1005.
Culliton, B. (1972): *Science, 178,* 138.
Dussault, J. H., Coulombe, P., Laberge, C., Letarte, J., Guyda, H. and Khoury, K. (1975): *J. Pediat., 86,* 670.
Dussault, J. H., Letarte, J., Guyda, H. and Laberge, C. (1976): *J. Pediat., 89,* 541.
Goldstein, J. L., Hazzard, W. R., Schrott, H. G., Bierman, E. L. and Motulsky, A. G. (1973): *J. clin. Invest., 52,* 1533.
Harris, H. and Hopkinson, D. A. (1972): *Ann. hum. Genet., 36,* 9.
Kaback, M. M., Becker, M. H. and Ruth, M. V. (1974): *Birth Defects: Orig. Art. Ser. X/6,* 145.
Laberge, C., Scriver, C. R., Clow, C. L. and Dufour, D. (1975): *Un. méd. Can., 104,* 428.
Levy, H. L. (1973): In: *Advances in Human Genetics, Vol. 4,* p. 1. Editors: H. Harris and K. Hirschhorn. Plenum Press.
Mentzer, W. C., Lubin, B. H. and Nathan D. G. (1970): *New Engl. J. Med., 282,* 1155.
Milunsky, A., Littlefield, J. W., Kanfer, J. N., Kolodny, E. H., Shih, V. E. and Atkins, L. (1970): *New Engl. J. Med., 283,* pt. I, 1370; pt. II, 1441; pt. III, 1498.
Motulsky, A. G. (1974): *Science, 185,* 653.
Nadler, H. L. (1968): *Pediatrics, 42,* 912.
National Academy of Sciences (1975a): *Genetic Screening. Programs, Principles and Research.* Washington. D.C.
National Academy of Sciences (1975b): *A Study of Knowledge and Attitudes of Physicians.* Washington, D.C.
Scriver, C. R. (1976): *Fed. Proc., 35,* 2286.
Scriver, C. R. (1977): In: *Genetic Counseling,* p. 253. Editors: H. A. Lubs and F. de la Cruz. Raven Press, New York.
Scriver, C. R., Laberge, C. and Clow, C. L. (1977): In: *Medico-Social Management of Inherited Metabolic Disease. Proceedings, 13th Symposium of the Society for Study of Inborn Errors of Metabolism,* p. 21. MTP Press, Lancaster. U.K.
Starfield, B. and Holtzman, N. A. (1975): *New Engl. J. Med., 293,* 118.
Wilson, J. M. G. and Jungner, G. (1968): *Public Health Papers No. 34.* World Health Organization, Geneva.

FUTURE PROSPECTS

Chairman: Victor A. McKusick, Baltimore, Md.

Human cytogenetics

M. A. FERGUSON-SMITH

Department of Medical Genetics, University of Glasgow, United Kingdom

Although human chromosomes have been known for almost 100 years (Arnold, 1879), human cytogenetics made its first real impact on clinical medicine in 1959 with the discovery of trisomy-21 and the sex chromosome abnormalities. In July, 1959 the 9th International Congress of Paediatrics was held in this city and one can recall the interest with which the implications of this new development were discussed. Human cytogenetics has lived up to the expectations of those days and now almost every major medical school in the world has at least one human cytogenetics laboratory engaged in the diagnosis and prevention of human chromosome disorders. The 1977 edition of the International Directory of Genetic Services published by the National Foundation lists 584 such laboratories and this list does not claim to be complete. With such an active interest in the field, it is not surprising that the karyotype and its normal and abnormal variations are now better known in man than in any other species. A great deal of the credit for this progress must be attributed to 2 important technical innovations, namely, the introduction of short-term lymphocyte cultures in 1960 (Moorhead et al., 1960) and, 10 years later, the development of banding techniques. The first meant that excellent chromosome preparations could be made easily from small blood samples taken with the minimum of discomfort to the subject, and the second provided the investigator with a reliable means of identifying each individual chromosome. Much of the literature in human cytogenetics in the past few years has been concerned with exploiting the advantages of these 2 techniques. Karyotype-phenotype correlations have been made in all manner of different chromosome duplications and deletions defined precisely by banding. This work has led to the characterisation of almost as many different clinically recognisable chromosomal syndromes as there are chromosome arms, and the possibilities are nowhere near being exhausted. The days are long past when one can review the chromosomal syndromes adequately in 25 minutes. The characterisation of these syndromes has been almost entirely on a morphological basis and one looks forward to the days when it will be possible to undertake a biochemical characterisation. It is unlikely that we will understand the pathogenesis of malformations associated with chromosome aberrations until this is achieved. Apart from a few speculations about the significance of abnormal dosage of several enzymes whose structural gene loci happen to have been located within the relevant duplicated or deleted chromosome segment, there is little progress in this direction to report to date.

349

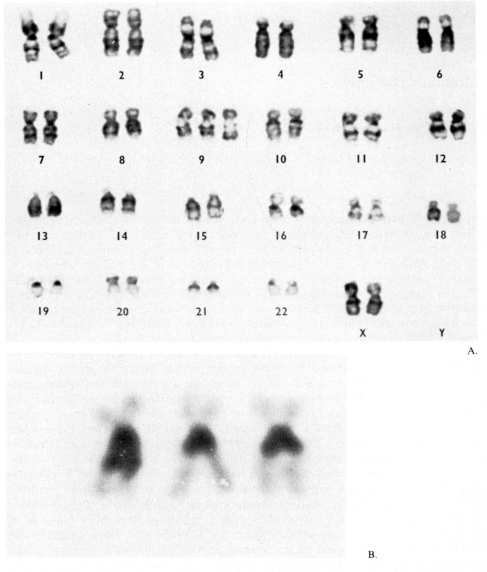

Fig. 1. Karyotype showing tetrasomy of the short arm of chromosome 9. A. Stained by G-banding to show the dicentric isochromosome. B. Stained by C-banding which reveals that 1 of the 2 centromeres is inactive.

The complexity and variety of aberrations detectable by banding and the precision of the method can be illustrated simply by looking at one short segment of the chromosome complement. For example, duplication of the short arm of chromosome 9 is one of the commonest of the so-called partial trisomy syndromes. Those affected show severe psychomotor retardation associated with a characteristic facies consisting of a large bulbous nose, prominent abnormal ears, antimongoloid slant, hypertelorism, and unusual forehead with bossing. A variant of the syndrome is produced by partial tetrasomy of the short arm of chromosome 9 (Fig. 1). A patient studied personally was found to be a mosaic with a normal cell line and a cell line in which there was an additional dicentric isochromosome for the short arm of chromosome 9; banding revealed that only one centromere was active in each cell. As far as I know, no one has given a satisfactory explanation for the mechanism which inactivates such centromeres, but more and more examples are being described each year.

The short arm of chromosome 9 is also involved in another syndrome, the 9p deletion syndrome, in which affected patients show quite different clinical features which in part may be considered a countertype to the 9p duplication syndrome.

In addition to defining chromosome aberrations most precisely, the banding methods have undoubtedly allowed the recognition of much smaller duplications and deletions than was possible previously. An excellent example is provided by the interesting 11/22 translocation (Fig. 2) which may turn out to be one of the commonest reciprocal translocations to be identified in man. The importance of this translocation is that heterozygotes frequently produce progeny with the partial trisomy-22 syndrome through 3:1 segregation in meiosis. Although the abnormal chromosome 22 translocation product is easy to identify, it is more difficult to distinguish the segment of chromosome 22 which has been translocated to the end of the long arm of chromosome 11, and there are examples published in the literature

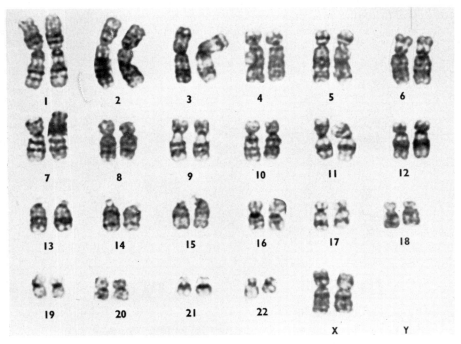

Fig. 2. Karyotype of individual heterozygous for the common 11/22 translocation. Breakpoints are at 11q25 and 22q13.

in which it has been missed. With the collaboration of many colleagues, in Europe and further afield (to whom I am most grateful), it has been possible to collect information on a series of 18 families in which the break points appear to be at almost if not identical sites namely at 11q25 and 22q13. It might be worth emphasising that although the abnormal chromosome 22 is very similar in appearance to the Philadelphia chromosome, chronic myeloid leukaemia has not yet been described in any of these families.

The extraordinary extent of normal variation in the human karyotype has been revealed largely by banding methods. The common chromosomal polymorphisms involve mainly the satellites and short arms of the acrocentric chromosomes, the centric regions of chromosomes 1, 9 and 16, and the fluorescent distal segment of the Y chromosome. Chromosome 9 provides an excellent example of a polymorphic chromosome as the amount of centric heterochromatin is extremely variable and complete and partial inversions of the centric region are very common (Fig. 3). Complete inversions occur in about 1% of cases referred to our chromosome diagnostic service. They do not appear to have much clinical significance because duplication deficiencies resulting from crossing-over within the inversion have never been described. It is possible that, very occasionally, they may be associated with other types of aberration resulting from mispairing at meiosis. Nevertheless, cytogeneticists often have difficulty in convincing their clinical colleagues that prenatal diagnosis is not indicated if a parent is found to carry the inverted 9. In general, the risk of abnormal progeny to individuals heterozygous for pericentric inversions increases with the length of the segment involved, the highest risk occurring when the break points of the inversion are near the ends of both chromosome arms (Ferguson-Smith, see: *Summary, Workshop VI*, p. 428).

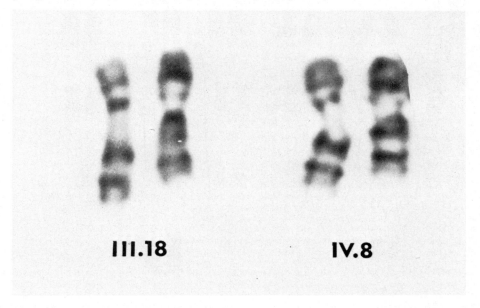

III.18   IV.8

Fig. 3. The pericentric inversion of chromosome 9 in father (III.18) and child (IV.8), the latter having failed to inherit the AK-1 allele carried by the inverted chromosome (see text).

Although new methods for chromosome banding continue to be published, it seems likely that the limit of resolution of the technique has probably already been reached. The detection of even smaller chromosome aberrations will require quite different methods. One possibility for the future is the hope that we may be able to define aberrations in terms of gene loci rather than Giemsa bands. This depends, of course, on the availability of sufficiently detailed chromosome maps and we have heard at this Congress much about the present high investment in human gene mapping and its achievements. In order to use the chromosome map for the type of genetic analysis I have in mind, it would probably be sufficient to know the location of about 500 of the postulated 50,000 structural gene loci in man; these 500 loci must of course be amenable to analysis. At present, we know the chromosomal assignment of about 150 loci and a more precise intrachromosomal location for about one third of this number. All this has been achieved in the past 9 years, particularly by the study of chromosome segregation in interspecific somatic cell hybrids, but also by other techniques such as family studies and duplication-deletion mapping using chromosome aberrations. Less developed techniques of considerable potential are in situ molecular hybridisation and interspecific gene transfer in somatic cells, and I am sure that we will hear more about these methods in the future. It is clear that a good start has been made on achieving a workable chromosome map and it may not be too optimistic to hope that in the foreseeable future we may be able to use these chromosome maps for such purposes as the prenatal diagnosis of abnormal genotypes by linkage, and to identify chromosome duplications and deletions beyond the resolution of the microscope.

How many clinical geneticists have not had the experience of confidently predicting a chromosome aberration on the basis of their clinical examination only to be disappointed later by finding an apparently normal karyotype with the most sophisticated banding techniques? There seems every chance that at least some of these unidentifiable dysmorphology syndromes may eventually be shown to be due to minute chromosome aberrations detectable only by genetic marker studies. In support of this view, I would like to quote an unusual observation made quite fortuitously in my own laboratory.

The proposita of the family in question presented with a dysmorphology syndrome which had many of the features of a chromosomal syndrome including profound psychomotor retardation, microcephaly, short stature, preaxial polydactyly of the right foot, hypertelorism, small low-set ears, kyphoscoliosis and hypertrichosis. Apart from a pericentric inversion of chromosome 9 which the patient shared with her father (Fig. 3) and other paternal relatives, no chromosome aberration could be demonstrated by a variety of banding techniques undertaken on several different samples. Routine genetic marker studies, however, unexpectedly revealed that the patient had only one allele at the red cell adenylate kinase (AK-1) locus having failed to inherit a gene from her father (Fig. 4). The child had inherited the inverted 9 from her father and genetic marker studies made non-paternity even more improbable. A familial silent allele was excluded by gene dosage studies which showed that the AK-1 activity in the child was 50 % of normal whereas both parents and all other family members had normal enzyme levels (Table 1). Previous studies in our laboratory have provided evidence that the structural gene for AK-1, and consequently the closely linked ABO blood group and nail patella syndrome loci, is

GO77MG

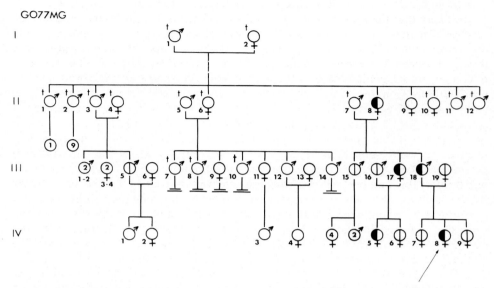

Fig. 4. Pedigree of child heterozygous for a pericentric inversion of chromosome 9 in which anomalous inheritance of AK-1 was discovered by chance. Half-shaded symbols indicate individuals carrying the inversion.

located precisely in the proximal half of band 9q34 (Ferguson-Smith et al., 1976). Is it possible that our patient has a submicroscopic deletion in the paternally derived inverted 9 at band 9q34? If so, the malformation syndrome might have resulted from deletion of loci closely linked to AK-1, for it is unlikely that deficiency of AK-1 in itself could have contributed to the clinical abnormality. The missing AK-1 allele may simply pinpoint the site of a more significant chromosomal lesion. If this supposition proves to be correct, this would appear to be the first example of a specific chromosome aberration detected by genetic marker studies.

In considering progress in the diagnosis and characterisation of a wide variety of chromosomal syndromes, one must not forget the extremely important responsi-

TABLE 1

A possible deletion at the AK-1 locus?

	9 inv.	AK type	Mean AK activity
Father III.18	+	11	107.1 ± 16.3
Mother III.19	—	21	85.3 ± 9.9
Sister IV.7	—	21	99.8 ± 16.5
Proposita IV.8	+	2	$42.1 \pm 11.1^*$
Sister IV.9	—	21	100.8 ± 22.8
Normal controls	n = 22	11	113.1 ± 13.3
	n = 9	21	105.8 ± 12.2

$^*p = < 0.001.$

bility that human cytogeneticists have in the prevention of birth defects due to chromosome aberrations. The ability to diagnose fetal chromosome aberrations early enough in pregnancy to allow parents the option of selective termination is one of the most important, if not the most important contributions made by human cytogenetics to clinical practice. The potential of the method for reducing the birth incidence of Down's syndrome and other common chromosome aberrations is considerable, for the majority of parents seem to accept that selective abortion is a humane approach to the problem of severe fetal abnormality. It is therefore extremely disappointing to have to admit that 10 years after amniotic cell culture was introduced, so few mothers at risk of having a chromosomally abnormal child are being offered the chance of amniocentesis. The most neglected and most important category of mothers are those 40 years of age and over, where the risk of fetal chromosome abnormality may be as high as 4%. The Clinical Genetics Society of Great Britain are currently considering the provision of prenatal diagnostic facilities in Britain and have estimated that in 1976 only about 1,200 of the 12,000 pregnancies in women 40 years of age and over were tested for a fetal chromosome abnormality. About 45 pregnancies were found to be affected and were terminated, whereas an estimated 400 other pregnancies in this category continued to the delivery of a chromosomally abnormal infant. The fact that only 10% of women who required it had prenatal diagnosis, indicates that we are not doing enough to educate our colleagues and the community. With the exception of Denmark, where it is

TABLE 2

Maternal age specific risks of fetal chromosome abnormality (West of Scotland Series, 1977)

Maternal age (yr)	Number of pregnancies	Trisomy 13	Trisomy 18	Trisomy 21	Sex chrom. aneuploidy XXX	Sex chrom. aneuploidy XXY	Sex chrom. aneuploidy Other	% Abnormal		% with Down's Observed	% with Down's Expected
35	45	·	·	·	·	·	·	0			
36	54	·	·	·	·	·	·	0			
37	74	·	·	3	·	·	·	4.0 } 1.2		0.9	0.37
38	86	·	·	·	·	·	·	0			
39	81	·	·	·	·	1	·	1.2			
40	90	·	·	·	·	·	·	0			
41	83	·	·	2	·	1	·	3.6 } 4.2		3.5	1.50
42	63	·	1	4	·	·	·	7.9			
43	36	·	·	1	·	·	·	2.8			
44	15	·	·	3	·	·	·	20.0			
45	9	·	·	·	·	·	·	0			
46	5	·	·	1	·	·	·	20.0 } 6.7		6.7	6.21
47	0	·	·	·	·	·	·	·			
48	1	·	·	·	·	·	·	0			
49	0	·	·	·	·	·	·	·			
Totals	642	0	1	14	0	2	0	2.65			

*Live birth prevalence after Lindsjö (1974).

believed that 30% of mothers in the age group 40 years and above were tested in 1976 (Mikkelsen, 1976), most countries seem to share this poor record.

Anxiety about the hazards of amniocentesis may have deterred some obstetricians from offering amniocentesis to their patients. The risks of amniocentesis have been studied in a number of countries, notably Canada and the United States, and the results show a reassuringly low risk of inducing abortion so this problem is unlikely to be an important deterrent in the future. More important perhaps is the tendency for obstetricians to discount the risk of chromosome abnormality in older mothers as being too small to warrant the risk of creating undue anxiety by mentioning it. Risks based on the maternal age specific prevalence rate of Down's syndrome among live births which are commonly used in counselling, tend to be much lower (less than 50%) than the risks estimated prospectively from the results of prenatal diagnosis (Table 2). The discrepancy between the 2 estimates is too great to be due solely to the loss of chromosomally abnormal pregnancies by spontaneous abortion or stillbirth between 16 weeks and the time of delivery. Further study is required to resolve this problem so that mothers and their obstetricians can be provided with reliable risk estimates on which they can make sensible decisions about whether or not to have amniocentesis. For our part, we must understand that there is little point in developing methods for reducing the incidence of birth defects if we cannot also provide the means for making these methods available and acceptable to the community.

SUMMARY

The interest generated by the discovery of trisomy-21 and the sex chromosome abnormalities in 1959 has led to the establishment of many hundreds of cytogenetics laboratories throughout the world engaged in the diagnosis and prevention of human chromosomal disorders. Progress on such a scale would not have been possible but for the introduction of short-term lymphocyte cultures in 1960, and, 10 years later, the development of banding techniques. The first provided a simple and readily available source of material for diagnostic chromosome analysis and the second permitted the unequivocal identification of each individual chromosome. It is not surprising that more is known about spontaneous chromosome aberration and chromosome polymorphism in man than in any other species. Karyotype-phenotype correlations in patients with chromosomal duplication and deletion, defined precisely by banding methods, have led to the recognition of almost as many chromosomal syndromes as there are chromosomal arms. Characterisation of these syndromes is almost entirely on a morphological basis and there is need for bio-chemical characterisation if the pathogenesis of malformations associated with chromosome aberration is to be fully understood. The limit of resolution of current banding techniques has probably already been reached, and the detection of smaller chromosome aberrations will require new methods. Future progress will depend on the availability of sufficiently detailed gene maps, which will define aberrations in terms of gene loci rather than Giemsa bands. It is therefore encouraging that techniques for gene mapping continue to improve so that the uncharted areas of the human karyotype gradually grow smaller. Every time an unbalanced karyotype is identified, an opportunity to contribute to the gene map can be taken or missed and so every human cytogenetics laboratory should consider their responsibility in this aspect of the development of their discipline.

Human cytogenetics have in recent years been given a new and heavy responsibility for a procedure capable of substantially reducing the incidence of severe birth defects. The potential benefits of prenatal diagnosis of fetal chromosome aberrations to the individual family and community are high, but the procedure requires 100% reliability. The signs are that prenatal diagnosis is making a disappointingly small impact, simply because it is being made available to only a small proportion of those families who require it. The development of new methods to prevent birth defects is surely wasted if insufficient effort is made to bring them to the community.

REFERENCES

Arnold, T. (1879): *Virchows Arch.*, *78*, 279.
Ferguson-Smith, M. A., Aitken, D. A., Turleau, C. and De Grouchy, J. (1976): *Hum. Genet.*, *34*, 35.
Mikkelsen, M. (1976): In: *Prenatal Diagnosis*, pp. 95–103. Editor: A. Boué. INSERM, Paris.
Moorhead, P. S., Nowell, P. C., Mellman, W. J., Batips, D. M. and Hungerford, D. A. (1960): *Exp. Cell Res.*, *20*, 613.

Future prospects in somatic cell genetics *

JOHN W. LITTLEFIELD

Department of Pediatrics, Johns Hopkins University School of Medicine, Baltimore, Md., U.S.A.

In this brief paper I would like to suggest one particular direction for somatic cell genetic research, which could well have relevance for common human problems, such as atherosclerosis, aging, diabetes, tumors, and congenital malformations. These conditions are generally regarded as multigenic as they usually present, but each also occurs occasionally in the form of single gene disorders. It is a common and reasonable speculation that the genetic loci involved in these single gene disorders are also involved when the inheritance is multigenic. The theme of this paper is that investigation of the less common disorders inherited as single genes should increase our understanding of the more common multigenic form of the same conditions. Perhaps such investigations would also illuminate the pathogenesis and even facilitate the prenatal diagnosis of these disorders.

It is now well-recognized that single gene disorders, as they occur naturally, are heterogeneous, with different alleles or even different loci responsible, each of which produces the same phenotype. If this phenotype is evident at the cellular level, cells cultured from individuals with the phenotype in different families will contain a variety of molecular lesions. Also, if normal cells can be mutated experimentally to give the same phenotype, additional molecular lesions will become available. Then, if it can be demonstrated that certain of the affected cells correct or 'complement' the defect in some of the other cells, sorting of the natural and experimental mutants into a series can begin. Such a search for genetic complementation of this nature is a classic genetic approach to dissect a biochemical mechanism or pathway. In regard to the common disorders under consideration, the pathways involved might be the synthesis of cholesterol, or of certain key proteins or nucleic acids involved in cell division, the regulation of certain cell surface constituents or topography, or the control of commitments made early in embryogenesis, or of differentiation later on, for example.

Indeed the dissection of DNA repair mechanisms by complementation analysis, using fibroblasts from individuals with certain rare disorders defective in DNA repair, is already being pursued actively as described by Dr. Cleaver *(This Volume)*. To extend this approach to single-gene inherited atherosclerosis, aging, diabetes,

* Research mentioned in this article was supported by U.S.P.H.S. grant no. CA-16754.

tumors and congenital malformations, one needs to answer 3 questions: Do human cells in culture express the phenotype of interest? Is it possible to induce more mutants than occur naturally? How can complementing and non-complementing mutants be distinguished?

Do human cells in culture express the phenotype of interest?

In regard to familial hypercholesterolemia, an autosomal dominant condition which predisposes to premature atherosclerosis, human skin fibroblasts clearly express the phenotype, as was discussed in detail by Drs. Brown and Goldstein *(This Volume)*. Likewise, the phenotype of aging is expressed in fibroblasts, indeed in all diploid cell types, and is being studied in increasing detail. Fibroblasts from patients with certain chromosomal or recessive conditions show premature aging (Littlefield, 1976). This appears to be true also for cells from patients with diabetes, and probably also from individuals with single gene conditions which predispose to diabetes (Goldstein et al., 1969, 1974; Vracko and Benditt, 1975).

However, fibroblasts from patients with inherited tumors do not express the tumor phenotype, at least spontaneously, nor do fibroblasts from patients with single-gene-determined congenital malformations show any recognizable abnormality.

Is it possible to enhance the expression of these phenotypes? Drs. Goldstein and Brown were the first to use cells from individuals homozygous for an autosomal dominant disorder in order to make the disorder more evident at the cellular level. The same approach should be tried with other, less common dominant diseases, such as achondroplasia or Marfan's syndrome, whenever a putative homozygote is recognized. Genetic 'compounds' can be expected, as has already probably been encountered in the case of familial hypercholesterolemia. Indeed, when unavailable naturally, it might be possible to induce the homozygous state in heterozygous cells with mutagenic agents, or alternatively by stimulation of a 'parasexual' genetic process, such as mitotic recombination, followed by selection of the homozygous cell (Pontecorvo, 1962).

In regard to other ways to enhance a cellular phenotype, some sort of metabolic stress might accelerate the premature aging of cells from patients with diabetes or other conditions. Also, in those chromosomal or single-gene-inherited conditions which predispose to neoplasia, such as Down's syndrome, Bloom's syndrome, and Fanconi's anemia, fibroblasts seem to be more easily transformed with SV40 virus (Todaro et al., 1966). This may be true for other disorders, such as Gardner's syndrome (Pfeffer et al., 1976) or bilateral retinoblastoma (Jensen and Miller, 1971), for example. Indeed the enhanced susceptibility of certain fibroblasts to transformation with SV40 virus is a fascinating phenomenon which needs to be confirmed and studied in much more detail. Recently, it has been reported that fibroblasts from the neurofibromas of patients with neurofibromatosis (Benedict et al., 1975), and perhaps even normal fibroblasts (Milo and DiPaolo, 1977), have been transformed with carcinogenic chemicals, a hitherto elusive achievement.

If skin fibroblasts from one site on the body do not express a phenotype, it is possible that fibroblasts from other sites may do so (Kaufman et al., 1977). Or only fibroblasts which are not growing may express the phenotype (McInnes et al., 1976). Also, if fibroblasts are not useful, several other types of human cells are now available, such as long-term lymphocyte cultures or 'lymphoblasts', epithelium, endothelium, muscle and blood stem cells. Indeed, to study congenital malformations in cell culture, it may be necessary to grow fibroblasts in combination with other cell types, in order for the defect to be evident. Or fusion of 2 cell types may be necessary to 'activate' a differentiated phenotype (Davidson, 1974).

Is it possible to induce more mutants than occur naturally?

Since the initial studies of Albertini and DeMars (1970) on experimental mutagenesis at the hypoxanthine-guanine phosphoribosyltransferase locus in diploid human fibroblasts, variation has been produced at several other loci, including that for adenine phosphoribosyltransferase (Rappaport and DeMars, 1973), that for the ability to utilize homocysteine (Hankinson and Jacoby, 1975), that for resistance to ouabain (Mankovitz et al., 1974), etc. Mutagenic agents such as X-rays, nitro-soguanidine (Albertini and DeMars, 1970), ethylmethane sulfonate, 5-bromodeoxy-uridine (Stark and Littlefield, 1974), and even SV40 virus (Marshak et al., 1973; Theile et al., 1976), have been effective. Also such work has been extended to long-term diploid human lymphoblasts. For example, a number of phosphoribosyl-transferase-deficient lymphoblast mutants have been induced, in addition to those mutants which occur naturally. Some of these contain immunologically cross-reacting material, and therefore probably represent structural gene mutations (Epstein et al., 1977).

To identify new mutations in human fibroblasts, lymphoblasts, or other cell types which are equivalent to those occurring naturally in the cells of patients with single-gene-inherited premature atherosclerosis, premature aging, diabetes, neo-plasms, or congenital malformations, the phenotype must be selectable, since probably no more than one mutant cell per 10^5 or 10^6 parental cells will be produced. This may be difficult to achieve. For example, Dr. David Valle and I have wondered if fibroblasts defective in the ability to make collagen could be detected by virtue of protection against anticollagen antibodies, as suggested by work elsewhere (Maoz et al., 1973). Were this possible, a collection of cells with different mutations in the collagen biosynthetic pathway might be obtained. We have encountered or anti-cipated several problems with this idea. These include the difficulty in obtaining potent clean antibody to collagen, the necessity for 2 mutations at the homologous loci in the case of autosomal genes, and the possibility that collagen produced in normal cells will migrate to collagen-deficient cells, making them a target for the antibody.

Nonetheless, possible selective systems come to mind for the phenotypes now being considered. For example, fibroblasts from patients with familial hyper-cholesterolemia overproduce cholesterol and cholesterol esters when exposed to concentrations of low density lipoprotein which inhibit cholesterol production in normal cells. Although this excess cholesterol is largely secreted into the culture medium, enough of it may be retained, or secretion might somehow be inhibited, so that the cholesterol-overproducing cells were lighter in density than normal cells similarly treated, and perhaps could be separated from them. Alternatively, if the newly induced mutant cells were not too rare, some non-toxic vital stain might serve to identify them in a culture of normal cells. These ideas could be tested presently, using mixtures of normal fibroblasts and those available from individuals homozygous for familial hypercholesterolemia.

For diabetes, as well as the other inherited conditions which cause premature aging, one needs to identify new mutations which produce either diminished growth potential relative to normal cells or a lethal effect. In somatic cell genetics just as in bacterial genetics, this problem can be approached through the use of conditional lethal techniques, such as auxotrophy or temperature sensitivity. Alternatively, it might be possible to rescue non-growing mutant cells in some novel way, for example, by fusion to heteroploid cells (Silagi et al., 1969), or by insertion of a chromosome containing the SV40 genome (Croce and Koprowski, 1974). These maneuvers may need to be carried out on single cells by means of micromanipulation.

The identification of new mutants exhibiting a neoplastic or 'transformed' phenotype should not be a problem, because of the selective advantage this phenotype confers.

In regard to the single gene conditions which cause congenital malformations, we may need to understand better the behavior and capabilities of individual cell types in normal development, as well as the interactions between cells, before we can devise selections for cells newly mutated in regard to their ability to participate in differentiation or morphogenesis. Still, some ideas come to mind. For example, various cells undergo terminal differentiation in culture, either spontaneously or when exposed to certain conditions. The selection of cells unable to terminally differentiate seems straightforward. For other situations, more complex selective systems involving two or more cell types could probably be designed, in which one of the cell types was selected for loss of ability to terminally differentiate, or to participate in the formation of a multicellular structure.

How can complementing and non-complementing mutants be distinguished?

The techniques to classify somatic cell mutants in regard to ability to complement one another are now fairly well advanced. Complementation can occur through cross-feeding, in heterokaryons, or in viable hybrid cells. When studying cross-feeding or heterokaryons, one must be able to identify the normal phenotype in an individual cell. In the case of viable hybrid cells, the normal phenotype must provide a selective growth advantage to the hybrid cell in which complementation has occurred.

For example, complementation between mutant fibroblasts which overproduce cholesterol and cholesterol esters should diminish the possible accumulation of these products in the hybrid cell. This might be utilized to separate such a hybrid cell from a background of mutant cells through a difference in cell density, as mentioned earlier. For the premature aging conditions, complementation by cross-feeding or in viable hybrids would have a strong selective advantage. Incidentally, it is interesting in this regard that complementation was not observed between several pairs of aged normal fibroblasts (Littlefield, 1973; Norwood et al., 1974). However, such studies should be extended to cells from individuals with the single-gene-determined premature aging conditions.

Complementation between 2 types of mutant cells both of which exhibit the neoplastic or transformed phenotype would require detection of cells at a disadvantage in regard to growth. It should be possible to achieve this through the use of conditional lethal techniques, or analogous maneuvers, as mentioned earlier. Likewise, in regard to mutants involving differentiation and morphogenesis, complementing cells might regain the ability to terminally differentiate, requiring rescue by conditional lethal or analogous techniques, or to form a structure which could be identified and separated.

SUMMARY

Somatic cell genetic experiments with fibroblasts or other cells from individuals with the single-gene-inherited forms of common multigenic conditions, such as athero-sclerosis, aging, diabetes, tumors, and congenital malformations, seem likely to be profitable in several ways. These studies should further increase our knowledge of the control of cholesterol biosynthesis, cell division, aspects of the cell surface, and cell differentiation. They should identify genetic loci participating in these processes which are particularly susceptible to mutation. Furthermore, identification of these loci might indicate the components which contribute to the more common multigenic inheritance of these disorders. Indeed, it is possible that one could proceed to create hybrid cells which would mimic multigenic inheritance! Next, such studies should increase our understanding of the pathogenesis of these conditions, especially when homozygous cells can be obtained or induced, as has been elegantly demonstrated in the case of familial hypercholesterolemia. Finally, if methods to enhance cellular phenotypes can be developed, genes presently not evident in cultured amniotic fluid cells might be made visible, increasing the scope of prenatal diagnosis. In general, many of the techniques required for this sort of work are now available, and what is needed is imaginative application to carefully selected experimental problems.

REFERENCES

Albertini, R. J. and DeMars, R. (1970): *Science, 169*, 482.
Benedict, W. F., Jones, P. A., Laug, W. E., Igel, H. J. and Freeman, A. E. (1975): *Nature (Lond.), 256*, 322.
Croce, C. M. and Koprowski, H. (1974): *J. exp. Med., 140*, 1221.
Davidson, R. L. (1974): In: *Somatic Cell Hybridization*, p. 131. Editors: R. L. Davidson and F. F. de la Cruz. Raven Press, New York.
Epstein, J., Leyva, A., Kelley, W. N. and Littlefield, J. W. (1977): *Somatic Cell Genet., 3*, 135.
Goldstein, S., Littlefield, J. W. and Soeldner, J. S. (1969): *Proc. nat. Acad. Sci. (Wash.), 64*, 155.
Goldstein, S., Moerman, E. J., Soeldner, J. S., Gleason, R. E. and Barnett, D. M. (1974): *J. clin. Invest., 53*, 27a.
Hankinson, O. and Jacoby, L. B. (1975): *Exp. Cell Res., 96*, 138.
Jensen, R. D. and Miller, R. W. (1971): *New Engl. J. Med., 285*, 307.
Kaufman, M., Straisfeld, C. and Pinsky, L. (1977): *Somatic Cell Genet., 3*, 17.
Littlefield, J. W. (1973): *J. Cell Physiol., 82*, 129.
Littlefield, J. W. (1976): *Variation, Senescence, and Neoplasia in Somatic Cells*, p. 73. Harvard University Press, Cambridge, Mass.
Mankovitz, R., Buchwald, M. and Baker, R. M. (1974): *Cell, 3*, 221.
Marshak, M. I., Varshaver, N. B. and Shapiro, N. I. (1973): *Genetika, 9*, 138.
Maoz, A., Dym, H., Fuchs, S. and Sela, M. (1973): *Europ. J. Immunol., 3*, 839.
McInnes, R. R., Shih, V. E. and Erbe, R. W. (1976): *Pediat. Res., 10*, 368.
Milo, G. E. and DiPaolo, J. A. (1977): *In Vitro, 13*, 193.

Norwood, T. H., Pendergrass, W. R., Sprague, C. A. and Martin, G. M. (1974): *Proc. nat. Acad. Sci. (Wash.)*, *71*, 2231.
Pfeffer, L., Lipkin, M., Stutman, O. and Kopelovich, L. (1976): *J. Cell Physiol.*, *89*, 29.
Pontecorvo, G. (1962): *Brit. med. Bull.*, *18*, 81.
Rappaport, H. and DeMars, R. (1973): *Genetics*, *75*, 335.
Silagi, S., Darlington, G. and Bruce, S. A. (1969): *Proc. nat. Acad. Sci. (Wash.)*, *62*, 1085.
Stark, R. M. and Littlefield, J. W. (1974): *Mutat. Res.*, *22*, 281.
Theile, M., Scherneck, S. and Geissler, E. (1976): *Mutat. Res.*, *37*, 111.
Todaro, G. J., Green, H. and Swift, M. R. (1966): *Science*, *153*, 1252.
Vracko, R. and Benditt, E. P. (1975): *Fed. Proc.*, *34*, 68.

Metabolic diseases: future directions

LEON E. ROSENBERG

Department of Human Genetics, Yale University School of Medicine, New Haven, Conn., U.S.A.

To make predictions about the future is easy. To make serious and intelligent predictions, however, is not particularly easy when a subject as broad, complex and fluid as the future of metabolic diseases is the topic, and a person more comfortable in the realm of facts than in the kingdom of fancy is the author. My discomfort is eased a bit by two things. First, by the origin of the word 'metabolic', which comes from two Greek roots, *meta* meaning beyond, and *ballein* meaning to throw. In an etymologic sense then, throwing ourselves beyond current understanding and into the future seems fitting. Second, by the realization that my predictions cannot be instantly disregarded as incorrect because no one else here can be certain about the future either.

Before attempting any 'fortune telling', I must accept 3 basic assumptions: that mankind has a future other than the bang of nuclear annihilation or the whimper of energy depletion; that society will continue to permit open and unfettered inquiry by its scientists; and that the combined scientific experience of the past and present provides a foundation upon which to project a future.

Having framed my assumptions, I must next delimit a pair of terms. For purposes of this discussion, the word, 'future', will refer to the next quarter century, thus to about the year 2000. This finiteness will prevent the kind of frivolous speculation that open-ended future-casting encourages, and may, if I am lucky, allow me to smile at the wisdom or frown at the ignorance of my projections. The phrase, 'metabolic diseases', too, requires constraints. All disease is metabolic in the sense that 'metabolism' considers the sum of all physical and chemical processes by which living, organized substance is built up and broken down. Therefore, I will restrict myself to those metabolic diseases in man which are birth defects, that is those in which inherited chemical disturbances are brought about by mutations at a single major genetic locus or small number of loci.

Let us look first at likely developments in our understanding of the basic mechanisms underlying inherited metabolic diseases. In this arena I feel confident that advances will be major and rapid. Currently, only those disorders characterized by abnormalities in the structure and function of hemoglobin can be approached at all 4 levels of sophistication: the gene; the gene product; the chemical consequences; and the clinical expression. We already know that mutant hemoglobins can result from gene deletions, base substitutions, base deletions and insertions, frame shift mutations, and non-homologous cross-overs, and we will almost surely find other defects in the hemoglobin system involving gene regulation, message initiation, and messenger processing and transport (Bunn et al., 1977). This elegant model system demonstrates conclusively that human disease can be understood in molecular terms and offers a road map to students of all other metabolic disorders. It seems certain that the hundreds of other known metabolic diseases like phenylketonuria, Tay-Sachs disease and hemophilia which are characterized by specific deficiency of circulating proteins or intracellular enzymes result from mutations analogous to those described for hemoglobin. For most of these conditions understanding is incomplete even at the level of the gene product, but I believe that improved methods of cell propagation, protein purification, immunochemical characterization and gene amplification will lead to the definition of the molecular basis for many other now partially understood metabolic disorders.

I am also optimistic about future progress in our understanding of such common and important conditions as cystic fibrosis, Huntington's disease, and muscular dystrophy, for which we currently have no good biochemical 'handle'. This optimism is based on the rapid advances currently being made in membrane chemistry, cell biology, and neurobiology and the belief that such advances will generate novel approaches to disorders like cystic fibrosis which, thus far, have frustrated workers by revealing a plethora of abnormalities but no underlying and unifying defect (Di Sant'Agnese and Davis, 1976).

Up to now, I have talked of new information about known diseases. Two other kinds of related discoveries seem certain. The first involves the continued description of currently unrecognized disorders. The number of known inborn errors has been increasing logarithmically for the past 20 years, and there is every reason to think this trend will persist for the foreseeable future (Childs, 1973). The second concerns discovery of additional monogenic lesions in disorders now classified as polygenic or multifactorial. Just as we have learned that familial hypercholesterolemia due to a defective cell surface receptor for the low density lipoprotein-cholesterol complex is an important cause of coronary artery disease (Brown and Goldstein, 1976) so will we find that other monogenic disturbances underlie that deadly disease state. Just as we have learned that α_1-antitrypsin deficiency predisposes to pulmonary emphysema (Talamo, 1975), so will we discover other enzymatic antecedents for that problem. And finally, just as methylenetetrahydrofolate reductase deficiency and cystathionine synthase deficiency can lead to schizophrenia (Rosenberg, 1976) so will other, as yet, unperceived inborn errors.

So much for this brief glimpse at advances in acquisition of information. What of its application to sick people? I shall look first at treatment of metabolic diseases around the year 2000, with the proviso that we are viewing the most advanced treatment programs available in the world at that time, and the caveat that such optimal therapy will not be uniformly, or even widely, available in all countries because major economic disparities will continue to dictate different sociologic structures and divergent health priorities. For the most part, therapeutic advances will reflect extension of current modalities, but I foresee some innovative developments as well. Avoidance therapy will have become widely recognized as a key therapeutic tool in many diseases: avoidance of tobacco smoke and other air pollutants in α_1-antitrypsin deficiency; avoidance of a number of drugs or anesthetics in acute intermittent porphyria, G6PD deficiency, pseudocholinesterase deficiency, and malignant hyperthermia; avoidance of ultraviolet light exposure in xeroderma pigmentosum or of X-rays in ataxia telangiectasia. These are but a few examples of the extent to which critical interaction between specific genetic and environmental factors will be appreciated. Nutritional restriction, taking PKU and galactosemia as the prototypic diseases, will be employed for a large number of disorders of amino acid and organic acid metabolism and will also have been proven to be highly efficacious in the treatment of certain hyperlipidemias and intestinal transport defects (Holliday et al., 1976). Nutritional supplementation, too, will be widely used. Specific vitamin supplements will have been shown to have long-term efficacy in a number of diseases caused by defects of vitamin metabolism or of enzymes dependent on specific vitamin-derived cofactors (Rosenberg, 1976). Supplements of other usual dietary constituents such as inorganic phosphate in hypophosphatemic rickets, uridine in orotic aciduria, and carbohydrate in Von Gierke's disease will have been refined far beyond current practice. Finally, I believe that administration of novel, 'tailor made' drugs will be much more widely employed to mitigate the consequences of such conditions as sickle cell anemia, hemochromatosis, Wilson's disease, cystinuria and cystinosis.

Thus far, I have dealt exclusively with modifying the chemical consequences of the disorder rather than attacking the gene or gene product. I believe that gene product replacement will have proceeded significantly, but unevenly. Conditions in which the gene product normally circulates in the blood (like hemophilia or diabetes) will be treated routinely with self-administered injections of the pure protein. Certain lysosomal storage diseases, which do not affect the brain (like adult Gaucher's disease), will also be managed by specific enzyme replacement owing to the natural tendency of such enzymes to find their way into the lysosomal particles where they function catalytically (Brady et al., 1974). Replacement of intracellular enzymes found in the cytosol, the mitochondrion, or the nucleus, however, presents far more formidable problems. Specific immunologic or chemical 'targeting' of such proteins may make it possible to direct them appropriately and even to pass such obstacles as the blood-brain barrier. Even so, rapid enzyme degradation, paucity of enzyme supplies and the possible need to administer enzymes in utero for conditions in which CNS pathology is already apparent in the fetal brain (like Tay-Sachs disease), suggests to me that enzyme replacement therapy will be far from routine. Where the enzyme itself cannot be replaced, I believe we shall hear more about replacing the cell type bearing the missing or defective enzyme. Pancreatic islet transplants in diabetes, partial hepatic grafts in ornithine transcarbamylase deficiency, red cell transfusions in adenosine deaminase deficiency (Polmar et al., 1976) are but a few of the conditions in which enzyme replacement via intact cells may prove useful.

My guarded optimism about gene product replacement does not extend to what might be termed the ultimate form of intervention – namely modification of the gene itself. Recent advances in our understanding of the eukaryotic genome, of its interactions with viruses, of virus biology, and of bacterial plasmids are startling. They suggest powerful means by which specific human genes could be inserted into human cells. However, I believe the formidable scientific problems of human gene isolation and of safe viral transduction, coupled with deeply felt concerns about viral oncogenicity, inadvertent mass human infection and the appropriate limits of experimentation will raise legal and ethical barriers that will not fall until well past our target date – the year 2000.

I have then projected that treatment programs will be aimed at several levels – the gene, the gene product, the metabolic milieu. Preventive measures, too, will be focused at different points. The first involves prevention of conception. In some instances this will involve choice of marriage partner. I foresee that broadly based and adolescent-oriented heterozygote detection programs for such disorders as sickle cell anemia, Tay-Sachs disease and cystic fibrosis will be generally accepted and that individuals found to be carriers for such disorders will use that information, along with more traditional inputs, in choosing a mate. In other instances prevention of conception will involve post-marital decisions. As genetic counselling becomes more widely used in disorders characterized by serious consequences in the adult but no significant impairment of reproductive fitness (like Huntington's disease or neurofibromatosis) some families will elect childless marriages or adoption. Others, in increasing numbers, will choose artificial insemination or its female counterpart, in vitro fertilization, to permit child bearing with much reduced genetic risk. Much of this activity will be voluntary, but problems posed by population growth and declining food and energy supplies will result in increased societal pressures for such reproductive options.

A second level of prevention will involve prevention of birth of a diseased fetus. Spurred by scientific advances in the ability to examine cultured amniotic fluid cells, to measure amniotic fluid metabolites, and to carry out determinations on fetal blood, and by a general acceptance of selective therapeutic abortion as a powerful and humane means of limiting the burden of genetic disease, prenatal diagnosis will be widely practiced for scores of metabolic diseases. Many of these disorders will still remain in the category of untreatable, progressive and ultimately lethal or incapacitating; others, however, will result in less serious, but still unacceptable, consequences as defined by the individuals who must bear the burden of child rearing – namely the parents.

A third, and already familiar, level of prevention (which merges with treatment) will be directed at preventing or minimizing the consequences of specific disorders by mass neonatal screening followed by early and effective treatment. PKU and galactosemia are the classic examples here, but they will be joined by congenital hypothyroidism and many other disorders involving defects in organic acid, amino acid, carbohydrate, and lipid metabolism (Childs et al., 1975).

Until this moment, I have written only of progress and of constructive developments. But, just as our concept of 'metabolism' involves the interplay of destructive (or catabolic) as well as constructive (or anabolic) events, so I believe must we discern some potentially destructive clouds on the horizon of the field concerned with metabolic disorders.

First, I am worried about our ability to continue to acquire the basic information needed to understand metabolic diseases of all sorts. I see the NIH and its counterpart in other countries being pushed further and further toward support of targetted or specific disease-related research. This trend, I believe, will act as a deterrent rather than a stimulant to unlocking the secrets to some of the most common and most serious metabolic disorders like cystic fibrosis or Huntington's disease. For those diseases and many more, targetted funds have not and will not buy fundamental answers. We need new questions and approaches and these, I believe, must still be sought in such seemingly unlikely places as laboratories studying basic molecular, cellular and neurobiology.

Second, I am increasingly concerned about certain aspects of health care delivery for inherited metabolic diseases. I see a very small number of research-oriented prenatal diagnosis laboratories being overwhelmed by service requests. I see a patchwork of institutional and state-run neonatal screening programs or enzyme reference laboratories with no national or international organization. I see children dying of ammonia intoxication in the newborn period because most hospitals have not yet added blood ammonia determinations to their clinical chemistry armamentaria. I see retarded children being discovered to have PKU at 2 years of age because they were dismissed from the newborn nursery too early for the results of their Guthrie neonatal screening tests to be meaningful (Starfield and Holtzman, 1975). And I see phenylalanine restriction in PKU children being relaxed at an earlier and earlier age without any rigorous or convincing evidence that such relaxation will not be followed in 5 or 10 years by deleterious intellectual or behavioral consequences. Wouldn't it be catastrophic to undo in the next 25 years what we have so laboriously done in the past 25 years!

Finally, I am anxious about how we disseminate information about metabolic diseases specifically, and about medical genetics generally. The pace of work in this field has been so rapid as to be intoxicating. Now, I think we're beginning to experience some of the hangover. Can it be surprising that a public which hears much more about 'cloning' than 'counselling', and about 'transduction' than 'treatment', distrusts our motives and fears our power? Can it be surprising that our medical colleagues, most of whom completed their formal education before the discipline of medical genetics even existed, understand neither our language nor our goals?

I do not mention these clouds to darken these sunny proceedings. On the contrary, all of the potentially destructive elements I've mentioned are eminently correctable if we are aware of them and offer them some of the attention they deserve, and if we try to narrow the gap between what we know and what we do. Then, and only then, can we look forward to a period of continuing, if less heady, progress in a field which has taught us about health as well as disease and which has the unusual attribute of linking knowledge about basic mechanisms with the means to modify disease consequences.

REFERENCES

Brady, R. O., Pentchev, P. G., Gal, A. E., Hibbert, S. R. and Dekaban, A. S. (1974): *New Engl. J. Med.*, *291*, 989.
Brown, M. S. and Goldstein, J. L. (1976): *Science, 191*, 150.
Bunn, F., Forget, B. and Ranney, H. (1977): *Human Hemoglobins.* Saunders, Philadelphia.
Childs, B. (1973): *Yale J. Biol. Med., 46*, 297.
Childs, B. (Chairman) and the Committee for the Study of Inborn Errors of Metabolism of the National Research Council (1975): *Genetic Screening.* National Academy of Science.
Di Sant'Agnese, P. A. and Davis, P. B. (1976): *New Engl. J. Med., 295*, 481.

Holliday, M. A. (Chairman) and the Committee on Nutrition of the American Academy of Pediatrics (1976): *Pediatrics, 57*, 783.

Polmar, S. H., Stern, R. C., Schwartz, A. L., Wetzler, E. M., Chase, P. A. and Hirschhorn, R. (1976): *New Engl. J. Med., 295*, 1337.

Rosenberg, L. E. (1976): In: *Advances in Human Genetics, Vol. 6*, Chapter 1, p. 1. Editors: H. Harris and K. Hirschhorn. Plenum Press, New York.

Starfield, B. and Holtzman, N. A. (1975): *New Engl. J. Med., 293*, 118.

Talamo, R. C. (1975): *Pediatrics, 56*, 91.

Future prospects: environmental factors

R. W. SMITHELLS

Department of Paediatrics and Child Health, University of Leeds, Leeds, United Kingdom

The most extraordinary thing about human development is that once the blastocyst is safety embedded in the uterine wall the rest usually proceeds normally. When we consider what a complex creature develops from something the size of a pinhead we should never cease to be amazed. The normal sequence of developmental events requires not only proper genetic programming but also a propitious environment. Historically, we have concentrated almost exclusively on adverse environmental factors capable of causing developmental harm – teratogenic viruses since the observations of Gregg (1941), teratogenic drugs since the observations of Lenz (1962) and McBride (1961), and before them all, the long mythology of antenatal influences. Perhaps we assume that environmental changes are likely to be for the worse, as we believe that genetic mutations are more likely to do harm than good. Perhaps mankind is not much interested in healthy living but prefers to await disaster and then apportion blame, in much the same way that sin, although we are against it on principle, is sometimes more fun than sanctity. And third, it is much more difficult to study the determinants of normality than to administer large doses of toxic substances to laboratory animals and to count, measure and record the adverse consequences.

But it should be possible to identify some aspects of the environment that are doing positive good to the embryo and fetus so that we may at least try to preserve them and possibly even enhance them. For example, Dalton (1976) gave progesterone to women with pre-eclamptic toxaemia of pregnancy and found that years later their children did better than controls in school examinations and were 6 times more likely to go to University. It sounds improbable and the controls are open to criticism, but more recently Reinisch (1977) reported that children exposed to synthetic progestin and oestrogen in utero showed personality traits which are associated with better school achievement although their IQ's did not differ significantly from those of their non-exposed siblings.

In my own department we have demonstrated a relationship between low maternal blood levels of folic acid and vitamin C in early pregnancy and neural tube defects in their infants (Smithells et al., 1976). To test the hypothesis that the association might be causal we are now recruiting mothers who have previously given birth to one or more children with neural tube defects and giving them appropriate vitamin supplementation before the next conception and through the first 2 months of pregnancy. Numbers are not yet large enough to draw even preliminary conclusions, but so far 3 of 34 controls have had either affected babies or raised alphafetoprotein in amniotic fluid but none of 29 supplemented mothers.

Neither of these connections – that between intrauterine hormone exposure and educational performance and that between vitamins and neural tube closure – rests yet on hard scientific data so far as man is concerned, although there is plenty of supporting evidence from animal studies. Nevertheless they encourage us to think in terms of defining and helping to supply a positively beneficial environment for the embryo and fetus rather than depending entirely upon a defensive strategy designed to detect and root out invading teratogens. The distinction is in fact artificial. The administration of a folic acid antagonist may have much the same effect as removal of folic acid from the diet. But it is always easier to recognise the presence of something that should not be present than the absence of something that should.

Another aspect of the intrauterine environment that deserves more attention is the mechanism whereby embryos with abnormal genotypes or phenotypes are recognised and aborted with remarkable efficiency. The birth defects which we see as clinicians, although numerous enough in all conscience, represent only the tip of an iceberg of malformation, most of which is lost as blighted ova, unimplanted blastocysts and spontaneous abortions. Autosomal trisomies of the A, B, C and F group chromosomes together with polyploids are totally rejected, as are more than 95 % of trisomies D and E and sex chromosome anomalies, 80 % of Down's syndrome, and 25 % of spina bifida. Zygotes which never establish vascular connections with the maternal organism must contain the seeds of their own destruction. Those which we recognise clinically as abortions may be discarded by some more subtle mechanism. Nature seems to have her eye on the next generation already, for although in our society a person with Down's syndrome might be considered at a greater disadvantage than one with Turner's syndrome, the XO embryo is rejected a good deal more ruthlessly than one with 21 trisomy. Mental handicap is less important than reproductive handicap. It is better to be well-bred than well-read. And yet infants with renal agenesis, doomed to die at birth, may be carried to term, and anencephalics with equally little future sometimes show an embarrassing reluctance to leave the womb.

It is important to unravel these discard mechanisms because the clinical and social problems of birth defects could be mitigated if we could increase their efficiency. There can be little doubt that the immunologists have a lot to offer in this field. Histocompatibility antigens may be important in the transplant business but I don't believe that was why the Almighty invented them.

Turning from the environment of the embryo to that of the parents, and remembering that fathers as well as mothers have environments, it may be helpful to distinguish between the three dimensions of epidemiology: the Where, the Who and the When. Some environmental factors belong to a place – the air we breathe, the water we drink, the stone we use to build our houses. Others belong to people – our personal habits of eating, drinking, smoking and drug consumption, our occupations, even our recreations. Yet other environmental factors belong to a time – an epidemic disease, the marketing of a new drug, the accidental or deliberate pollution of air or water. We are interested in all three aspects of the environment but rather different approaches may be needed both in the detection and in the elimination of teratogenic agents.

A surveillance programme which records accurately all malformed births in a defined population over several years will only be sensitive to one of the three dimensions I have described – that of time. A significant increase in one or more malformations suggests the recent arrival of a teratogenic factor in that community and should trigger off an intensive search. I should like to emphasise that a significant decrease in malformation rates is of equal importance. One of the difficulties, familiar to everybody who has played the monitoring game, is to know what is significant. 5 % of phenomena will be significant at the 5 % level, but most of them will be of no consequence.

If the surveillance programme is designed to study human subgroups within the defined population a second dimension – the personal – is opened up. The pattern of birth defects in the offspring of people of different racial or ethnic groups, different social classes and different occupations has already yielded important clues.

To study the third dimension, that of place, comparisons must be made between cities, between nations, between continents. This requires some agreement about methodology and it requires international co-operation. It is good that the National Foundation–March of Dimes is actively promoting such co-operation. However, even within quite small territories there may be striking geographical variations. In the north-west of England, for example, neural tube defects are about 3 times as common as they are in the south-east, the distance between averaging about 250 miles.

Most of the important lessons of birth defects surveillance have been well learned and well recorded. I would just like to make 3 points regarding their further exploitation.

1. It is time we paid a little more attention to the occupational hazards of parents of both sexes. Occupational cancers have been recognised for a very long time. Carcinogenesis, teratogenesis and mutagenesis are first cousins. Recent work on the reproductive problems of people employed in hospital operating theatres has underlined the relevance of the working environment (Vaisman, 1967; American Society of Anaesthesiologists, 1974).

2. Exceptionally low malformation rates deserve as much attention as the high. In the British Isles almost all the publications on the epidemiology of neural tube defects have come from Ireland, South Wales and north-west England, the areas of highest incidence, and very little from the south-east and East Anglia. We may be looking in the wrong place.

3. A specific epidemiological question may need a specific surveillance programme. When rubella vaccine was introduced to the United Kingdom a National Congenital Rubella Surveillance Programme was set up (Sheppard et al., 1977) to answer, in due course, the specific question, 'Has vaccine reduced the incidence of congenital rubella?'. The variable manifestations of congenital rubella and the need for laboratory confirmation of the diagnosis make it impossible for a routine surveillance programme to answer this question.

So much for the systematic search for new teratogens, remembering that the odds favour the next new one being detected by an astute clinician and not by a monitoring service. What more can be done to diminish the effects of environmental teratogens which we already know about or strongly suspect? They can only gain access to the embryo directly by irradiation or by sound waves, and via the mother by ingestion, inhalation or infection.

The only form of ionising radiation likely to be met by many people is medical X-rays. It is normal practice to avoid non-urgent X-ray examination of women of child-bearing age in the fortnight prior to an expected menstrual period, and this makes sense. It is also good sense to shield the gonads so far as possible when the pelvis or hips are being X-rayed at any age, and this is not always remembered.

The widespread use of ultrasound, both to obtain information about the fetus and to localise the placenta prior to amniocentesis, has tended to gallop ahead of safety testing. There can be little doubt that it is a useful clinical tool, and despite some frights engendered by chromosome breakages induced by ultrasound in vitro, and some fears about shaking up delicate structures like the organ of Corti, there is so far no evidence that the various forms of ultrasound in clinical use are harmful to the unborn baby. It would be more satisfactory to have positive evidence that it was safe.

Risks from ingestion are most likely to come from food, water or drugs. Quite apart from additives used to affect the taste, colour and keeping qualities of food (Lloyd and Drake, 1975) natural food substances may contain a frightening number of potentially carcinogenic or teratogenic toxins (Crampton and Charlesworth, 1975) including aflatoxins, nitrosamines, mycotoxins (Austwick, 1975) and trace metals. The potato blight hypothesis of Renwick (1972) in relation to neural tube defects did not survive testing, but it would be a great pity if this was allowed to divert all attention from the more general thesis that naturally occurring food toxins might be teratogenic.

Drinking water could at one time be regarded as safe for human consumption if it was free from pathogenic organisms. The habit of dumping industrial effluents in the nearest river or lake creates new and complex problems, and the lesson of methylmercury and Minamata disease must be remembered. Man's apparently insatiable demand for water will soon necessitate recycling of water where demand outstrips supply (Martin, 1975) and this will compound the problems. Continuous chemical monitoring is likely to be expensive. In some of the states of the Arabian Gulf water costs more than petrol. I hope this paradoxical situation will not become more widespread.

So far as drugs are concerned, thalidomide taught us a lesson we are unlikely to forget. Many nations have set up machinery for controlling the manufacture and marketing of drugs. Animal testing in regard to several aspects of reproduction, including teratogenesis, is now mandatory. Nevertheless it is important to remember that no amount of animal testing will tell us whether a new drug is teratogenic in man. The weakness of the system, in my own country at least, is that once a new drug has been released for human consumption there is no systematic attempt to find out about the offspring of women who happened to be pregnant when they took it. Human teratogenicity testing is, in effect, going on whenever a pregnant woman takes a drug, but the experiment is without design or control and the experimenters, not recognising themselves as such, have their eyes tightly shut.

Turning to infections, we already have a good vaccine against rubella though we may not yet know the best way to use it. However, I think we are all learning something from one another and that a common policy will emerge during the next few years. The only other organisms which are undoubtedly capable of harming the unborn baby are cytomegalovirus, herpesvirus hominis and *Toxoplasma gondii*. There are considerable technical problems involved in developing a vaccine against either virus, and there is a lot we do not understand about the pathogenesis of congenital toxoplasmosis (Dudgeon, 1973). But I doubt if these problems will defeat for ever a technology which can put a man on the moon and bring him home again.

In concluding, I should like to consider briefly future prospects in that field where genetic and environmental factors interact. Environmental factors can clearly influence genetic structure – of individuals by mutagenesis, of populations by natural selection. Genetic factors can influence environment, as we see in the migrations of birds, butterflies and caribou, and in the individual's response to the environment in terms of metabolic behaviour. Man has acquired the ability to modify his environment to such an extent that he can almost opt out of natural selection, but he has become so clever at educating electrons and manipulating molecules that the possibility of mutagenic accidents must increase each year. There has been no shortage of chemical disasters in recent years which may not have been mutagenic but nevertheless had far-reaching biological effects. The disposal of increasing quantities of radioactive waste increases the chances that a similar and perhaps more serious mishap may occur.

On a more constructive note, man is continually learning new ways of modifying his environment to accommodate unhelpful genes. Until such time as genetic engineering in man is a reality the best we can do is to dodge the consequences of our less desirable genes. The best examples are in the field of metabolic disease, where we can either exclude from the personal environment factors which cause genetic indigestion (for example, phenylalanine in phenylketonuria) or we can satisfy a genetic hunger for something missing (for example, cortisol in the adrenogenital syndrome). Historically, of course, many food taboos have for millenia been playing the same game, protecting people from, for example, a deficiency of glucose-6-phosphate dehydrogenase in their red blood cells.

What has this to do with birth defects? Petter et al. (1977) have recently reported a fascinating observation in brachydactylous rabbits. Animals homozygous for the br gene all have congenital amputations of the limbs and an associated macrocytosis of the red blood cells, but with polycythaemia, not anaemia. The administration of folic acid and vitamin B_{12} to the pregnant does on days 9–16 not only corrected the red blood cell abnormality but also prevented the congenital amputations in about half the offspring and reduced the severity of the defects in the other half. Whether this observation will prove to have any bearing on the human malformation syndromes in which haematological abnormalities are associated with limb defects, time will tell. But it serves to remind us that genes can only exert their effects through biochemical mechanisms, and therein lies man's opportunity to intervene.

If an atheist was invited to translate the Bible, the book of Genesis might start: 'In the beginning was the Environment'. It has the same potential for good as the creatures with genes that arrived on the scene later. By all means let us continue to keep watch for any environmental malevolence that may molest us in the dark, but let us also regard the environment as something that we have been given power to manipulate for the good of mankind. And especially for the good of mankind as yet unborn.

REFERENCES

American Society of Anaesthesiologists (1974): *Anaesthesiology, 41*, 321.

Austwick, P. K. C. (1975): *Brit. med. Bull., 31*, 222.

Crampton, R. F. and Charlesworth, F. A. (1975): *Brit. med. Bull., 31*, 209.

Dalton, K. (1976): *Brit. J. Psychiat., 129*, 438.

Dudgeon, J. A. (1973): In: *Intrauterine Infections, Ciba Foundation Symposium 10 (New Series)*, p. 179. Editors: K. Elliott and J. Knight. Elsevier–Excerpta Medica–North-Holland, Amsterdam–London–New York.

Gregg, N. M. (1941): *Trans. ophthal. Soc. Aust., 3*, 35.

Lenz, W. (1962): *Lancet, 1*, 45.

Lloyd, A. G. and Drake, J. J. P. (1975): *Brit. med. Bull., 31*, 214.

Martin, A. E. (1975): *Brit. med. Bull., 31*, 251.

McBride, W. G. (1961): *Lancet, 2*, 1358.

Petter, C., Bourbon, J., Maltier, J-P. and Jost, A. (1977): *Teratology, 15*, 149.

Reinisch, J. M. (1977): *Nature (Lond.), 266*, 561.

Renwick, J. H. (1972): *Brit. J. prev. soc. Med., 26*, 67.

Sheppard, S., Smithells, R. W., Peckham, C., Dudgeon, J. A. and Marshall, W. C. (1977): *Hlth Trends, 2*, 38.

Smithells, R. W., Sheppard, S. and Schorah, C. J. (1976): *Arch. Dis. Childh., 51*, 944.

Vaisman, A. I. (1967): *Eksp. Khir. Anesteziol., 3*, 44.

Pre-natal and perinatal factors

J. P. M. TIZARD

University Department of Paediatrics, John Radcliffe Hospital, Oxford, United Kingdom

My assignment is to discuss foetopathies and perinatal hazards, topics which have rightly occupied a relatively small part of the conference, since these conditions are outnumbered by the embryopathies. However, the possibilities for prevention in the near future seem somewhat greater than in cases of defects originating in the embryonic period.

Foetopathies, causing deformity of organs that have undergone normal differentiation, have, unlike most of the embryopathies, relatively well understood explanations. Ultimately, avoidance of the damaging environmental factors will be necessary since screening followed by selective abortion is not, for obvious reasons, as practical a proposition as it is in the case of the embryopathies. In any case one has to consider the cost and question if the money involved could not be more profitably – in terms of health – used in other ways. Here local considerations are important. For instance, I doubt if the screening of all mothers for certain infections during pregnancy would really be worthwhile in Oxford. Dr. Nicholas Wald has kindly provided me with the results of testing cord blood samples in Oxford for IgM-specific cytomegalovirus and toxoplasma antibodies (Table 1).

Also on the grounds of expense, and for other rather different reasons, routine screening for the large number of rare metabolic diseases of the foetus now detectable by means of amniocentesis is also clearly impracticable. Routine screening of new-born babies is another matter as is that of screening pregnant women. The importance of detecting diabetes has long been recognised both from the standpoint of embryopathies and also of perinatal hazards. But it is by no means always efficiently carried out.

TABLE 1

IgM-specific antibodies in cord blood (Oxford 1973–1976, N. Wald)

	Tested	Positive
Cytomegalovirus	10,800	5*
Toxoplasma	10,800	0

*Only 1 of the 5 babies has shown developmental retardation.

From the original observations of Mabry et al. (1966) it seems likely that mental retardation – and also malformation (Stevenson and Huntley, 1967) – due to transplacental hyperphenylalaninaemia-induced brain damage in non-phenylketonuric children may be commoner than might be supposed. Institutionalised phenylketonuric women are not likely to reproduce, but phenylketonuric women who have been successfully treated in infancy and childhood, unsuspected phenylketonurics of normal intelligence and even heterozygotes may subject their foetuses to dangerously high levels of phenylalanine. I wonder to what extent this condition is now searched for routinely in pregnant women at first booking – in time to prevent the very high consumption of milk which some women (and their doctors) regard as desirable during pregnancy. Urine testing has the advantage of simplicity but may not be an entirely effective screen. Nevertheless it would be easy, and not too expensive, simply to add to the routine Guthrie testing of blood samples in the newborn.

In the past 2 years we have had 3 cases of what I think must be regarded as a maternal metabolic effect, that of severe hypotonia and weakness, especially of muscles of deglutition and respiration, plus talipes equinovarus in babies born to mothers who, unknown to themselves, had dystrophia myotonica. As far as I am aware no such cases have been reported in babies of fathers with the condition, but the nature of the abnormal intra-uterine environment is as yet unknown.

I will not attempt to list the drugs that are known adversely to effect the embryo or foetus when taken by the mother. They do, of course, include the drugs to which mankind is most addicted – tobacco and alcohol. The extent to which even moderate alcohol intake is responsible for foetal damage is convincingly demonstrated by the studies of Streissgath and colleagues (1977). The possibilities of prevention are obvious.

I now wish to turn to my principal topic, that of the prevention of brain damage – largely or at least most obviously manifest as cerebral palsy – as a consequence of perinatal hazards.

TABLE 2

Cerebral palsy in Denmark, east of the Little Belt

	Number of cases per 10,000 live births (total live births 825,263)			
	1950/54	1955/59	1960/64	1965/69
All	25.9	26.9	21.9	20.0
Spastic	19.4	18.9	16.3	14.9
Dyskinetic	3.6	4.4	2.9	2.8
Others	2.9	3.5	2.6	2.3

(From Glenting (1976a,b), by courtesy of the Editor of *Ugeskrift for Laeger*.)

There is now reliable evidence that the incidence of cerebral palsy has fallen in certain countries and in certain districts in other countries. A long-term survey was carried out in that part of Denmark that lies east of the Little Belt – for practical purposes all the islands including Zealand on which Copenhagen is situated. It comprises over half the total population of Denmark of 5 million. Dr. Paul Glenting ascertained all cases of cerebral palsy in children born over a 20-year period – 1950 to 1969 (Glenting, 1976a,b). Cases originating prenatally or perinatally numbered 1945 and represented 89% of all cases of cerebral palsy in children born in these 20 years, the remaining 11% being of post-neonatal origin (Table 2). It is probable that ascertainment was not complete in the first 5-year period, but since then there has been a steady fall in total cases and in each subdivision of spastic, dyskinetic and other cases.

It has frequently been said in the past that reduction in perinatal deaths would lead to an increase in the numbers of chronically handicapped children. This is, of course, untrue as a generalisation. Hagberg et al. (1975a,b) have ascertained all cases of cerebral palsy in children born in the Gothenburg region of Sweden (population 1.8 million) over a period in which perinatal mortality has fallen and, again, there has been a remarkable fall in incidence (Fig. 1). The total incidence has fallen from over 2.2 to under 1.4 per 1000 live births and this is principally due to a fall in the number of cases of diplegia, whether or not associated with low birthweight. In Hagberg's series, about 50% of all cases of cerebral palsy were associated with adverse perinatal factors and it seems likely that a high proportion of these are preventible in the light of existing knowledge.

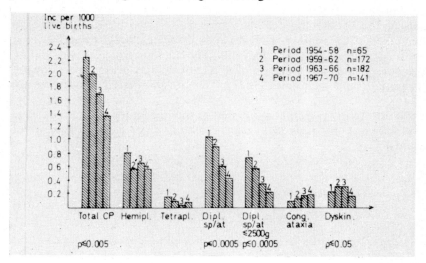

Fig. 1. Incidence of cerebral palsy according to syndrome. Sp/at = spastic/ataxic. (Reproduced from Hagberg et al. (1975a), by courtesy of the Editor of the *Acta paediatrica Scandinavica*.)

Although no type of cerebral palsy, except perhaps choreoathetosis, has a clear-cut aetiology, there are 2 situations in which associations, if not pathogeneses, are fairly obvious. The first is the association between pre-term delivery and spastic diplegia, usually spastic paraplegia. The second is the association of foetal and intrapartum asphyxia with dyskinetic syndromes, both athetosis and dystonia, with spastic tetraplegia and some cases of hemiplegia.

TABLE 3

Spastic diplegia in survivors of very low birthweight

Authors	Year of birth	Sample number	Spastic diplegia (%)
Lubchenco et al. (1972)	1947–1950	133	32
Drillien (1964)	1948–1960	91	20
McDonald (1967)	1951–1953	560	7
Wright et al. (1972)	1952–1956	65	9
Davies and Tizard (1975)	1961–1964	58	10
Davies and Tizard (1975)	1965–1970	107	0

There has been a marked decline in recent years in the incidence of spastic diplegia in survivors of very low birthweight. The outcome in certain follow-up studies is shown in Table 3. It is tempting to think that better care of the pre-term baby has been responsible, better temperature control, rational oxygen therapy and early feeding, but the fact is that we have no idea as to why this improvement has taken place. The only difference approaching a low level of significance in the Hammersmith series was that the spastic babies born in the period 1961–1964 had a lower rectal temperature on the first postnatal day than their contemporaries who survived without cerebral palsy. Obviously the best solution to this problem would be the prevention of pre-term labour, which is too large and complex a topic to be discussed in this paper (see Wynn and Wynn, 1977).

I now turn to the problem of babies whose cerebral palsy is in some way related to birth asphyxia. There is much circumstantial evidence to suggest that acute asphyxia, even of a severe degree, does not usually result in serious chronic brain damage in survivors. When it does the resultant damage differs from that produced by chronic or recurrent foetal asphyxia, as shown by R. E. Myers (1968) in his experiments on Rhesus monkeys.

Dr. Hilary Scott (1976) has studied the outcome of severe birth asphyxia in babies born over a 7-year period in the Hammersmith Hospital. There were 48 babies in all: no less than 15 of these were apparently fresh stillbirths, while the remaining 33 did not breathe spontaneously until more than 20 minutes after delivery. All were resuscitated at least temporarily and all were treated promptly with alkalis, which as Dawes et al. (1964) have shown will protect against brain damage in experimental asphyxia in newborn Rhesus monkeys. Half of these babies died within a few hours or days of birth, but of the 23 long-term survivors all but 6 have escaped severe brain damage (Fig. 2). Figure 3 shows a histogram of intelligence quotients at follow-up. All but 3 have IQ's above 70, including 3 of the cerebral palsy children. Table 4 shows the relationship between the outcome and the presence or absence of evidence of foetal distress.

It will not have escaped your notice that this work raises a complex ethical and possibly medico-legal problem. It seems clear to me from this evidence that one should try to resuscitate the freshly stillborn child, especially if there has been no evidence of foetal asphyxia. But this will result in the survival of some chronically brain damaged children.

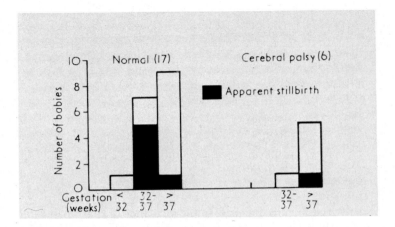

Fig. 2. Gestational age in relation to outcome (survivors). (Reproduced from Scott (1976), by courtesy of the Editors of the *Archives of Disease in Childhood*.)

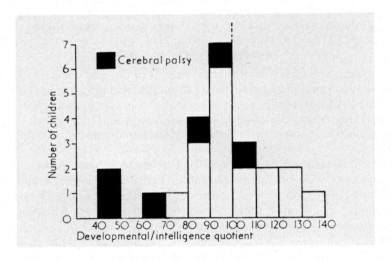

Fig. 3. Severe birth asphyxia and later intelligence. (Reproduced from Scott (1976), by courtesy of the Editors of the *Archives of Disease in Childhood*.)

Thus, while the prompt and effective treatment of acute asphyxia is undoubtedly of importance, of even greater importance is the detection of chronic or recurrent foetal asphyxia. This does, of course, bring us into the field of perinatal death, but I do not think that this is outside my terms of reference since many cases of cerebral palsy can be regarded as near fatalities.

TABLE 4

Ante- and intrapartum factors in relation to outcome

	Normal (n = 17)	Cerebral palsy (n = 6)	Death from asphyxia (n = 13)
Acute stress	8	1	4
Prolonged stress	2	4	13
Persistent foetal bradycardia	1	5	6

(From Scott (1976), by courtesy of the Editors of the *Archives of Disease in Childhood*.)

There is not time to discuss the detection of intrauterine growth failure, nor of the indirect pointers to placental insufficiency such as falling maternal oestriol outputs or, more recently from the work of Redman et al. (1976) in Oxford, the more promising sign of raised maternal serum levels of uric acid. Of some considerable interest is the recent finding in Oxford and Edinburgh of maternal serum alpha-fetoprotein levels as an indicator of perinatal mortality, quite apart from the detection of anencephaly and myelomeningocoele. The work of Brock et al. (1977) and Wald et al. (1977) was in fact concerned with maternal alphafetoprotein levels as an early indicator of low birthweight.

There is now routine examination of maternal serum alphafetoprotein levels between 10 and 22 weeks gestation in Oxford. Of a total of 3114 women screened in 1976 125 had levels more than 3 times the median for single pregnancies at the same period of gestation. A break-down of the 125 is shown in Table 5. The important finding is that, even when CNS deformities were excluded, the total perinatal deaths in these 125 pregnancies amounted to about one quarter of the perinatal deaths in the 3114 women. This was partly due to the detection of multiple pregnancy and partly due to the fact that the singleton babies had a smaller head circumference, lower birthweight and lower gestational age than babies born to mothers whose serum alphafetoprotein levels were within the range of 0.7 to 1.3 times the median.

In passing I would like to mention the problem of multiple pregnancy. Table 6 is derived from the findings of the British Births Surveys of 1958–1970 (Chamberlain et al., 1975) and shows the change in perinatal mortality rates for singletons and multiple births over this 13-year period. The latter survey and our own experience in Oxford suggests that pre-term birth rather than intrapartum asphyxia in the full-time baby is the principal hazard in multiple pregnancy.

TABLE 5

Outcome of pregnancies with high maternal serum AFP levels

Spontaneous abortion[a]	5	(4%)
Terminations[b]	11	(9%)
Multiple live birth[c]	15	(12%)
Singleton birth[d]	94	(75%)
Total	125	

[a]Includes 1 twin pregnancy. [b]6 with anencephaly, 3 with spina bifida, 1 termination on psychiatric grounds, and another on account of a high amniotic fluid AFP. [c]12 twins, 2 triplets, 1 quadruplet, 3 neonatal deaths. [d]3 neonatal deaths, 1 stillbirth.

(From Wald et al. (1977), by courtesy of the Editors of the *Lancet*.)

TABLE 6

British births 1970 – perinatal mortality

Year	Singletons	Multiple	Total
1958	32	115	33
1970	21	111	23

All the screening methods I have mentioned may enable one to concentrate the prediction of a high proportion of all hazardous deliveries in a small proportion of total pregnancies. But all are indirect indications of foetal ill health and the link between them and methods of foetal monitoring in labour should be provided by direct observation of the foetus. The most obvious is that of foetal movements. Obstetricians are, at long last, paying respectful attention to mothers' observations, but clearly further studies are needed. The next promising approach lies, I believe, in measurements of foetal breathing movements. Professor Geoffrey Dawes and his colleagues at the Nuffield Institute for Medical Research in Oxford have shown convincingly that disturbances of foetal breathing movements occur many days before the death of lamb foetuses from hypoxia, asphyxia, hypoglycaemia, infection and other causes – and well before changes in foetal heart rate, other possibly than beat-to-beat variation, have become manifest (Dawes, 1973).

It is disappointing that, although this work began in 1970, its human applications have not produced results of more than anecdotal significance. This has been in part due to the necessity of establishing normal variation in man, for instance diurnal variation and changes with maternal blood sugar levels, but also because it is only very recently that the technology has improved to the point of our being able to obtain continuous and, most important, quantitative measurements in women.

This brings me to my last topic, that of selection of mothers for delivery in what one might call Special Care Maternity Hospitals, where facilities for measurements of foetal breathing and other direct indices of foetal well-being exist. It is not, in my opinion, a case of providing all maternity hospitals with these facilities, not on the grounds of expense of personnel and equipment, but because of the importance of concentrating experience. No one, for example, would advocate the setting of heart transplant teams in every general hospital.

TABLE 7

Neonatal mortality by unit

Unit	Total live births (≤ 2000 g)	Neonatal deaths	Neonatal mortality rate (%)
1	118	47	398
2*	265	61	230
4	85	28	329
5	116	34	293
6	91	23	253
Died before admission	17	17	---
Total	692	210	303

*All babies from Unit 3 were transferred immediately to Unit 2. (From Stanley and Alberman (1978). by courtesy of the Editors of *Developmental Medicine and Child Neurology*.)

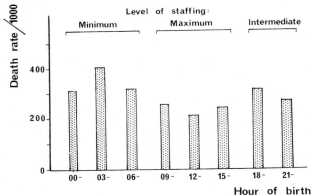

Fig. 4. Influence of time of birth on survival rate. (Reproduced from Stanley and Alberman (1978), by courtesy of the Editors of *Developmental Medicine and Child Neurology*.)

Exactly the same considerations apply to intensive care nurseries, which should of course exist in each, special care, but not in all maternity hospitals. Usher (1970) was the first to prove the advantage of the intensive care nursery in reducing neonatal mortality. His findings have recently been confirmed by Stanley and Alberman (1978). They studied the survival of infants of a birthweight of 2000 grams or less born in 6 hospitals in a district in South East London. There was a total of 699 such births over the study period. Of course the difficulty inherent in such studies is that of ensuring comparability of the populations at risk. But Stanley and Alberman have some indirect evidence of a novel type to strengthen the view that intensive care does indeed save life. Table 7 shows the neonatal mortality rate for each unit. Unit 2 was the only maternity hospital with a fully staffed and equipped intensive care nursery. Figure 4 shows the influence of time of birth on survival rate; when the low birthweight baby was born at a time when staff/patient ratios were highest survival rates were also at their highest; Table 8 shows the influence of the day of birth on survival rates. In

TABLE 8

Neonatal mortality rate by day of week of birth and unit (≤ 2000 g)

Unit	Total live births		Deaths		Neonatal mortality rate (%)	
	WE	WD	WE	WD	WE	WD
1	41	77	21	25	500	325
2*	92	173	17	39	185	225
4	35	54	13	18	371	333
5	31	79	10	20	323	253
6	36	57	13	17	361	298
Died before admission	3	14	3	14		
Total	692		210			

*All babies from Unit 3 were transferred immediately to Unit 2. WE = 'weekend' from 6 p.m. on Fridays to 9 a.m. on Mondays. (From Stanley and Alberman (1978), by courtesy of the Editors of *Developmental Medicine and Child Neurology*.)

all but Unit 2 mortality rates were higher at weekends; however, only in the case of Unit 1 is the difference statistically significant. Table 9 shows the staffing ratios in Unit 1 and 2 and you will notice that, compared with Unit 2, Unit 1 was understaffed at night and at weekends.

Another of the findings of Stanley and Alberman illustrates a very important aspect of intensive care of the very low birthweight baby (Table 10). It shows the direct relationship between survival rates and body temperature on admission to the special care baby unit. The case that fatality rate was 80.5 % when the temperature was below 33°C and nil when over 37°. There was a marked relationship between the incidence of the respiratory distress syndrome (RDS) and body temperature on admission to the Special Care Nursery even when maturity was allowed for. It is true that the illest babies are likely to lose heat most rapidly after birth but discriminant function analysis showed that body temperature was, with five other factors, an independent predictor of the risk of developing RDS. The other factors were

TABLE 9

Staffing in Units 1 and 2

	Cot: staff ratio (all year)	
	Unit 1	Unit 2
A. Nursing		
Total	3.6	2.0
Trained	8.3	5.0
Day	6.25	4.0
Night	12.5	5.0
Weekend	12.5	4.0
B. Medical		
Total (= day)	6.25	2.5
Night	13.9	5.0
Weekend	13.9	5.0

(From Stanley and Alberman (1978), by courtesy of the Editors of *Developmental Medicine and Child Neurology*.)

TABLE 10

Neonatal mortality and temperature of infant on admission to Unit

Temperature (°C)	≥ 1500 g			1500 g–2000 g			All birthweights* (≤ 2000 g)		
	Number at risk	Deaths	Rate (%)	Number at risk	Deaths	Rate (%)	Number at risk	Deaths	Rate (%)
≥ 32.9	22	19	864	11	7	636	36	29	805
33–	82	34	415	98	15	153	181	51	282
35–	67	25	373	240	9	38	309	35	113
≤ 37	0	0	0	15	0	0	15	0	0
Unknown	82	69	(750)	67	24	(358)	151	95	(629)
Total	253	147	581	431	55	128	692	210	303

*Includes 8 with unknown birthweights (but < 2001 g). (From Stanley and Alberman (1978), by courtesy of the Editors of *Developmental Medicine and Child Neurology*.)

gestational age, sex, antepartum haemorrhage before the 28th week, Caesarean section and condition at birth. Quite apart from the effect of temperature on surfactant synthesis, recent research suggests that the effect of surfactant in lowering surface tension is directly related to temperature. Thus the promptness and efficiency with which resuscitative measures are carried out will have an important effect on chances of survival and possibly, as I have already suggested, on the risk of cerebral palsy.

All that I have said surely points not only to the necessity but also to the growing practicability of concentrating potentially hazardous pregnancies in Regional Maternity Hospitals with special facilities for foetal monitoring and intensive care of the newborn. This seems to have been achieved with greater success in the Province of Quebec than anywhere else. There are nevertheless formidable logistic and human problems to be faced in doing so. Logistic problems include those of distances and population densities and will be very different in, say, Canada than in the United Kingdom.

Human problems apply to doctors and nurses as well as to mothers. The obstetrician understandably does not want to lose his 'interesting' cases. And we all know of 1 kg babies who have survived sound in mind, wind and limb skilfully nursed in a cottage hospital with a total lack of intensive care equipment. But in the words of my friend Professor John Davis doctors and nurses should remember that they are 'running a service and not a hobby' and acquiesce in measures to benefit their patients. From the mother's point of view there may be problems of quickly getting to know and feel confidence in a strange medical and nursing staff, of separation from her family, of difficulties in being visited. From the baby's point of view there may be additional hazards to emotional development of prolonged separation from their mothers and the horrors of intensive care. But perhaps I am straying too far from my topic. Is juvenile delinquency a birth defect?! According to Dr. Peter Dunn's definition it might be – and I am inclined to agree with him!

I would summarize as follows. Cerebral palsy is becoming less common in countries with high living standards. Nevertheless about half of all cases now occurring could probably be prevented by application of existing knowledge. To achieve this it is necessary to apply clinical and laboratory screening methods to all mothers in early pregnancy to select a minority for antenatal care and confinement in Special Care Maternity Hospitals, with facilities for direct foetal monitoring and Intensive Care Nurseries.

Finally, I must acknowledge that what I have said applies to countries with already high standards of living, which are probably of much greater importance than any medical considerations.

REFERENCES

Brock, D. J. H., Barron, L., Jelen, P., Watt, M. and Scrimgeour, J. B. (1977): *Lancet, 2,* 267.
Chamberlain, R., Chamberlain, G., Howlett, B. and Claireaux, A. (1975): *British Births 1970, Vol. 1. The First Week of Life.* Wm. Heinemann Medical Books Ltd., London.
Davies, P. A. and Tizard, J. P. M. (1975): *Develop. Med. Child Neurol., 17,* 3.
Dawes, G. S. (1973): *Pediatrics, 51,* 965.

Dawes, G. S., Hibbard, E. and Windle, W. F. (1964): *J. Pediat.*, 65, 801.

Drillien, C. M. (1964): *The Growth and Development of the Prematurely Born Infant*. Livingstone, Edinburgh and London.

Glenting, P. (1976a): *Ugeskr. Laeg.*, 138, 2984.

Glenting, P. (1976b): *Ugeskr. Laeg.*, 138, 1356.

Hagberg, B., Hagberg, G. and Olow, I. (1975a): *Acta paediat. scand.*, 64, 187.

Hagberg, B., Hagberg, G. and Olow, I. (1975b): *Acta paediat. scand.*, 64, 193.

Lubchenco, L. O., Horner, F. A., Reed, L. H., Hix, I. E., Metcalf, D., Cohig, R., Elliott, H. C. and Bourg, M. (1963): *Amer. J. Dis. Child.*, 106, 101.

Mabry, C. C., Denniston, J. C. and Coldwell, J. G. (1966): *New Engl. J. Med.*, 275, 1331.

McDonald, A. (1967): *Children of Very Low Birth Weight. M.E.I.U. Research Monograph No. 1*. Heinemann, London.

Myers, R. E. (1968): In: *Diagnosis and Treatment of Fetal Disorders*, p. 226. Editor: Karlis Adamson. Springer-Verlag, Berlin–Heidelberg–New York.

Redman, C. W. G., Beilin, L. J., Bonnar, J. and Wilkinson, R. H. (1976): *Lancet*, 1, 1370.

Scott, H. (1976): *Arch. Dis. Childh.*, 51, 712.

Stanley, F. J. and Alberman, E. D. (1978): *Develop. Med. Child Neurol.*, in press.

Stevenson, R. E. and Huntley, C. C. (1967): *Pediatrics*, 40, 33.

Streissguth et al. (1977): In: *Abstract Volume, V International Conference on Birth Defects, Montreal, 1977*, Abstr. nrs. 146, 147, 247, 305 and 306. Excerpta Medica, Amsterdam.

Usher, R. H. (1970): *Pediat. Clin. N. Amer.*, 17, 199.

Wald, N., Cuckle, H., Stirrat, G. M., Bennett, M. J. and Turnbull, A. C. (1977): *Lancet*, 2, 268.

Wright, F. H., Blough, R. R., Chamberlin, A., Ernest, T., Halstead, W. C., Meier, P., Moore, R. Y., Naunton, R. F. and Newell, F. W. (1972): *Amer. J. Dis. Child.*, 124, 506.

Wynn, M. and Wynn, A. (1977): *The Prevention of Preterm Birth*. Foundation for Education and Research in Child Bearing, London.

Developmental mechanisms and abnormalities: toward a developmental genetics of man*

CHARLES J. EPSTEIN

Department of Pediatrics and Division of Genetics, Department of Biochemistry and Biophysics, University of California, San Francisco, Calif., U.S.A.

As you have read this volume, I suspect that you, like I, have been struck by the great dichotomy between our knowledge of some of the fundamental aspects of genetic regulation and developmental processes and our understanding of the mechanisms which underlie many of the developmental abnormalities which we recognize clinically. Progress is rapidly being made in working out the organization of the genome. The structure of the cell surface is gradually being defined, as is its role in a large number of developmentally and physiologically important functions. The clonal development of cells and tissues during the embryogenesis of organisms as complex as mammals is under intensive analysis. Yet, when we consider the developmental abnormalities which afflict man and his most useful mammalian experimental counterpart, the mouse, we find ourselves operating at a highly descriptive level. In man, in particular, we are still very much concerned with nosology – with attempts to delineate specific disorders and to determine what, in McKusick's (1969) terminology, should be 'lumped' and what should be 'split'. Because of the difficulties in doing the types of genetically manipulative experiments that are possible in the mouse and lower organisms, the clear separation of apparently related disorders into etiologically distinct entities is not always possible and sometimes degenerates into semantic disputations that severely strain one's logical faculties. However, the importance of these efforts, both clinically and for more basic purposes, should not be underestimated. From the purely clinical point of view, accurate delineation is essential for appropriate counseling – and here I define counseling in the broadest sense, including treatment, prognosis, and calculation and communication of genetic risks. I would only remind you that it remains a fundamental tenet of genetic counseling that accurate diagnosis is the basis of effective counseling (Ad Hoc Committee, 1975). But the value of clinical classification goes far beyond these primarily pragmatic goals. If, as I discuss below, the clinical disorders are to provide useful material for the study of the fundamental mechanisms of development, these entities must be as clearly defined as possible, both genetically and

*The studies reported here were supported in part by N.I.H. grants GM-19527 and HD-03132.
The author is an Investigator of the Howard Hughes Medical Institute.

clinically. From the point of view of trying to learn about underlying mechanisms, it will make a great deal of difference whether a single mutant gene is involved, as in a 'dominantly' inherited disorder, as opposed to both genes in a pair being abnormal, as in a 'recessively' inherited condition (Epstein, 1977); whether a single locus is involved, as in a point mutation, or a series of loci are aberrant, as in a macroscopically visible chromosome abnormality; or whether a genetic aberration or an environmental insult alone results in maldevelopment, or interaction of the two is required. Sometimes the distinctions will be difficult to make. How much of the variability in the more common dominantly inherited disorders, such as neurofibromatosis and the Marfan syndrome, is genetic in origin and how much is environmental?

When is a genetic lesion big enough to be considered a chromosomal abnormality rather than a point mutation? Although α-thalassemia results from the deletion of the entire hemoglobin α-chain (Taylor et al., 1974), few would, I think, consider it a gross chromosomal abnormality. Conversely, although many inherited multiple malformation syndromes follow the rules for autosomal dominant inheritance, how do we know that they do not actually represent substantial but not yet visualizable chromosome aberrations? Likewise, I would be quite surprised if some ill-understood sporadic conditions, such as the Cornelia de Lange and Rubenstein-Taybi syndromes, do not turn out to result from just this type of lesion. Hopefully, advances in both the quantitative (Mendelsohn and Mayall, 1974) and qualitative (Yunis, 1976) analysis of human chromosomes will permit this notion to be tested.

THE ANALOGY OF HUMAN BIOCHEMICAL GENETICS

Coming back to my assertion that more extensive knowledge of the clinical and genetic aspects of developmental abnormalities will further our understanding of the fundamental mechanisms involved, it is now necessary to explain more explicitly what I mean. This is perhaps best done by analogy. One of the great accomplishments of the past century has been the exploitation of human biochemical genetics for the elucidation of many of the intricate details of intermediary metabolism. Starting with a general knowledge of biochemical processes, the analysis of a large number of metabolic defects has led to the discovery and investigation of many previously unsuspected pathways. Once this had occurred, knowledge of these pathways permitted the explanation of still other genetic abnormalities. The important aspect of this process, and the one which I would like to see extended into the areas of development and developmental abnormalities, is that it is a reciprocal one. Knowledge of normal biochemical processes and of their genetic control has permitted an understanding of how a genetic abnormality results in metabolic abnormalities. Reciprocally, analyses of situations in which metabolism is abnormal has increased our understanding of the normal biochemical processes. Changing the wording slightly, what I would suggest is that knowledge of normal developmental phenomena and of their genetic control should permit an understanding of how a genetic abnormality or environmental insult results in aberrant development. Reciprocally, analysis of situations in which development is aberrant should increase our understanding of normal development.

Archibald Garrod is generally regarded as the founder of human biochemical genetics, and a perusal of his works easily leads one to agree with this appellation. As early as 1902 (Harris, 1963) and more extensively in his classic 'Inborn Errors of Metabolism' which was delivered as lectures in 1908 and published in 1909 (Harris, 1963), he clearly demonstrated the usefulness of the reciprocal process of explaining disease by an understanding of biochemistry, and the reverse. It is somewhat ironic, but perhaps even the greater tribute to Garrod's foresight, that the classical Garrodian inborn errors are not completely understood even to this day – witness the difficulty in pinpointing the biochemical lesion or lesions in the several types of albinism (Witkop et al., 1974) or in understanding the pathogenesis of ochronotic arthropathy in alkaptonuria (Murray et al., 1977). Nevertheless, the earlier successes with the various pathways of amino acid and carbohydrate metabolism and the more recent achievements with purine metabolism (Seegmiller, 1976), and, to me the most impressive of all, with the catabolism of complex sphingolipids (Brady, 1976) and mucopolysaccharides (Neufeld, 1974; Dorfman and Matalon, 1976), certainly testify to the power of studying diseases to understand normal processes. If the point needs further emphasis, just lift up an edition of Stanbury, Wyngaarden, and Fredrickson's (1978) 'The Metabolic Basis of Inherited Diseases' which now weighs close to 2.9 kilograms.

On re-reading Garrod, I was delighted but not surprised to find that he was not unaware of the problem of structural or developmental abnormalities. In discussing the inborn errors of metabolism he points out that

> "...they are characterized by wide departures from the normal of the species far more conspicuous than any ordinary individual variations, and one is tempted to regard them as metabolic sports, the *chemical analogues of structural malformation.*" (italics mine)
> "...At first sight there appears to be little in common between inborn derangements of function and structural defects, but on further consideration the difference is seen to be rather apparent than real. Almost any structural defect will entail some disorder of function; sometimes this is almost inappreciable, but, on the other hand, the resulting functional disorder may be so conspicuous that it clearly overshadows the defect to which it is due.....
> "By selective breeding there has been produced a race of waltzing mice, but their bizarre dance is merely the functional manifestation of an inborn and hereditary malformation of the semi-circular canals. In the same way beneath each chemical sport may well exist some abnormality of structure, so slight that it has hitherto escaped detection. Among the complex metabolic process of which the human body is the seat there is room for an almost countless variety of such sports..."

Of course, Garrod was, for the most part, referring to the structural basis of functional (or biochemical) disease, and we now know that the structures he was referring to are macromolecules and organelles of various types – the enzymes and transport molecules, the membranes, the messenger RNAs, the genes themselves. However, if we now understand 'structural malformations' to refer to malformations in the conventional developmental sense and 'function' to refer to molecular processes, and if we rearrange the wording a bit when necessary, we arrive at what I feel is a reasonable conceptual basis for approaching the 'inborn errors of development'. Thus, with apologies to Garrod, I think we can regard

> "...structural malformations as the structural analogues of the metabolic sports"

and assume that

> "almost any structural defect will entail some disorder of function,"

not as a result but as a cause. Therefore,

> "beneath every structural sport of malformation will exist some abnormality of chemistry, so slight that it has hitherto escaped detection"

And finally,

> "among the complex structural processes of which the human body is the seat there is room for an almost countless variety of such sports."

What has just been expressed is, of course, essentially a reductionist philosophy of development and developmental aberrations. Stated more explicitly, development is controlled by molecular processes which operate through the medium of macromolecules and related substances and are basically under genetic control. Aberrations of development should, therefore, like the inborn errors of metabolism, be ultimately explainable in molecular terms. This formulation is not intended to negate the importance of epigenetic or environmental factors, but even these are presumed to be mediated by molecular events (Wright, 1973).

Before leaving the analogy with biochemical genetics, one additional point should be made. As Garrod indicated, the distinction between metabolic disorders and structural defects is sometimes more apparent than real, and we already have many examples of structural aberrations resulting from well-defined enzyme defects of the classical type. Consider just two – homocystinuria and the Hurler syndrome. The first, a defect in the sulfur amino acid pathway between methionine and cysteine, is associated with an abnormal skeletal habitus which includes many of the features of the Marfan syndrome (McKusick, 1972). Similarly, the Hurler syndrome, which results from a deficiency of α-iduronidase in the mucopolysaccharide degradation pathway, causes gross structural abnormalities of the skeleton, the so-called dysostosis multiplex (McKusick, 1972). If such conventional enzyme defects can result even secondarily in structural abnormalities, it is not difficult to visualize how defects in biochemical mechanisms more directly related to developmental processes could result in developmental abnormalities.

THE RECIPROCAL PROCESS OF STUDYING HUMAN AND OTHER MAMMALIAN MUTATIONS WHICH AFFECT DEVELOPMENT

Lest all of these ideas seem only hypothetical, a few examples which illustrate the nature of the reciprocal process of studying human and other mammalian mutations which affect development will be presented. A great deal of very important work on development has and continues to be carried out with species as diverse as sea urchins, round worms, fruit flies, and slime molds. However, I have deliberately chosen examples from work with mammals, human or otherwise, in an attempt to dispel the notion that mammals are so complex as to make them unsuitable for molecular investigation. None of these examples represents a definitive solution of a developmental problem and some presently accepted conclusions might not hold up in the long run. But, collectively they form a precedent for how the study of disease might shed light on developmental processes, and visa versa.

The pallid mutation and otolith formation

Perhaps the most intensively studied developmental mutants in the mouse are those associated with the T-locus, and this area has already been discussed in detail in an earlier article (Bennett, *This Volume*). It is generally expected that an understanding of these t-alleles will shed light on a variety of developmental events from the pre-implantation period on. But there are many other mutations of developmental interest in the mouse, and one which is particularly intriguing to me is caused by the mutant gene, *pallid*. Animals homozygous for this mutant gene have, in addition to pigmentary and growth abnormalities, an ataxia which results from defective formation or absence of the otoliths of the inner ear (Lyon, 1953). Since the same phenotype occurs when genetically normal animals are born to mothers who are deficient in manganese, Erway and coworkers (1966) determined whether manganese administration during pregnancy could prevent the occurrence of the otolith defect in the pallid mice. They observed that high concentrations of manganese administered prior to the 4th day of gestation resulted in normal otolith formation. The precise nature of the gene product which is affected by *pallid* is unknown. However, both this mutation and manganese deficiency result in an absence of incorporation of $^{35}SO_4$ into the mucopolysaccharide matrix of the otolithic membrane, and this defect in mucopolysaccharide synthesis is presumably responsible for the abnormalities of otolith formation (Shrader et al., 1973). Thus, analysis of the *pallid* mutation has provided insight into the basic requisites for normal otolith differentiation. Further investigation of the role of manganese in mucopolysaccharide synthesis should define the precise nature of the mutation itself, although the corrective effect of high concentrations of manganese suggests, by analogy with the several vitamin-dependent metabolic disorders (Rosenberg, 1976), that the mutation may affect the binding of this metal to a required enzyme.

Facial clefting and glucocorticoid receptors

The *pallid* example is of interest because it is concerned with the relationship between an exogenous agent, in this case manganese, and a genetically altered morphogenetic process. Another example of a similar type, but this time more related to the group of multifactorial disorders exemplified by facial clefting, is concerned with the binding of glucocorticoids to receptors in the cells of the facial mesenchyme. These studies, by Salomon and Pratt (1976), were prompted by the well-established observation that certain strains of mice, such as A/J, are much more susceptible to glucocorticoid-induced cleft palate than are mice of other strains – for example, C57BL/6J. In an attempt to assess the nature of this genetically determined difference in susceptibility, the specific binding of ^{3}H-dexamethasone to cytoplasmic glucocorticoid receptors in mesenchymal cells was determined. A/J cells were found to have about twice as many receptors as C57 cells, a biochemical difference which the investigators feel 'might partially account for the variation in observations observed in vivo in the ability of these 2 strains of mice to respond differentially to the teratogenic effect of glucocorticoids'. How this might actually work remains unclear, although glucocorticoids are known to be capable of inhibiting cell proliferation.

Brachypodism and the cell surface

While the facial clefting example does not relate to an inherited disease per se, but rather to the mechanism by which a teratogenic agent affects normal development, it is relevant to the present discussion because it is an illustration of how other teratogenically and multifactorially determined developmental abnormalities might be approached. However, back to back in *Nature* with the report just discussed is one which more directly illustrates the use of genetic mutations to study molecular factors affecting development. One of the many mouse mutations which affect skeletal development is brachypodism *(bp^H)*. Animals homozygous for this mutation have marked abnormalities of the limbs, with the 'hands' and 'feet' being most severely affected (Grüneberg and Lee, 1973). On the supposition that surface-mediated events are involved in cell interactions which are of morphogenetic importance, experiments were carried out to determine whether there are significant surface differences between mesenchymal cells from normal and mutant animals. Using ^{3}H-concanavalin A (con-A) as a probe, Hewitt and Elmer (1976) showed that the cell surface binding of this lectin is 2.6 times as great with mutant as with normal cells obtained from 12-day embryonic limb mesoblast. Similarly, agglutination of mutant cells by con-A is also increased. Although the relationships between agglutination, con-A binding, limb development and the brachypodism mutation are not known, and these data are clearly preliminary, it seems safe to assume that analysis of mutants such as these will ultimately lead to a more thorough understanding of the molecular aspects of limb morphogenesis.

Conradi syndrome and γ-carboxyglutamate

Another example, perhaps even more conjectural, relates to the human disorder, Conradi disease, which is sometimes also known as stippled epiphyses or chondrodysplasia punctata. This generalized skeletal disorder occurs genetically, inherited either in a severe autosomal recessive or a milder autosomal dominant form (Spranger et al., 1971). In addition, however, a phenocopy occurs when anticoagulants of the dicumarol type, such as warfarin, are administered during the first trimester of pregnancy (Warkany, 1976). Vitamin K has recently been shown to be a cofactor for an enzyme or enzyme system which carboxylates protein glutamic acid residues to form a new amino acid, γ-carboxyglutamate (Esmon et al., 1975). This amino acid has been found not only in the vitamin-K-dependent clotting factors, where it is required for calcium binding, but also in bone of various types (Hauschka et al., 1971). The precise role of γ-carboxyglutamate in bone is not known, but it is presumed to be involved in the process of calcification, either as an initiator or as an inhibitor. The phenotypic similarity between the teratogenically produced disorder, which is presumed to be due to interference with γ-carboxyglutamate formation (Perutz, 1976), and the genetically caused Conradi disease suggests that the mutation may also affect the same process, either by altering the carboxylating enzyme system or by affecting the protein substrate itself. With regard to the present discussion, the important point again is that knowledge of normal developmental processes may make it possible to understand genetically and teratogenetically produced developmental malformations, and the reverse.

Chromosomal aneuploidy and gene dosage

As a final example, I shall turn to a subject of great interest to me personally – chromosomal aneuploidy. Some of the work in this field has already been discussed in an earlier article (Rethoré, *This Volume*). If the multifactorially determined common congenital malformations, which affect about 1.0 to 1.5% of newborns (Carter, 1969), are taken as a group, chromosomal abnormalities, which affect about 0.5% (Hook and Hamerton, 1977), are the second major cause of developmental abnormalities. However, if we consider all known conceptions, then chromosomal abnormalities are clearly the principal cause of developmental defects which, for the most part, result in embryonic or fetal death. Conservative estimates indicate that about 10% of conceptuses are chromosomally abnormal and that about 95% of these are inviable (Carr and Gedeon, 1977). Of those that do survive with autosomal abnormalities, mental retardation and other developmental defects are the rule, while sex chromosome aberrations may be associated with these problems as well as with sterility. The challenging question is, of course, why? Why does the presence of an extra chromosome or chromosome segment, or the deletion of chromosomal material, have such devastating effects on development and viability? The answers – and there must be a multiplicity of answers – are not known, mainly because of an understanding of what is happening requires a detailed knowledge of mammalian genetic regulation and developmental mechanisms which we do not yet possess. However, it is my belief that the study of the effects of aneuploidy can add appreciably to just this type of knowledge.

In our own work we have been particularly concerned with the question of dosage effects – with whether changes in chromosome number are accompanied by proportional changes in the quantities or activities of gene products coded for by the aberrant chromosome. Three experimental approaches have been particularly useful. One is the establishment of aneuploid cell cultures, primarily from human sources. With such cultures we have been able to demonstrate dosage effects for the enzyme, superoxide dismutase-1 (SOD-1), in cells aneuploid for chromosome 21 (Feaster et al., 1977). In addition, we have found that cells trisomic for chromosome 21, the chromosome which carries a gene *(AVG)* governing the ability of cells to respond to interferon, are much more sensitive to the antiviral effects of this agent than are normal cells (Epstein and Epstein, 1976). This enhanced sensitivity, which ranges from 2- to 10-fold in magnitude, is considerably greater than the 50% increase which would be expected if we could directly measure the *AVG* gene product and indicates that small changes in the quantities of primary gene products may have greatly amplified effects on complex physiological processes.

The second experimental approach we have used is to generate, in a deliberate manner, mouse embryos aneuploid for specific chromosomes. Production of such embryos is accomplished by utilization of breeding stocks carrying induced or naturally occurring Robertsonian translocation chromosomes and makes it possible to study the effects of aneuploidy on a variety of gene products and the functions which they control. With this method we have been able to demonstrate, for example, that the specific activity of isocitrate dehydrogenase in embryos trisomic for mouse chromosome 1, which carries the locus *(Id-1)* for this enzyme, is exactly 1.5 times that in normal embryos (Epstein et al., 1977). Again, as with superoxide dismutase-1 a process of strict dosage appears to be operating.

We have also used the gene dosage approach in another way, and this constitutes our third general approach – one directed at the study of X-chromosome function. By measuring the activities of several X-linked enzymes in eggs derived from normal XX (40,XX) female mice and from XO females with only a single X (39,X) it was demonstrated that both female X chromosomes normally function during oogenesis (Epstein, 1972). A consequence of this is that oogenesis in XO females is genetically unbalanced with regard to the X-chromosome products which are made. This may, in turn, explain the reduced survival of oocytes in the ovaries of both human (Weiss, 1971) and mouse (Lyon, 1972) XO females, as well as the greatly reduced viability of zygotes, again human (Carr and Gedeon, 1977) and mouse (Burgoyne and Biggers, 1976), derived from such eggs. At the present time we are using a similar methodology to examine the questions of when the X-chromosome is functionally inactivated and whether both X-chromosomes actually do function prior to the time of inactivation. A clonal line of cultured mouse teratocarcinoma stem cells, designated LT, has been found to have 2 X chromosomes. Both appear, by gene dosage criteria, to be functional when the cells are in the undifferentiated state (Martin et al., 1978). However, as differentiation in vitro occurs, one of these X chromosomes is functionally inactivated, and there are no longer the 2-fold quantitative differences between XX and XO cell lines in the activities of X-linked enzymes. Once again, the use of genetically abnormal material, this time chromosomally aneuploid, is giving us new information about normal developmental and regulatory processes – information which, ultimately, should help us better understand the nature of the defects which result from the aneuploid state.

CONCLUSION

These examples, as diverse and preliminary as they may be, should indicate what can be accomplished by studying developmental mechanisms and genetically determined developmental abnormalities in mammals and, more particularly, in man. *Human developmental genetics*, if I can coin a phrase, appears to be ready to enter a period of considerable activity and growth. Knowledge of the cellular and molecular processes of development and morphogenesis and of their genetic control has been relatively limited to this point in time, especially with reference to man. However, as the material presented in this volume clearly indicates, the pace of research in these areas is gradually increasing and considerable progress can be expected in the coming years. Conversely, there already exists a substantial body of information about the effects of human and other mammalian genetic abnormalities on the grosser aspects of development, and numerous syndromes of chromosomal and genic origin with highly specific effects on various morphogenetic events have already been defined. What is now required is the establishment of the reciprocal process whereby studies of the genetic control and other aspects of normal development and of the genetically caused defects of human and mammalian development interact to foster expansion of knowledge of both spheres.

REFERENCES

Ad Hoc Committee on Genetic Counseling (1975): *Amer. J. hum. Genet.*, *27*, 240.
Brady, R. O. (1976): *Arch. Neurol. (Chic.)*, *33*, 145.
Burgoyne, P. S. and Biggers, J. D. (1976): *Develop. Biol.*, *51*, 109.
Carr, D. H. and Gedeon, M. (1977): In: *Population Cytogenetics Studies in Humans*, p. 1. Editors: E. B. Hook and I. H. Porter. Academic Press, New York.
Carter, C. O. (1969): *Brit. med. Bull.*, *25*, 52.
Dorfman, A. and Matalon, R. (1976): *Proc. nat. Acad. Sci. (Wash.)*, *73*, 630.
Epstein, C. J. (1972): *Science*, *175*, 1467.
Epstein, C. J. (1977): In: *Proceedings, 5th International Scientific Conference of the MDA*, p. 9. Editor: L. P. Rowland. Excerpta Medica, Amsterdam–Oxford.
Epstein, L. B. and Epstein, C. J. (1976): *J. infect. Dis.*, *133 Suppl.*, A56.
Epstein, C. J., Tucker, G., Travis, B. and Gropp, A. (1977): *Nature (Lond.)*, *267*, 615.
Erway, L., Hurley, L. S. and Fraser, A. (1966): *Science*, *152*, 1766.
Esmon, C. T., Sadowski, J. A. and Suttie, J. W. (1975): *J. biol. Chem.*, *250*, 4744.
Feaster, W. W., Kwok, L. W. and Epstein, C. J. (1977): *Amer. J. hum. Genet.*, *29*, 563.
Grüneberg, H. and Lee, A. J. (1973): *J. Embryol. exp. Morphol.*, *30*, 119.
Harris, H. (1963): *Garrod's Inborn Errors of Metabolism*. Oxford University Press, London.
Hauschka, P. V., Lian, J. B. and Gallop, P. M. (1975): *Proc. nat. Acad. Sci. (Wash.)*, *72*, 3925.
Hewitt, A. T. and Elmer, W. A. (1976): *Nature (Lond.)*, *264*, 177.
Hook, E. B. and Hamerton, J. L. (1977): In: *Population Cytogenetics Studies in Humans*, p. 63. Editors: E. B. Hook and I. H. Porter. Academic Press, New York.
Lyon, M. F. (1953): *J. Genet.*, *51*, 638.
Lyon, M. F. (1972): *Biol. Rev.*, *47*, 1.
Martin, G. R., Epstein, C. J., Travis, B., Tucker, G., Yatziv, S., Martin Jr, D. W., Clift, S. and Cohen, S. (1978): *Nature (Lond.)*, *271*, 329.
McKusick, V. A. (1969): *Perspect. Biol. Med.*, *12*, 298.
McKusick, V. A. (1972): *Heritable Disorders of Connective Tissue*, 4th Ed. C. V. Mosby Company, St. Louis.
Mendelsohn, M. L. and Mayall, B. H. (1974): In: *Human Chromosome Methodology*, 2nd Ed., p. 311. Editor: E. J. Yunis. Academic Press, New York.
Murray, J. C., Lindberg, K. A. and Pinnell, S. R. (1977): *J. clin. Invest.*, *59*, 1071.
Neufeld, E. F. (1974): *Progr. med. Genet.*, *10*, 81.
Perutz, M. (1976): *Nature (Lond.)*, *262*, 449.
Rosenberg, L. E. (1976): *Advanc. hum. Genet.*, *6*, 1.
Salomon, D. S. and Pratt, R. M. (1976): *Nature (Lond.)*, *264*, 174.
Seegmiller, J. E. (1976): *Advanc. hum. Genet.*, *6*, 75.
Shrader, R. E., Erway, L. C. and Hurley, L. S. (1973): *Teratology*, *8*, 257.
Spranger, J. W., Opitz, J. M. and Bidder, V. (1971): *Humangenetik*, *11*, 190.
Stanbury, J. B., Wyngaarden, J. B. and Fredrickson, D. S. (Eds.) (1978): *The Metabolic Basis of Inherited Disease*, 4th Ed. McGraw-Hill Book Company, New York.
Taylor, J. M., Dozy, A., Kan, Y. W., Varmus, H. E., Lie-Injo, L. E., Ganesan, J. and Todd, D. (1974): *Nature (Lond.)*, *251*, 392.
Warkany, J. (1976): *Teratology*, *14*, 205.
Weiss, L. (1971): *J. med. Genet.*, *8*, 540.
Witkop Jr, C. J., White, J. G. and King, R. A. (1974): In: *Heritable Disorders of Amino Acid Metabolism: Patterns of Clinical Expression and Genetic Variation*, Chapter 11, p. 177. Editor: W. L. Nyhan. John Wiley and Sons, New York.
Wright, B. E. (1973): *Critical Variables in Differentiation*. Prentice-Hall, Inc., Englewood Cliffs, N.J.
Yunis, J. J. (1976): *Science*, *191*, 1268.

Future prospects – clinical

F. CLARKE FRASER

Department of Biology, McGill University, Montreal, Canada

The previous authors have provided excellent reviews of what may, should or will happen in a variety of disciplines relevant to birth defects, all of them with an obvious bearing on the clinical aspects. I will just try to present an overview, by means of this simple-minded diagram (Fig. 1). The baby represents the babies of the world, both in and ex utero, and the bundle, of course, is the burden of birth defects. It should be represented as heterogeneous, composed of packages of various sizes (frequency) and weights (severity).

The weights on the bar, on the opposite side of the fulcrum are some of the various factors that tend to decrease the burden. The most important of these is surely 'natural' selection. There is no doubt that there is a major genetic component in the burden, and that there is strong selection against the relevant genes. It seems likely, however, that at least the 'common' congenital malformations are so common that there must be factors holding the underlying genes in the population – presumably because they are doing useful things, of which the occasional malformation is an unfortunate by-product (Neel, 1958). This implies that there may be an *irreducible minimum* frequency of these defects, and that increasing negative selection any further may have unforeseen unfortunate effects. But it may be that natural selection is so strong compared to what we can do to reinforce it, that this possibility should

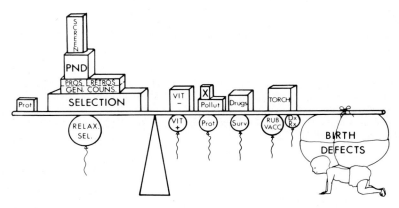

Fig. 1.

not be a matter of concern. Perhaps as we come to a better understanding of these balances we will at least know whether to be worried – or rather what to be worried about.

The next weight, reinforcing natural selection, is 'genetic counseling', which should more properly be called 'family counseling' or 'birth defect counseling', since families with non-genetic birth defect problems need counseling too. Most genetic counseling today is retrospective, that is, occurring after the birth of an affected child. That means that even if (a big if) all affected families were counseled, and if they chose not to have further children, the reduction in the number of affected children would be comparatively small – about 10–15% for autosomal recessive conditions and less for 'multifactorial' conditions (Smith, 1970). Furthermore, even in our society, comparatively few families who would benefit from counseling actually get it, either because of ignorance that they have a problem, unawareness that there is a source of help, or indolence. And, of course, even in the face of a 'risk' that may seem high (to us), parents may have further children, after reaching a responsible decision, or a state of non-decision, or neither (Lippman-Hand, 1977).

Until recently, very few disorders were exposed to *prospective* counseling, in which the high-risk couples are identified before conception occurs. With the advent of prenatal diagnosis the picture has changed somewhat, in particular with respect to mothers at risk because of their age. We are about to experience a sudden increase in the population eligible for PND as it becomes practicable to obtain blood from fetuses, and to screen appropriate populations for elevated α-fetoprotein in maternal serum (Brock, *This Volume*). It is time to take another look at the demands imposed on our health care services if we actually applied prospective screening, genetic counseling and prenatal diagnosis to its full extent. When we are able to detect cystic fibrosis, for example, we would need to monitor the pregnancies of about 1 couple in every 400, by amniocentesis. I think we are in the position of the small boy, running down a grassy slope, who fell, picked himself up, laughing and said 'me run faster than me can'. Already we are in a position where our potential for birth defect prevention far exceeds our capacity. Of women over 40 in this country about 4% are receiving amniocentesis for their pregnancies (Simpson et al., 1976). If we reached even half of the eligible women over 40 and more so if we use age 35 as the cut-off point, we would need a major expansion of resources. Not overwhelming, but major enough to cause problems in deciding how to enlarge or re-allocate health care funds, as we would need to monitor well over 1% of pregnancies. If we add to these the facilities for prenatal diagnosis for hemoglobinopathies, thalassemias and (very likely) cystic fibrosis, as well as prospectively ascertained neural tube defects – plus the necessary screening programs and counseling services there would have to be a vast expansion or re-allocation of resources. These would all be justifiable on a cost/benefit basis, in the appropriate populations, but those who allocate funds will have to be persuaded, and will have to find the funds.

Under the bar is a balloon, relaxed selection, which refers to the fact that improved medical care allows more individuals with genes of deleterious effect to survive and reproduce, and to the recent reduction in average family size, which gives selection less chance to operate. The consensus is that these changes will have comparatively small effects on the birth defect burden (Fraser, 1972), but it is interesting to think that demographic changes over which we have virtually no control, and know very little about, such as changing maternal age and family size, are probably changing the birth defect frequency more than any of our preventive programs will.

On the other side of the lever are nutritional deficiencies, environmental pollutants, X-rays, drugs, and infections, and these have been covered so well by previous authors that I will say nothing about them except that no one of them accounts for a major portion of birth defects, so no one preventive measure will bring about a dramatic drop in frequency (Fraser, 1978). We must not be discouraged by this – we are making good progress in identifying environmental teratogens, developing preventive measures and even understanding mechanisms. We must keep on chipping away at each of them; each small decrease in the burden will be vitally important to some families, and the cumulative effect will eventually be visible.

To reinforce one of the things Barton Childs said, let me emphasize that maternal alcohol, for example, probably the most important environmental teratogen known to us, should be represented not by a weight, but a pot, with a shrub in it (or perhaps a baobab tree) – the branches of the tree representing the many factors that determine why some mothers drink too much during pregnancy and others do not. The alcohol is not the teratogen, but the whole psycho-socio-economic problem of drinking.

And so we come to look (briefly) at the burden itself, as it is seen by the birth defects counselor. We see a frustratingly large number of dysmorphogenic retarded babies that we cannot diagnose, even nosologically, much less etiologically. Many of them seem to represent syndromes, still unclassified. Syndromology is struggling manfully (or rather personfully) to sort them out, and the recent application of the techniques of numerical taxonomy to syndromology may help (Preus and McGibbon, 1977). Classification is a necessary prerequisite to determining etiology, so we certainly need progress in this area. My personal hunch is that some of the syndromes of unknown causes will turn out to result from chromosomal rearrangements, not so far identified, that by crossing over occasionally lead to unbalanced gametes. They certainly behave that way.

We see frustratingly large gaps in our knowledge of frequencies of birth defects (Leck, 1977; Fraser, 1978). We see curious epidemiological variations, for example, in the frequencies of neural tube defects, that provide tantalizing hints of relevant environmental factors, but they remain stubbornly elusive (Leck, 1977). Perhaps this is because the real variations are occurring *prenatally*, and the variations we see at birth are the 'negative', so to speak, of the real variations. Are neural tube defects more frequent in N.W. England than in S.E. England because fewer die in utero in N.W. England? Is cleft lip more frequent in males because relatively more cleft lip females die in early pregnancy? If so, this would change radically our interpretation of the demographic data, and the hypotheses we would form. Prenatal epidemiology is one of our biggest blind spots, and urgently needs pursuit, yet it is difficult to get support for such studies, as grant review committees tend to think that this is service, rather than research – and (to continue Dr. Kinch's comparison) 'counting' is even more boring than 'preventing'. Yet counting is absolutely necessary for the construction of useful hypotheses (Poland and Lowry, 1974).

It has also been suggested that, if there is selective prenatal loss (and there undoubtedly is), one might capitalize on this to reduce the burden. Diana Juriloff, in our department, has shown that thyroxin, given to pregnant A/Jax mice, selectively kills embryos with cleft lip (Juriloff and Fraser, 1977). We are still far from a practical application, but the potential is there. Dr. Josef Warkany has coined a term for this: 'terathanasia', and suggests that we should devote more effort to understanding the factors that selectively abort abnormal fetuses (Warkany, 1978). This would be an attractive alternative to prenatal diagnosis and induced abortion.

Probably the most dramatic development in the near future with respect to the burden of birth defects is prenatal detection. There has been little emphasis at this conference on the moral, ethical and legal problems raised by these developments, but I think the next conference will have, because by then they will not be nearly so hypothetical. Our attitudes towards abortion have changed radically, and our regard for human life is doing so as well. Will this change our attitude to the deformed child in an adverse way? We must guard against this.

There are respected members of this gathering who feel that the 'right' to have children is not a right, but a privilege, and that parents should not be allowed to take a high risk of having a severely defective child. How high? How severe? What degree of severity of β-thalassemia, for example, justifies abortion? Surely the factors involved are so complex, and so personally individual, that the decision should be reached personally and individually, and cannot be done from a set of predetermined rules.

There are groups that would stop all research on prenatal diagnosis because it imperils the rights of the fetus, or because abortion is immoral. I find it much easier to disagree with the latter group than the former, but both imply legislated restrictions of what are now considered rights, and I feel very uncomfortable about this. I would also feel uncomfortable about basing health insurance premiums (much less laws) on our genetic risks, though I can see that Ministers of Health might see some benefits in this. But we are not responsible for the genes we carry and this would be a dangerous trend.

What we can do is improve public awareness of genetic risks and thus diminish the number who unknowingly take them. Social pressures will undoubtedly mount against those who choose to go ahead in the face of bad odds, whether we like it or not. These trends will provide a far better approach than penalties or legislated restrictions of liberties imposed on those who have been revealed to carry abnormal genes, in contrast to those who also carry them but don't know it. Restrictions of liberty imposed on some by others demean society as a whole. So let us continue to strive for means to lighten the baby's burden, without putting any fetters on the parents, and even by the time of the next conference perhaps the baby's expression will be distinctly happier!

REFERENCES

Fraser, G. R. (1972): *J. Génét. hum.*, *20*, 185.

Fraser, F. C. (1978): *Teratology*, *17*, in press.

Juriloff, D. M. and Fraser, F. C. (1977): *Teratology*, *15/2*, 18A.

Leck, I. (1977): In: *Handbook of Teratology, Vol. III*, p. 243. Editors: J. G. Wilson and F. C. Fraser. Plenum Press, New York.

Lippman-Hand, A. (1977): In: *Abstracts, Vth International Conference on Birth Defects, Montreal*, Abstr. Nr. 253. Excerpta Medica, Amsterdam.

Neel, J. V. (1958): *Amer. J. hum. Genet.*, *10/4*, 398.

Poland, B. J. and Lowry, R. B. (1974): *Amer. J. Obstet. Gynec.*, *118/3*, 322.

Preus, M. and MacGibbon, B. (1977): *Birth Defects: Orig. Art. Ser.*, *XIII/3*, 31.

Simpson, N., Dallaire, L., Miller, J. R., Siminovich, L., Hamerton, J. L., Miller, J. and McKeen, C. (1976): *Canad. med. Ass. J.*, *115*, 739.

Smith, C. (1970): In: *Modern Trends in Human Genetics-1*. Editor: A. Emery. Butterworths, London.

Warkany, J. (1978): *Teratology*, *17*, in press.

WORKSHOP SUMMARIES

What's new in genetic counselling

Chairman:

CEDRIC O. CARTER, MRC Clinical Genetics Unit, Institute of Child Health, London, U.K.

Speakers:

ELIZABETH IVES, University Hospital, Saskatoon, Saskatchewan, Canada
Genetic counseling for prereproductive married couples

ELSPETH WILLIAMSON, Southampton Children's Hospital, Southampton, U.K.
The combined genetic-obstetric clinic

MARY VOWLES, Paediatric Research Unit, Royal Devon and Exeter Hospital, Exeter, U.K.
Genetic counseling in schools for the physically handicapped

ANDREW CZEIZEL, National Institute of Hygiene, Budapest, Hungary
Advantages and disadvantages of genetic TV-programme for genetic counseling

E. ANTHONY MURPHY, Johns Hopkins Hospital, Baltimore, Maryland, U.S.A.
Estimating probabilities in genetic counseling

AIDA DE VARGAS, Hospital Vargas, Caracas, Venezuela
Vesico-ureteral reflux

GRAZIANO PESCIA, Hôpital Cantonal Universitaire, Lausanne, Switzerland
The risk of recurrence for bilateral renal agenesis

ELIZABETH IVES, University Hospital, Saskatoon, Saskatchewan, Canada
Exstrophy of the bladder – A family study

What's new in genetic counselling

C. O. CARTER

A. Provision of counselling

The first 4 papers were devoted to advances in methods of alerting couples to their need for genetic counselling.

There has been controversy as to the value of premarital and early postmarital genetic counselling. Dr. Elizabeth Ives described a study of a large and random sample of couples in Saskatchewan, who were visited within 6 months of their marriage in 1974 and 1975. The study was designed to estimate the need for and value of prereproductive counselling. Couples were visited in their own homes and a full family history taken with, wherever possible, verification of the diseases recorded from hospital and other records. Blood and urine samples were taken for chromosome analysis, plasma aminoacid levels and cholesterol levels. The total of couples visited was 528. The chromosome analysis showed only clinically non-significant polymorphisms, but 10 women were over the age of 35 and so candidates for prenatal screening by amniocentesis. Eight husbands and 5 wives had dominant conditions (including 1 each with probable monogenic hypercholesterolaemia), 1 husband had an X-linked condition and 1 wife had a recessive condition (hitherto unsuspected classical phenylketonuria), 4 husbands and 1 wife had a congenital malformation, 10 husbands and 7 wives other presumed multifactorial conditions (including 3 husbands and 1 wife with diabetes). In about 11 % of marriages there was a condition implying significant extra risk to their children and in 2 % a high risk of a severe condition in their children. Few of them were aware of this risk. In addition 10 dominant conditions were recognised in parents of the couple, few of which had been previously recognised. Three dominant, 3 recessive and 1 X-linked condition were also recognised for the first time among sibs of the index couples as well as 4 monogenic conditions that were previously recognised. In sum, 12 couples had at least a 1 in 2 risk of monogenic conditions in their children, 12 couples a 1 in 4 risk and 33 had a lower but significant risk of a multifactorial condition in their children. Dr. Ives concluded that there is a clear case for premarital, or at least prereproductive, family history taking to detect those who need genetic counselling because of a significant risk to their offspring.

The new developments in prenatal screening have created a need in many instances for the cooperation of obstetrician with a medical geneticist or paediatrician in genetic counselling. Dr. Elspeth Williamson described such a clinic in Southampton based on a district hospital which serves some 400,000 people and draws patients from

404

a population of some 2 million. The combined clinic is used especially for the counselling of patients who have had an unsuccessful outcome of pregnancy. There were 312 couples seen in the last 2 years, the largest single group being women who had had a previous child with a neural tube defect. There were firm indications for amniocentesis in 129 of these women. The obstetrician present was able to describe in detail the indications, risks, technical methods of the procedure, and the methods available for the termination of the pregnancy should this prove desirable. The combined counselling clinic was also valuable in giving firm support to patients where the indications for amniocentesis were insufficient to justify the procedure. The obstetrician was also able to contribute when there was a question of A.I.D., sterilisation or long-term contraception. The obstetrician also had a particular contribution to make where there had been repeated abortions and no obvious genetic reason for this was found, the risk of recurrence of abortion depending largely on obstetric factors.

The advantages of the combined clinic included that: (1) the couple could be counselled on both genetic and obstetric recurrence risk at a single consultation; (2) there is improved communication between the clinical genetic and obstetric services; (3) the clinical geneticist and obstetrician are able to educate each other in areas of common interest.

A special group who need prereproductive counselling are those in special schools for the physically handicapped, the deaf and the blind. Dr. Mary Vowles described a project to effect this in the City of Exeter and the surrounding district. The project began in 1973 with the physically handicapped and some 5 years after the genetic counselling clinic had been set up in the city. The project has now been extended to the 2 adjacent centres of population in the County of Devon, Plymouth and Torquay. At 4 of the schools Dr. Vowles sees all school leavers, irrespective of whether their handicap is thought to be genetic or acquired. At the other 2, after initial discussion with the medical officer to the school, she sees those in whom the handicap is likely to be genetic or part genetic. Cooperation of headmasters and medical officers of the schools has been excellent. Parents are informed of the intention to counsel, their permission is sought and they are invited to be present. Less than 2% of parents fail to give permission, though many are unable to attend because of the distances of the school from the home. Medical records are examined prior to the interview and at interview all the necessary further investigations are arranged. At the schools for the deaf, where communication with the patients is specially difficult, a teacher who has a close relationship with the patient attends and can help as an expert interpreter. The information given is recorded in the patient's National Health Service records which in Britain go with the patient for life. The patients are advised to seek further counselling before marriage if, as is often the case, they plan to marry another similarly handicapped person. On enquiry 70% of patients said that they had had anxieties about transmission of their handicap. In many instances the patients had sibs who are also at risk and they are referred for genetic counselling. It is intended to carry out a follow-up of these patients seen hitherto, starting in 1978, when the pedigree already obtained will be updated. The proportion of children being educated at special schools in the United Kingdom is about 3 per 1000 aged 5 to 16 years.

For genetic counselling to be successful depends in large part on adequate background knowledge of its possibilities and principles among the general public. Perhaps the most effective medium for such education presently is television. Dr. A. Czeizel described the response to the 2 series of lecture demonstrations he had given on the single Hungarian television channel to inform the general public about family planning and genetic counselling. It was estimated that the final lectures were watched by nearly half the population and the appreciation rating was higher than that for the standard programmes. The number of couples coming for genetic counselling rose from 54 in 1973 to 1216 in 1976 at the Budapest clinic, and similar though lesser increases were noted in other clinics in Hungary. This was accompanied by a substantial increase and interest in genetic research, an increase in the understanding of family histories on the part of the general public and the new discovery of a number of new cases of rare hereditary conditions. A disadvantage of the series was some increase in the proportion of inappropriate requests for genetic counselling and prenatal screening. Overall, however, the objects of the series have clearly been achieved.

B. Methodology

There is still much misunderstanding among medical practitioners and even among medical geneticists about the estimation of risks to future children. Dr. A. Murphy outlined the principles of making such estimates. Rational genetic counselling, he said, like all diagnosis, uses both the probabilities of the possible explanations for what is observed and the plausibilities of each as explaining the findings in the family. The products of these pairs of quantities are the joint probabilities, and since one of the explanations must be true, the joint probabilities are rescaled so that their sum is unity. Thus a single son with Duchenne muscular dystrophy may be explained by a new mutation in his normal mother, or inheritance from a carrier mother. Under certain assumptions explicitly discussed, the relative probabilities are the mutation rate and twice it, so the final probabilities are 1/3 and 2/3, respectively.

Probabilities which incorporate information on the carrier state are more accurate. Becker muscular dystrophy and Tay-Sachs disease are used as illustrations of univariate and bivariate data sets respectively. However, the main information may lie, not in the level of the measurement, but how it changes over time. Some unpublished data of Dr. H. L. Lau on levels of alphafetoprotein in maternal blood are used as an illustration. Unfavourable outcomes tend to occur where the regression line over time cuts across 'streamlines' for normal cases: the best index is probably not the level but the gradient over time.

C. Recurrence risks for renal malformations

Because these malformations are internal and therefore more difficult to recognise, there have hitherto been few family studies on which to base recurrence risk figures for malformations of the genito-urinary tract. Four contributors from the Clinical Genetics Unit in London described 3 such studies: on renal agenesis, vesico-ureteric reflux and bladder exstrophy. Dr. G. Pescia had found that 109 index patients with bilateral renal agenesis had 190 sibs and of these 7 (3.7%) were also affected. The sex ratio of the condition was 3.4 and the proportion of sibs affected was higher when the index patient was a female than when the index patient was male, 3 in 40 compared with 4 in 150. The birth frequency of bilateral renal agenesis is estimated to be between 0.01 and 0.03 %.

Mrs. K. Evans reported a study with Dr. Aida de Vargas based on 186 index patients with confirmed vesico-ureteric reflux (178 treated operatively). For the 39 sibs below the age of 4 years the parents were offered investigation by micturating cystogram, and 3 of the 20 so investigated were found to have reflux and 2 of these also had renal scarring. For the 214 sibs over the age of 4 the parents were offered investigation, by intravenous pyelogram, only where the sib had a history of repeated urinary tract infection. If scarring was found on the pyelogram there was further investigation by micturating cystogram. By this method renal scarring was found in 2 of the 104 brothers and 3 of the 110 sisters, 2 further sisters had previously been shown to have renal scarring (1 was on haemodialysis). The parents were treated in the same way as the sibs over the age of 4 years. Of 181 fathers 1 was found in this survey to have renal scarring and 2 had previously been shown to have renal scarring, both had been treated operatively for reflux. Of 183 mothers 1 in this survey was found to have scarring and 6 had previously been shown to have scarring (1 was on haemodialysis). It was estimated that the prevalence in these first degree relatives of the index patients was 10 to 20 times that in the general population. The nature of the anomaly and these family findings are compatible with polygenic inheritance.

It is known that bladder exstrophy occasionally occurs in sibs, but no recurrence risk figure has hitherto been available. Dr. Elizabeth Ives reported a family study based on 90 index patients treated operatively at The Hospital for Sick Children, London. The sex ratio was 2·3. Of 152 sibs (including 3 stillbirths) none were similarly affected, indicating that the recurrence risk must be low.

Detection of environmental teratogens

Chairman:

JOSEPHINE A. C. WEATHERALL, Office of Population Censuses and Surveys, Medical Statistics Division, London, U.K.

Speakers:

RINA CHEN, The Prime Minister's Office, Israel Institute for Biological Research, Ness Ziona, Israel
Statistical techniques in surveillance systems of birth defects

LEIV S. BAKKETEIG, Institute of Hygiene and Social Medicine, University of Bergen, Norway
Detecting teratogens by watching human births

CARL J. MARIENFELD, Department of Family and Community Medicine, University of Missouri, Columbia, Missouri, U.S.A.
Detecting teratogenic substances by watching the animal populations

PATRICIA BUFFLER, Department of Preventive Medicine and Community Health, University of Texas, Medical Branch, Galveston, Texas, U.S.A.
Some problems involved in recognizing teratogens used in industry

RICHARD JOHNSON, Johns Hopkins University, Baltimore, Maryland, U.S.A.
Problems in relating viral infections to malformations in man

GILLIAN GREENBERG, Committee on Safety of Medicines, London, U.K.
Maternal drug histories and congenital abnormalities

Detection of environmental teratogens

JOSEPHINE A. C. WEATHERALL

The Chairman outlined the problems and the objectives of the Workshop. It was planned to consider some of the technical difficulties in recognising and establishing the teratogenic nature of substances present in man's environment be it in air, radiation, water, food, social habits or other aspects relevant to ways of living.

In order to establish the teratogenic nature of any factor it must be shown that more malformed infants are born to parents exposed to the factor than to parents not exposed and that removal of the factor leads to a reduction in the numbers of malformed infants born.

Some teratogenic substances in mammals have been discovered in the context of animal breeding. But substances which are teratogenic to animals are not necessarily so to humans. So far, teratogenic substances present in the environment have been discovered by clinicians, through their intelligent observation of cases and their collection and analysis of epidemiological data about these cases; as was carried out by Gregg in discovering maternal rubella to be the cause of formerly rare eye defects in a particular community and by several clinicians observing the gross reduction deformities in babies whose mothers had been treated with thalidomide.

Congenital malformations, some severe some trivial, are found in about 2.0% of all births in most countries where records have been kept. Sometimes a family predisposition to a particular type of malformation can be recognised but for many malformations no cause is known and environmental factors may be playing a part in their causation. Many substances have been suspected to be teratogenic and have been or are being investigated, so far without establishing any relationship. These substances include tea, alcohol, diseased potatoes, nitrites, fluorides and lead.

No national system for counting all kinds of malformed babies or babies with birth defects existed in any country until 1955, when Sweden set up a system to record malformations among all births. However, in Sweden the system was not exploited as an on-going monitoring system so that the increase in babies with gross limb malformations was not recognised until thalidomide had already been established as a teratogenic drug and it is probable that more timely analysis of the Swedish data between 1958 and 1961 would have led to an earlier recognition of the increase in severe limb deformities and to analysis of causes of the increase.

The recognition of environmental factors in causing malformations requires therefore a system for counting the occurrence of malformed children and a system for investigation of possible causal factors.

Statistical techniques used in surveillance systems

In considering the statistical systems needed to conduct surveillance of birth defects on an on-going basis R. Chen described surveillance techniques used to distinguish random from systematic changes in occurrence. The prerequisites for a satisfactory technique are: (1) it should be powerful enough to detect a small increase or change in the frequency of the event; (2) a small increase or change in frequency observed in consecutive data sets will be taken into account and will lead to a significant result; (3) it should be adaptable, within the same framework, to surveillance of a large area or country and to the smaller constituent sub-areas of the whole area.

Three techniques which are currently used do not all comply with all of the above requirements. Two techniques are based on the assumption that the events (births of malformed babies) are distributed as a Poisson variate. The first considers malformed babies as a proportion of all babies born in unit time and an increase is declared at 2 or at 3 standard deviations from an expected level. The second (the Cusum method) – also Poisson based – considers the distribution of the events in unit time periods. The difference between observed and expected events in consecutive periods are summed until the value of the sum reaches a predetermined level, at which an increase is declared. In the third technique the random variable considered is the number of births occurring between 2 consecutive births of children with a particular malformation. The size of such a set is a geometric variate and an increase is declared when each set in a certain sequence of sets is less than a predetermined size. The second and third methods were shown to be of equivalent efficiency but the third involved less computing and was useful, particularly for small blocks of data.

Watching human births

L. S. Bakketeig reviewed the systems being used to watch birth defects and malformations among human births and pointed out that watching the changes in frequency of malformations alone would not provide clues to the association with environmental factors unless the environmental factors are measured simultaneously. There is a need to record routinely for all pregnancies details of antenatal care and of contact during pregnancy with potential teratogenic agents such as drugs or infections. Such data is invaluable for retrospective case/control type enquiries as these can be easily mounted and suspected associations quickly investigated without encountering the bias in the collecting of unrecorded data through the recollections of patients or doctors. The exchange of data internationally through the International Clearing House for Birth Defects was also seen as an essential procedure to provide data wherewith to help to interpret the variations in local rates, to help to distinguish the population background rates from those caused by new environmental factors, and to encourage international collaboration in studies of causation of malformations.

Watching animal populations

C. J. Marienfeld reviewed the problems and value of watching the breeding performance of animals which share the human environment and he described the study of birth defects of swine in the farms of Missouri. Variations in incidence of defects on each farm were mapped which have allowed the identification of plants eaten by pigs which influenced fertility and/or caused malformations. The advantages of using farm animals over human populations to study environmental factors are that the fertility of the animals as well as the malformations among the offspring can be easily studied for small areas; also preventive experimentation is more possible. Information about human births is usually available for only relatively large areas and not for individual homesteads or even for villages.

Industry and human teratogens

Some of the problems of looking for or establishing the relation between substances used in industrial processes and the reproductive health of workers having contact with particular substances were discussed by P. Buffler.

Three basic approaches have been made: (1) the assessment of reproductive outcomes among the wives of exposed male or among exposed female employees; (2) the assessment of foetal loss, congenitally malformed infants and infant death rates in communities where the particular industry forms the major employer; (3) cytogenetic monitoring for chromosomal aberrations in circulating lymphocytes of exposed employees.

The possible outcome of attempted family formation which can be measured are: infertility, foetal loss, or birth of malformed children. Type and time of exposure may influence the type of outcome according to whether mothers are exposed before conception, at conception or during pregnancy or whether the father is exposed before conception.

As the epidemiology of spontaneous abortion suggests that 90% occur before the 11th week of gestation and more than half have chromosomal anomalies, and of the 'recognised' pregnancies (i.e. those which reach 6–8 weeks gestation) 15% end in spontaneous abortion, it is probable that loss among all conceptions is as high as 78%. With such high proportion of normal loss it is desirable for industries to develop methods which will allow the recording, at the time of the events, of reproductive outcome for all their male and female staff. Such records will be more reliable than surveys conducted later in life involving recollected events. In some cases research has involved a recall period of up to 20 years of employees who can still be traced, and although such studies of family building and foetal loss allow analysis of employees by cohorts, they carry all the potential unreliability of recollected data.

Which viral infections are teratogenic?

In considering the problem of the relation of infections to malformations R. T. Johnson pointed out that infections of the mother with viruses which result in a chronic inflammatory lesion in the child such as rubella infection or cytomegaly virus infection make the causal association between infection and malformation relatively easy. However, in some animals natural and experimental infection with various viruses lead to a variety of malformations none of which give any clue to suggest the occurrence of an antecedent infection, and the absence of persistent virus make studies of individual cases futile.

The benign nature of the infection of the mother makes clinical recognition unlikely and the possibility of studying changes in immunity pattern by serology to detect the fact and time of infection would be very costly. It should be remembered that a virus used for immunisation and presumably therefore benign to the mother may prove hazardous to the foetus as has been shown with immunisation of sheep for Blue Tongue disease.

What drugs are used in pregnancy and which are teratogenic?

J. Weatherall (reading G. Greenberg's paper) gave an account of the concern felt by the Committee of Safety of Medicines of the United Kingdom at the very low reporting of malformations as suspected adverse reactions to drugs consumed in pregnancy. In order to maintain better surveillance, an on-going study was devised to compare records of drugs used before and in the first 3 months of pregnancy for mothers who later gave birth to malformed children with records of drugs used by mothers of normal children. Mothers of 836 malformed babies were matched by date of birth and by general practitioner/doctor with mothers of control babies. In addition to drugs prescribed, information about previous obstetric history and illnesses treated and family history were collected.

Drugs administered were analysed by their active ingredients and about 300 active ingredients had been prescribed. Only 31 ingredients had been used for either or both mothers of more than 20 out of the 836 pairs of mothers analysed.

Positive association of drugs with abnormal babies was found for hormone pregnancy testing drugs. However, where hormones had been used as oral contraceptives or in support of pregnancy no association was found. The association with hormone pregnancy testing drugs persisted when mothers with a family history of malformations had been eliminated. Benzodiazepines and antibiotic drugs were both used slightly more for cases than controls, but in each case differences were not significant. Barbiturates, which were used particularly in epileptic mothers and had been prescribed more for case mothers than for control mothers, but there was no significant difference between the figures for these 2 groups after mothers with a family history of malformed children had been eliminated. Most epileptic mothers were receiving a mixture of anti-epileptic drugs.

The most commonly used drugs were preparations of iron, with or without folic acid, and the anti-emetic drugs: there were no significant differences for either groups. Other drug groups reported in sufficient case pairs to allow testing included phenothiazine tranquillisers (40 pairs) and monoamine oxidase inhibitors (23 pairs). No significant differences were found. There remain some 285 active ingredients or groups of ingredients which were used too infrequently to allow a valid comparison of use to be made. It is hoped that the continuation of this study will allow the accumulation of enough cases treated by newly marketed drugs and some of the more rarely used drugs and will permit adequate measurement of their teratogenic risk when used in pregnancy.

Discussion

In the ensuing discussion it was pointed out that none of the methods reported in the workshop have exposed new environmental teratogens beyond those already reported by clinical observers. This view was countered by reference to the growing bodies of data now available which allow relatively rapid investigation of specific causal hypotheses. Much work has been done to confirm or refute clinical reports, such as the teratogenic nature of tricyclic antidepressant drugs, and of oral contraceptives – both of which are cleared by the United Kingdom Survey. Other allegedly teratogenic hazards are atomic power stations and preventive health procedures such as fluoridation of drinking water.

It was also stressed in the discussions that methods used for surveillance must allow rapid interpretation and that any scheme should be developed so that doctors are not required to fill in extensive records, and so that information needed to conduct surveillance is gathered from source documents needed for the proper care of each mother and baby.

An additional and essential need in the health information system was recognised to be the recording of spontaneous abortions and the conducting of karyotype analysis of aborted foetal material. Perhaps also, this sort of analysis is needed for foetal material from legal abortions or for a sample therefrom. It was emphasised that in any monitoring system, detailed examination of stillborn children (late foetal deaths) as well as competent post-mortem examination of all perinatal deaths is desirable.

Finally it was emphasised that data systems which are capable of providing information about family building and failure of reproduction are needed for the proper care of persons employed in industry and indeed for all families covered by a health information system which will be sensitive enough to allow the recognition of environmental teratogens.

Advances in biochemical genetics and screening

Chairman:

HARRY HARRIS, Department of Human Genetics, School of Medicine, University of Pennsylvania, Philadelphia, Pennsylvania, U.S.A.

Speakers:

DAVID A. HOPKINSON, Medical Research Council, Human Biochemical Genetics Unit, The Galton Laboratory, University College London, London, U.K.
Changes in tissues isozyme patterns during human development

CHARLES R. SCRIVER, McGill University, Montreal Children's Hospital Research Institute, Montreal, Canada
Genetics of transepithelial transport

MICHAEL S. BROWN, Department of Internal Medicine, University of Texas Health Science Center, Dallas, Texas, U.S.A.
Screening for genetic defects in metabolic regulation: lessons learned from the hyperlipedemias

JOHN S. O'BRIEN, School of Medicine, University of California, San Diego, La Jolla, California, U.S.A.
Lysosomal storage disorders

Advances in biochemical genetics and screening

HARRY HARRIS

This Workshop was concerned with 4 different areas in human biochemical genetics.

Dr. David A. Hopkinson discussed the changes which occur in tissue isozyme patterns during the course of human development. He gave an account of systematic studies on the isozyme patterns found in the tissues of fetuses (about 10–20 weeks gestation), young infants and children, and adults (20–80 years). A wide range of tissues were studied, and included liver, kidney, brain (cerebral cortex), placenta, lung, intestine (jejunum), heart and skeletal muscle. More than 50 different enzymes were examined. These included oxidoreductases, transferases, hydrolases, lyases and isomerases. Some of the enzymes are determined by single structural gene loci. Others, however, are determined by 2 or more structural loci, each coding for a structurally distinct polypeptide chain. The series of enzymes investigated appeared to be the products of at least a hundred different gene loci.

The so-called single locus enzymes showed the least developmental changes. In general, these enzymes were detected in a wide range of fetal and adult tissues and there was usually little variation from one tissue to another. It was noted, however, that secondary isozyme formation due to post-translational modifications was less marked in fetal life than later on.

In contrast, extensive developmental changes were found among many of the enzymes determined by multiple locus enzymes and there was much more marked tissue differentiation in their expression. Most of the developmental changes appear to occur in the second part of gestation and in early infancy so that the normal adult patterns of enzyme synthesis are established in the major organs by the end of the first year of post-uterine life.

Early on in fetal life, there is a tendency toward uniformity, so that the isozyme patterns of one tissue tend to resemble those of another. As development proceeds, the patterns gradually become more complex and dissimilar in the various tissues. Developmental changes appear to be particularly marked in the cardiac and skeletal muscle isozymes during the second and third trimesters. In contrast, there are relatively few changes in the brain (cerebral cortex) during this period.

Relatively few examples of what could be regarded as specifically fetal isozymes were identified among the very extensive series of enzymes that were studied. One striking example was an acetylesterase, known as A-7, which was found only in fetal brain. Most isozymes found in fetal life however normally persist to varying degrees in at least one type of adult tissue. No differences were detected between the tissue isozyme pattern of young (less than 20 years) and old (more than 60 years) adults.

Dr. Charles R. Scriver discussed recent work on the genetics of membrane transport. He pointed out that transepithelial transport, in tissue such as kidney and intestine, is a vectorial process. Consequently, asymmetry of structure at opposite poles of these epithelial cells is to be expected. In vivo studies on human mutants suffering from conditions such as cystinuria, iminoglycinuria, X-linked hypophosphatemia and Hartnup disease have provided information about the nature of these processes. More recently, new in vitro methods have assisted in their delineation. In addition, detailed studies of renal transport mutants in mice have proved of considerable value in defining many features of transepithelial transport.

Transient postnatal renal hyperiminoglycinuria is a normal phenomenon in man. In subjects homozygous for renal iminoglycinuria there is almost no transport function for proline and glycine in the neonatal period. However, during the first years of life, a partial proline transport process emerges first, followed by a partial glycine transport process. These findings reveal that 3 different mediations for proline and glycine in kidney epithelium occur. Complementary studies in the PRO/Re mouse (proline oxidase activity in renal cortex < of normal) indicate that epithelial (metabolic 'runout') strongly influences net reabsorption of proline. Since proline oxidation is apparently normal in renal iminoglycinuria and since renal proline concentration is normal in mammalian newborn kidney, it follows that the defective 'carrier' in the Mendelian iminoglycinuria trait resides in the luminal membrane.

Studies on a mutant in mice which causes hypertaurinuria have revealed that deficient net reabsorption in vivo is a function of defective β-amino acid transport at the luminal membrane. This interpretation was made possible by in vitro techniques which take into account the particular topology and asymmetry of the cortex slices.

Studies of X-linked hypophosphatemia in man suggest that this mutation allows abnormal backflux of phosphate anion from cell to lumen. Investigations of Hyp/Y mice, a murine analogue of the human trait, reveal a similar impairment of net reabsorption of phosphate anion in vivo, but no impairment whatsoever of phosphate permeation at the basolateral membrane of Hyp/Y renal epithelium.

Recent work with renal epithelium cultured in vitro has revealed a physiological transepithelial potential difference. It is anticipated that this preparation will make it possible to delineate more precisely the asymmetry of the transport function and the 'sidedness' of mutations which modify transepithelial transport.

Dr. Michael S. Brown discussed some recent work from which it is hoped that a practical and reliable procedure for screening for individuals who are heterozygous for a gene determining familial hypercholesterolemia will emerge. In recent years, considerable advances in our knowledge of familial hypercholesterolemia has been brought about by studies on the low density lipoprotein (LDL) receptor sites on fibroblasts grown in tissue culture. At least 3 different mutants affecting these LDL binding sites have been clearly defined. It would not, however, be practical to use fibroblasts in tissue culture for routine screening. Circulating mononuclear cells, however, which are more readily available on a routine basis might be the tissue of choice. An extensive study has therefore been carried out to see whether the receptor defects can be identified using mononuclear cells.

LDL receptor activity was assayed in blood mononuclear cells under 2 sets of conditions. First, ^{125}I-LDL degradation was measured in purified lymphocytes that had been incubated for 3 days in the absence of lipoproteins so as to induce a high level of LDL receptor activity. Phase-contrast autoradiograms of cells incubated with ^{125}I-LDL and electron micrographs of cells incubated with ferritin-labeled LDL confirmed the existence of LDL receptors on lymphocytes. Second, ^{125}I-LDL degradation was measured in mixed mononuclear cells (85 to 95% lymphocytes and 5 to 15% monocytes) immediately after their isolation from the bloodstream so as to assess the number of receptors actually expressed on the cells when they were in the circulation. Under both sets of conditions, cells from the familial hypercholesterolemia heterozygotes expressed an average of about one-half the normal number of LDL receptors.

These results make it clear that the receptor defects can be detected in circulating mononuclear cells. However, much more work will be required before the methodology can be made sufficiently secure and discriminative in order for it to be applied in routine screening.

Dr. John S. O'Brien discussed the genetic heterogeneity of G_{M1} gangliosidosis and the cause of the differences in phenotype which different mutants produce. He first reviewed the molecular genetics of G_{M1} β-galactosidase, whose defective activity is the cause of these diseases. This enzyme exists in 2 forms, A and B. Form A is monomeric with a molecular weight of 72,000 and appears to be coded by a single autosomal locus. Form B is polymeric and cross-reacts with anti-A antibodies; it is coded wholly or in part by the same locus that codes for A. This explains the simultaneous loss of A and B activity in G_{M1} gangliosidosis.

G_{M1} β-galactosidase A is heterocatalytic, cleaving β-D-galactose from ganglioside G_{M1}, lactose N-acetyllactosamine, and galactose-containing glycoproteins such as asialofetuin, red cell stromal glycoproteins and keratan sulfate. The pleiotropic effects of a single mutation affecting the locus for β-galactosidase A can thus be accounted for by a 'one gene:one polypeptide:many substrates' model.

Phenotypic variability among β-galactosidase A mutants probably results from better residual activity of the mutant enzyme for one substrate than for another. Certain patients with normal intelligence but severe bony deformities, and who are homozygous for a particular mutation affecting the enzyme, provide a clear illustration of this point.

Thus far, it has been found that all human mutants for G_{M1} β-galactosidase studied are structural mutants, synthesizing nearly normal quantities of mutant enzyme protein, but having abnormal and defective catalytic activities.

New developments in rehabilitation

Chairman:

MAURICE MONGEAU, Rehabilitation Institute of Montreal, Montreal, Canada

Speakers.

ALLAN S. BENSMAN, Department of Physical Medicine and Rehabilitation, Methodist Hospital, Minneapolis, Minnesota, U.S.A.
Habilitation of the person with myelomeningocele

YOSHIO SETOGUCHI, Medical Director of the Child Amputee Prosthetic Project, University of California, Los Angeles, California, U.S.A.
Total rehabilitation of the congenital amputee

Discussants:

PATRICIA LABOUTIN, Rehabilitation Institute of Montreal, Montreal, Canada

PIERRE LETOURNEAU, Chief of the Department of Psychology, Rehabilitation Institute of Montreal, Montreal, Canada

CAMILLE CORRIVEAU, Chief of the Prosthetics and Orthotics Department, Rehabilitation Institute of Montreal, Montreal, Canada

MAURICE MONGEAU, Rehabilitation Institute of Montreal, Montreal, Canada
Total approach in the rehabililation of the child born with congenital malformations

New developments in rehabilitation

MAURICE MONGEAU

Until the time comes when prevention of the birth defects of the spine and of the extremities can occur, maximum effort should be done in order that the children, born with malformations, who live, be provided with a full opportunity to function.

In only one clinic in Montreal, 1271 children with malformations of the spine and the extremities have been evaluated and treated in the past 15 years: 464 with malformations of the upper extremities, 452 with malformations of the lower extremities and 355 with defects of the spine. We know the necessity of establishing special clinics for each type of disability in children if we want to obtain the total rehabilitation of the physically disabled. The habilitation programs should start at birth and should be continued until adult age. There should be a total approach in the habilitation of the child born with congenital malformations. Those children should be evaluated and followed in multidisciplinary clinics which are essential to obtain a better and functional result. The rehabilitation team of those comprehensive clinics should include a physician in charge of the clinic with medical and surgical consultants, a nurse, an occupational therapist, a physiotherapist, a prosthetist and orthotist, a psycho-educator, a psychologist, a social worker and others who may be needed. The parents and the patient should also be very important members of the rehabilitation team.

A habilitation program is divided into 4 stages. The first phase: *the habilitation program at birth*. The program should start very early after birth in order that a complete evaluation of the child and the family be performed by a medical and paramedical team with good expertise. The results of a positive, realistic, individual and functional evaluation are then presented to both parents, who are the ones who should take responsabilities regarding the present and future habilitation program of their child. At that stage, the parents usually need more help than the child and the members of the rehabilitation team should be ready to help the parents to see objectively their child with his potential and his limitations, to answer the questions regarding the etiology of the malformations, to help the parents to accept the child as he is and to propose a long-standing rehabilitation program which they will have to accept and to which they will have to cooperate very actively.

The second phase would be *the habilitation program during the first 5 years at home*. The child with birth defects should be accepted in his own family. If it is impossible, he should be placed with foster parents because we should not keep in a hospital a child with malformation unless it is absolutely essential for special evaluation and/or treatment. The parents should cooperate to an active, positive and functional program to help the physical, psychological and intellectual development of their child.

If the child suffers from malformations of the upper extremities, we should try to develop a mode of prehension with the existing limbs. If prehension is impossible on account of congenital amputations, the child should then be fitted with prosthetic appliances as soon as he has developed sitting balance, i.e. between the age of 6 to 8 months. We should use simple prosthesis and the use of externally powered systems is needed only if conventional prosthesis does not give enough function. The prosthesis has to be accepted by the parents before being accepted by the child. The child and the family have to be trained with the prosthesis in the occupational therapy department to have a good understanding and good cooperation by the family as the training with the prosthesis will be continued at home for a few years.

If the child has an impaired function of the lower extremities consisting of paralysis in myelomeningocele or of congenital amputations, he should be helped and fitted with simple prosthetic or orthotic devices to develop standing balance around the age of 10, 11 or 12 months and generally the child who has developed good balance with a prosthesis or an orthesis will gradually be able to walk, sometimes with very little training.

During that period, the child and the parents should continue to be seen for reevaluation and regular follow-ups by different members of the rehabilitation team in a well-organized and special clinic. The parents and the disabled child should learn to spend some time outside the family surroundings to meet other parents and other children. The child with any disability should start very early to compete with normal children.

The third phase: *the habilitation at school.* It is essential that the child with birth defects compete early with normal children and for this reason, it is important that he be accepted in a normal school. Though the child may suffer from physical disabilities and though he may have to wear prosthetic or orthotic devices, he should attend normal schools if he can mentally and intellectually compete with normal children. The schools for crippled children should be reserved for the disabled children who, after a good evaluation and trial in a normal school, are unable to attend ordinary schools. Any child is entitled to education, it is a must that the disabled child with normal intelligence be accepted in a normal school by the administration and by the teaching staff. If needed, the personnel of the special clinic may go to the school to present the child as he is with all his potential and his capabilities with different types of prosthetic or orthotic devices.

The parents and the child should continue to attend regularly the multidisciplinary clinic for follow-up and reevaluation. Function of both upper extremities are reevaluated regularly and if needed, the orthotic and prosthetic appliances may be modified or improved to make the child completely independent for all the activities of daily living. For the lower extremities, orthotic or prosthetic devices are also adjusted, lengthened or changed during the growing period to let the child continue to walk and if possible, to give possibility of participating in some sports.

If the child with birth defects has been well accepted as a child in his own familial milieu and if he has been accepted in a normal school, being able to compete with normal children, he should be accepted and integrated in our society as any other citizen in the community, he should learn to compete with normal people and he should become completely independent as a fully fledged member of the society.

Delineation of malformation syndromes

Chairman:

PAUL E. POLANI, Paediatric Research Unit, Guy's Hospital Medical School, London, U.K.

Speakers:

PETER M. DUNN, Department of Child Health, University of Bristol, Southmead Hospital, Bristol, U.K.
The classification of birth defects: problems and proposals

DAVID W. SMITH, University of Washington, Seattle, Washington, U.S.A.
Delineation of patterns of malformation: especially anomalads

JAIME L. FRIAS, Department of Pediatrics, University of Florida, Gainesville, Florida, U.S.A.
Categorization of malformation patterns in the Collaborative Perinatal Project

Delineation of malformation syndromes

PAUL E. POLANI

In clinical work it may be important to lump conditions together or to split them apart just as in general it can be eminently suitable to believe or critically relevant to doubt. In the clinical activities involved in lumping or splitting – or better lumping *and* splitting because most of us neither fully follow one path nor the other – the objective may superficially look like just trying to achieve an orderly tidiness which ties together and relates to each other seemingly disconnected facts. But behind this apparent quest for tidiness we aim at achieving a deeper objective, that of classifying and systematizing: though not as exercises *per se* but in the hope of arriving at some useful generalisations; useful, that is, in an immediately practical way, or for a more distant theoretical aim. Thus the recognition of characteristic clusters of signs and symptoms in individual patients with a disease, a malformation or other develop-mental deviation serves a number of purposes in medicine. For example it is essential for arriving at a forecast of the natural history of a condition, in other words, it is essential to formulate its prognosis, and thus, to the planning of management and treatment. It is essential for the particular form of management which is genetic counselling based on an empirical or other assessment of recurrence risk. It is equally essential as a preliminary to the collection of epidemiological information about clinical conditions and the study and comparison of their clustering in space and time. It also provides an essential basis for causation studies whose ultimate aim, generally, is prevention.

Such were the guiding thoughts of the organisers of this Workshop, which was introduced by 3 main speakers.

Peter M. Dunn introduced his presentation on the classification of birth defects by defining birth defect as an imperfection or impairment of normal development. The current classification of birth defects is mainly based on their anatomical characteristics. This methodology has the advantage of simplicity. However, the oversimplification of a complex subject is likely to impede progress towards a better understanding of the aetiology, significance and interrelationship of different congenital anomalies. It may also be responsible for the mis-interpretation of malformation statistics, and this may have serious implications. At the same time there is a lack of standardisation and definition of the terms and nomenclature used in this field. Congenital defects can present as 'anomalies' or in other ways, for example as the presence of foetal disease, perinatal illness, birth trauma, biochemical derangement, etc. Anomalies in turn can be 'malformations', i.e. defects originating during the period of organogenesis (embryopathies) or 'deformations', defects arising after completion of major organogenesis (foetopathies). These are, therefore, alterations in form or structure of a previously normally formed part. Approximately one-third of congenital anomalies are congenital postural (musculo-skeletal) deformities. The distinction is important. Thus clearly malformations have a higher incidence during the first 20 weeks of intrauterine life compared with deformations, the perinatal mortality of malformations is about 40 %, compared with just over 5 % in the case of deformations. In the former but not in the latter structural changes are common and recovery (spontaneously or after suitable postural treatment) is common in deformations and very rare in malformations. Two further concepts can be usefully introduced in the field of birth defects: abnormalities of structure or form due to delay or error of transitional state from foetal to postnatal life (for example persistent ductus arteriosus or undescended testis). These may be called misformations. Then there is unusual variation in size, structure or function, perhaps to be called 'variformations'. All in all there are 3 different methods of classifying birth defects. The first is based on the clinical significance of the defect in terms of survival, handicap and correctability. A second method depends on the prenatal time at which the defect is likely to have arisen. The third depends on the cause of the defect. The simultaneous use of some or all of these guidelines of classifications may help to clarify studies on birth defects.

In his presentation on patterns of malformations, especially anomalads, David W. Smith considered the general problem of classifying an infant with a defect in morphogenesis. There are essentially 3 clinical sub-categories into which the patient may fit. First, as emphasized by Peter Dunn, is the more benign *deformation* category due to extrinsic forces, most commonly the consequence of late uterine constraint. Second is the intrinsic *malformation* group in which a birth defect is interpreted as being the consequence of a single localized defect in morphogenesis, an *anomaly*. This, in turn, may result in a single defect by birth, or one in which there has been a cascade of additional defects by birth – an *anomalad* (alternative names have been suggested for this such as polyanomaly, anomaly complex, malformation complex, developmental field defect, etc.). The third category comprises patients with multiple anomalies and/or anomalads: *malformation syndromes*. The merit of such a distinction can be simply emphasized by an example. The recurrence risk for common postural deformities is seemingly quite low; for an anomaly or anomalad the risk is most commonly in the 1 to 5 % range; and for malformation syndromes the risk differs in relation to the specific aetiology of the particular syndrome. The constraints on the foetus as it outgrows its uterus underlie the origin of deformations. Thus these constraints are more likely in the firstborn, in twins, in prolonged breech presentations and/or in oligo-hydramnios. Incidentally the clue to treatment is the clue to the origin of the deformations.

The anomalad concept is an important one. Otherwise normal patients with an anomalad share similar types of findings with patients having a single anomaly. For example each anomaly or anomalad is more likely to occur in one sex than the other. Also, though concordance is greater in monozygotic twins than in dizygotic twins, the majority of affected monozygotic twins are non-concordant for a given anomaly or anomalad, and there is variability of expression of the anomalad between twins. An important issue is whether a given defect can be explained as secondary to a more primary abnormality. Examples of minor anomalies which are generally *secondary* to another defect in morphogenesis, are inner canthal folds secondary to a low nasal bridge, or upslanting palpebral fissures due to small frontal lobes of the brain. Though of little direct consequence to the patient, such minor anomalies can be valuable clues to the nature and timing of the problem in development.

Much more data should be obtained on the recurrence risk for specific anomalads and the predominant cause or causes responsible for them. In doing so relatives must be evaluated for the whole spectrum of a particular anomalad, from mild to severe. Preferably measurement data should be gathered. The data should be obtained in much the same fashion as has been done for cleft lip with or without cleft palate. Examples of anomalads include the Robin anomalad, Klippel-Feil anomalad, Sturge-Weber anomalad, holoprosencephaly anomalad, exstrophy of bladder anomalad, and many other patterns of malformation.

An anomalad may occur in an otherwise normal individual, in which case the recurrence risk is usually of low magnitude, or it may occur as a part of a syndrome of multiple anomalies in which case the recurrence risk is dependent on the specific diagnosis. For example, though the Robin anomalad most commonly occurs as an isolated problem in an otherwise normal individual, in at least 25 % of the cases it is part of a syndrome. In this case the recurrence risk depends on a complete diagnosis, including aetiology.

As his contribution to the Workshop Jaime L. Frias presented a classification of the malformations encountered in the Collaborative Perinatal Project of the Institute, now known as The National Institute of Neurological Disease and Stroke of the National Institutes of Health. The study, which ran from 1959 to 1965, recorded 54,452 pregnancies, of which 1,195 were multiple, and included 1,017 foetal and 1,416 infant deaths. Dr. Frias with D. W. Smith, N. C. Myrianthopoulos and C. S. Chung reviewed the clinical records of 1,488 subjects with malformations. 1413 had been initially identified as having multiple anomalies; among those classified as having a single malformation, there were some diagnoses that suggested the presence of multiple errors (e.g. Down's syndrome, neural tube defect).

587 among these 1,488 cases were considered to have significant multiple malformations, an incidence of 10.7 per 1,000 births. The remaining had either normal variants, single malformations or multiple minor anomalies and for this reason were excluded from further consideration.

Analysis of the 587 cases with multiple malformations showed that:
1. In 251 patients (43 %) the condition could be interpreted as the result of a single localised error in morphogenesis culminating in multiple defects *(anomalad)*. Among these, the most common were closure defects of the neural tube, cleft lip with and without cleft palate, the Smith-Töndury anomalad, the oligo-hydramnios tetrad and the amniotic bands anomalad (73 involved the central nervous system, 48 the genito-urinary tract, 33 the cardiovascular system, 31 the gastro-intestinal system, for example).
2. In 143 (24 %) a specific syndrome was identified, caused either by chromosomal abnormalities (74 cases), single gene defects (24 cases), environmental (34 cases) or unknown factors (11 cases). There were 59 examples of Down's syndrome (1.08 per

1,000 total births), 6 examples of trisomy 18 (0.11 per 1,000), 5 of trisomy 13 (0.09 per 1,000) and 3 of 45,X Turner's syndrome (0.05 per 1,000). Among the single gene defects there were 3 examples of the Meckel-Gruber syndrome and 2 each of achondroplasia, the Holt-Oram syndrome and osteogenesis imperfecta, etc. There were 14 examples of rubella, 11 of foetal hydantoin, 6 of foetal alcohol syndromes and 3 of other foetal infection. In the group of unknown origin there were 3 examples of Noonan and 1 each of the de Lange, Prader-Willi, Rubinstein-Taybi syndromes, as well as others.

3. In 193 cases (33%) the pattern of malformation could not be readily interpreted as an anomalad or as a recognizable syndrome.

Anomalads as a category are responsible for nearly one half of all multiple defect cases. This underscores the importance of a developmental approach to the evaluation of patients with patterns of malformation. It is clear that a system of classification based on clinical and morbid anatomical features and leaning on an appreciation of developmental mechanisms has much to recommend itself for epidemiological and aetiological studies. Equally clear is the emphasis laid on causation, first to bring uniformity into the method of classification and secondly to direct ideas at better methods of diagnosis and at prevention. It is also important to stress that adherence to clinical descriptions should be as strict as possible, while acknowledging the variability of expression of many anomalies, often discovered from the study of close relatives or when varied anomalies share a common cause. Eponyms in general retain their usefulness and when used should respect historical priorities.

Advances in cytogenetics

Chairman:

BERNARD DUTRILLAUX, Institut de Progenèse, Faculté de Médecine, Paris, France

Speakers:

K. SPERLING, Freie Universität Berlin, Berlin, Federal Republic of Germany
Premature chromosome condensation

ORLANDO J. MILLER, College of Physicians and Surgeons, New York, New York, U.S.A.
A silver staining technique for studying ribosomal RNA gene location, multiplicity, and function

JEAN DE GROUCHY, Hôpital des Enfants-Malades, Paris, France
Chromosome evolution of the primates

BERNARD DUTRILLAUX, Institut de Progenèse, Faculté de Médecine, Paris, France
The impact of BrdU incorporation techniques in human cytogenetics

MARIE-ODILE RETHORÉ, Hôpital des Enfants-Malades, Paris, France
Chromosome 8 anomalies

MALCOLM A. FERGUSON-SMITH, Department of Medical Genetics, University of Glasgow, U.K.
Human pericentric inversions: their behaviour in meiosis and implications for genetic counseling

CLAUDE-LISE RICHER, Département d'Anatomie, Université de Montréal, Montréal, Canada
Usefulness of R- and T-banding for meiotic bivalents

Advances in cytogenetics

BERNARD DUTRILLAUX

Important technical improvements since 1970 have led to a real revolution in human cytogenetics. Its applications have become more numerous, and above all its results much more precise. Furthermore, entirely new fields of research have opened up. Neither human cytogenetics nor that of mammals in general is any longer a purely descriptive technology. The loci of many genes are now assigned and the role, the replication, and the inactivation of segments of chromosomes have lost much of their secret.

The aim of this workshop was to review to date some of these recent developments.

Dr. K. Sperling introduced the phenomenon of 'premature chromosome condensation' (pcc): fusion between metaphasic and interphasic cells resulting in a condensation of the interphasic chromatin. The same phenomenon can be observed for single chromosomes in micronuclei. It thus has become possible to visualize interphasic chromosomes by light microscopy, their morphology varying according to the cell cycle: single stranded at G1, double stranded at G2, and apparently pulverized at S. Furthermore, it is postulated that the differential condensation of the chromatids, and some of their staining properties, are related to their physiological activity during interphase. This technique also offers, among other advantages, the possibility of visualizing chromosomal damage immediately after a mutagenic treatment.

Dr. O. J. Miller reported some recent applications of the silver staining technique in the study of the mapping and function of the ribosomal RNA genes. The nucleolus organizer regions (NORs), which are the sites of 18S and 28S ribosomal RNA genes, are localized in the short arm of the acrocentric chromosomes in man. The amount of Ag-stain is relatively constant for a given chromosome in a given individual, but varies between individuals.

The amount of Ag-stain on each acrocentric is correlated with the frequency with which it is involved in satellite association. In interspecific hybrids, there is evidence for regulation of the NORs, and Ag-staining can detect only functional NORs. Thus in mouse–human somatic cell hybrids, where human chromosomes are preferentially lost, and where human 28S rRNA is absent, there is no Ag-staining of the human NORs. On the other hand, in mouse–human reverse hybrids, where mouse chromosomes are eliminated and where mouse 28S rRNA is absent, there is no Ag-staining of mouse NORs while human NORs are stained.

The Ag-staining method is at present the only method which characterizes a precise genic function.

Dr. J. de Grouchy discussed chromosomal evolution in the primates. Comparative karyotype analysis and gene mapping yield convergent results: man, the Pongidae (chimpanzee, gorilla and orangoutan) and more distantly related species such as the African green monkey and the baboon have a certain number of chromosomes or chromosome segments in common. This is particularly clear for the chromosome corresponding to the human 1, and the successive modifications undergone by this chromosome may be traced back to a common ancestor living some 50 million years ago.

Dr. B. Dutrillaux presented a variety of chromosomal modifications, all obtained after treatment by BrdU and staining with acridine orange. One of the major applications of the technique is the study of DNA replication time in the R- and Q-bands. This provides a new criterion in chromosome analysis. It appears that all R-bands replicate their DNA in the early S-phase. In each group of bands, variations in replication time may be observed. For instance, some R-bands are very early replicating, and some relatively late. There appears to be a correlation between replication time and gene dosage effect in the case of trisomy or monosomy: for segments of equivalent length, the deleterious effect of the imbalanced state seems to be so much more severe than the replication time is earlier. Thus, a kind of 'hierarchy' in chromosome bands can be established.

  The BrdU technique is also suitable for studying chromosome X anomalies, and several cases of position effect have been demonstrated in man.

  Finally, chromatid asymmetries and sister chromatid exchanges, as revealed by the BrdU techniques, appear to be a good indication of the toxicity of physical or chemical agents.

Dr. M.-O. Rethoré discussed recent findings in human chromosome pathology, and more particularly the anomalies of chromosome 8. In cases of trisomy for a segment of this chromosome, resulting from malsegregation of a parental translocation, it is worth noting that the breakage point is often the same, 8q23, and that chromosome 22 is most often involved in the rearrangement.

  A comparison of clinical and cytogenetic data allows the identification of different syndromes resulting from trisomy for different segments of chromosome 8.

  Trisomy 8p is responsible for mental retardation, facial dysmorphia, nail dystrophies, and excess of digital arches.

  Trisomy for the proximal part of the long arm induces an abnormal shape of the helices, excess of ribs and deep palmar creases.

  Trisomy for the distal part of the long arm induces macrocephaly, stiffening of the joints, hydronephrosis and a palmar axial triradius in t' or t''.

  These different features are generally found in association in complete trisomy 8. This example shows that with the increasing refinement of techniques, it becomes possible to 'split up' a cytogenetic syndrome into 'sub-syndromes'.

Dr. M. Ferguson-Smith dealt with another aspect of clinical cytogenetics: the behaviour of pericentric inversions at meiosis and their implications for genetic counselling. A series of pericentric inversions involving chromosomes 2, 7, 8, 9, 10, 16 and 17 was described. Inversion heterozygotes usually have a normal phenotype; they transmit the inversion to approximately half of their progeny, and may have abnormal children, with partial deficiency of duplication of the inverted chromosome when crossing-over occurs within the inverted segment during meiosis. A general rule may be provided for assessing the risk of abnormal progeny: the risk increases according to the proportion of the chromosome length involved in the inversion.

Lastly, Dr. C. L. Richer revealed her recent results of the analysis of meiotic cells using chromosome banding techniques. The use of T-banding appears useful in the identification of bivalents at the first meiotic division metaphase.

Experimental animal models
for the study of human birth defects

Chairman:

ROBERT M. HERNDON, Center for Brain Research, The University of Rochester Medical Center, Rochester, New York, U.S.A.

Speakers:

PAUL B. SELBY, Biology Division, Oak Ridge National Laboratory, Oak Ridge, Tennessee, U.S.A.
A rich new source of dominant mutations causing skeletal abnormalities in mice

DONALD PATTERSON, University of Pennsylvania, School of Veterinary Medicine, Philadelphia, Pennsylvania, U.S.A.
Models of human birth defects in domestic animals

RONALD MYERS, Laboratory of Perinatal Physiology, National Institutes of Health, Bethesda, Maryland, U.S.A.
Models of developmental brain pathology caused by oxygen deficiency

MARY LOU OSTER-GRANITE, University of Maryland, School of Medicine, Baltimore, Maryland, U.S.A.
Toxic effects of drugs during neurogenesis

ROBERT M. HERNDON, Department of Neurology, Johns Hopkins Hospital, Baltimore, Maryland, U.S.A.
Viral models for the study of birth defects

KENNETH P. JOHNSON, Department of Neurology, Veterans Administration Hospital, San Francisco, California, U.S.A.
Animal models for cytomegalovirus infection

Experimental animal models
for the study of human birth defects

ROBERT M. HERNDON

The purpose of the workshop on animal models was to describe a variety of animal models which are suitable for the study of birth defects and to discuss the kinds of questions which can be answered regarding mechanisms and pathogenesis of disease states in these models. The models described included genetic, hypoxic, toxic and infectious disorders.

Paul B. Selby described a series of dominantly transmitted skeletal abnormalities which were induced by exposing spermatogonia of mice to high-dose gamma irradiation. The male offspring of these irradiated mice were allowed to breed and were then killed. Alizarin clearance preparations were made allowing detailed study of their skeletal structure. In this way 31 dominantly transmitted skeletal malformations were identified. Eighteen of these mutant strains have been established at the Oak Ridge Laboratories. These skeletal malformations were only rarely visible externally in the living animal. They consisted of alterations in the number or shape of bones, fusion of bones and changes in the relative positions of bones. Of the 31 mutants, 5 caused only one identifiable anomaly each, 19 caused 2–5 anomalies, 5 caused 6–10 anomalies and 2 caused 11–13 anomalies. Several of the skeletal malformations resembled known human disorders. One in particular resembled cleido-cranial dysplasia (cleido-cranial dysostosis).

Essentially all of these anomalies exhibited incomplete penetrance for some or all of their effects. Thus they might prove particularly useful in attempts to understand the pathogenesis of some of the dominantly inherited human disorders which display incomplete penetrance.

Ronald Myers discussed the current status of his studies of fetal hypoxia. Of particular relevance to human disease is his demonstration that the distribution of the pathology and its severity is dependent on fetal glycogen stores as well as the severity of the hypoxia. Oxygen tension must drop to about 10% of normal before obvious pathology occurs. In the presence of abundant glycogen stores, the fetal nervous system continues respiratory efforts for a longer time than it does in their absence, but the presence of these stores and the pH changes consequent to the anaerobic metabolism ultimately cause much more severe damage to the nervous system than occurs in the presence of limited glycogen stores. This suggests that hyperglycemia in the mother due to the infusion of glucose prior to delivery may cause severe adverse effects in the human infant, should severe hypoxia occur in the perinatal period.

Donald F. Patterson discussed several genetic anomalies in domestic animals and outlined the following advantages of domestic animals for the study of birth defects.

1. A high level of medical scrutiny at the level of the individual (veterinary medicine).

2. A favorable population structure. (a) Large 'free living' population of diverse species. (b) Breeds are genetic isolates, not geographically isolated. (c) Inbreeding is common enough to reveal recessive deleterious genes by production of homozygotes. (d) A cross-bred or 'mongrel' population is available for comparison with more inbred pure breeds.

3. Their size and docility are advantageous for physiologic and embryologic studies.

Among the conditions described were a sexual anomaly (XX male) syndrome in dogs, hereditary hyperextensibility and fragility of the skin in cats, which is transmitted as an autosomal dominant disease and closely resembles Ehler-Danlos syndrome and a mucopolysaccharidosis which closely resembles the Maroteaux-Lamy syndrome.

M. L. Oster-Granite discussed the effects of both licit and illicit pharmacologic agents on fetal development. The central nervous system is particularly susceptible to injury by drugs as well as other agents because of its prolonged development relative to most other organs or organ systems which in general go through a relatively short period of organogenesis. In addition, most of the drugs of abuse associated with fetal disorders are abused because of their neurologic and neurotoxic effects. Some of the drugs which produce relatively discrete developmental syndromes are diphenylhydantoin, cyclophosphamide, floxuridine, diazepam, antithyroid drugs, nicotine, barbiturates, and ethanol. These drugs act by a variety of mechanisms but in most instances, their effects in humans can be reproduced in animals. Thus, good animal models are available for the study of most, though not all, of the drug-induced fetal malformations seen in human infants.

Robert Herndon discussed 5 experimental animal models which illustrate the range of viral effects on the developing nervous system. These were:

1. Parvovirus infection which produces cerebellar maldevelopment by selectively destroying the granule cell precursors. This virus also induces communicating hydrocephalus in some animals. This malformation which occurs spontaneously in cats was believed to have a hereditary basis for over half a century.

2. Bluetongue virus which infects the subventricular zone of the developing cerebrum can result in porencephaly and neuronal heterotopia or hydranencephaly. The possibility that such malformation in humans could result from viral infection rather than from vascular causes has received relatively little attention.

3. Mumps virus infection which can produce acqueductal atresia in experimental animals and in man. This malformation which may occur postnatally produces changes indistinguishable from those occurring prenatally.

4. Influenza infection of the chick embryo which results in failure of closure of the neural tube.

5. Coxsackie B virus infection in the chick which causes muscle necrosis and resulting arthrogryposis.

These conditions serve to illustrate both the variety of effects produced by viruses and the absence of the usual stigmata of viral infection. As a result of the latter, it is often virtually impossible to establish the cause of a virus-induced malformation retrospectively.

Finally Kenneth P. Johnson discussed a New Guinea pig model of cytomegalovirus (CMV) infection which in a number of respects closely resembles human CMV infection. This model is of particular relevance since CMV is one of the most common viral infections of the human fetus and the similarity of the model to the human disease should make it possible to clarify a number of aspects of the pathogenesis of the human fetal infection.

The workshop was too short to cover more than a sampling of the available animal models, and due to the last minute withdrawal of one speaker we were unable to cover the large number of valuable neurological mutants available in inbred mice most of which are being maintained by the Jackson Laboratories.

Index of authors

Subject index